I0055053

Essentials of Mechanical Ventilation

Essentials of Mechanical Ventilation

Edited by June Hendricks

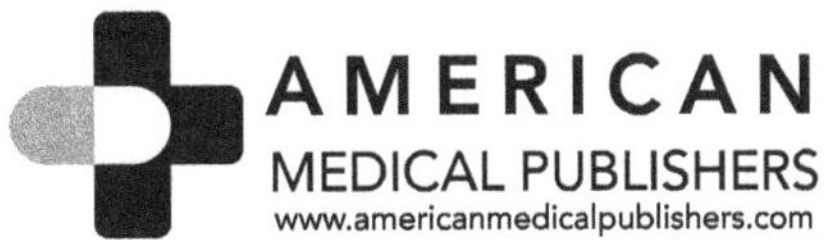

American Medical Publishers,
41 Flatbush Avenue,
1st Floor, New York,
NY 11217, USA

Visit us on the World Wide Web at:
www.americanmedicalpublishers.com

© American Medical Publishers, 2022

This book contains information obtained from authentic and highly regarded sources. Copyright for all individual chapters remain with the respective authors as indicated. All chapters are published with permission under the Creative Commons Attribution License or equivalent. A wide variety of references are listed. Permission and sources are indicated; for detailed attributions, please refer to the permissions page and list of contributors. Reasonable efforts have been made to publish reliable data and information, but the authors, editors and publisher cannot assume any responsibility for the validity of all materials or the consequences of their use.

ISBN: 978-1-63927-100-9

Trademark Notice: Registered trademark of products or corporate names are used only for explanation and identification without intent to infringe.

Cataloging-in-Publication Data

Essentials of mechanical ventilation / edited by June Hendricks.
p. cm.
Includes bibliographical references and index.
ISBN 978-1-63927-100-9
1. Artificial respiration. 2. Respiratory therapy. 3. Resuscitation. I. Hendricks, June.
RC87.9 .E77 2022
615.836 2--dc23

Table of Contents

Preface

This book has been a concerted effort by a group of academicians, researchers and scientists, who have contributed their research works for the realization of the book. This book has materialized in the wake of emerging advancements and innovations in this field. Therefore, the need of the hour was to compile all the required researches and disseminate the knowledge to a broad spectrum of people comprising of students, researchers and specialists of the field.

Mechanical ventilation or artificial ventilation refers to the mechanical means that are used in assisting or replacing spontaneous breathing. It is generally carried out by a machine called ventilator or by a qualified anesthesiologist and respiratory therapist. The four types of mechanical ventilators are transport ventilators, intensive-care ventilators, neonatal ventilators and positive airway pressure ventilators. Mechanical ventilation can be classified into invasive and non-invasive ventilation. Invasive ventilation involves the use of an instrument inside the trachea through mouth. Non-invasive ventilation includes usage of masks and is done in conscious patients. The two main types of mechanical ventilation include positive pressure ventilation and negative pressure ventilation. In positive pressure ventilation, air is pushed into lungs through airways whereas negative pressure ventilation involves sucking of air into lungs by stimulating movement of the chest. Mechanical ventilation is used in cases of acute severe asthma, acute lung injury, apnea, hypoxemia, etc. The topics covered in this extensive book deal with the core subject of mechanical ventilation. It provides significant information of this discipline to help develop a good understanding of various types that fall under mechanical ventilation. This book will serve as a reference to a broad spectrum of readers.

At the end of the preface, I would like to thank the authors for their brilliant chapters and the publisher for guiding us all-through the making of the book till its final stage. Also, I would like to thank my family for providing the support and encouragement throughout my academic career and research projects.

Editor

1

Accuracy of delivered airway pressure and work of breathing estimation during proportional assist ventilation: a bench study

Francois Beloncle[1,2], Evangelia Akoumianaki[3], Nuttapol Rittayamai[1,4], Aissam Lyazidi[5] and Laurent Brochard[1,6*]

Abstract

Background: Proportional assist ventilation+ (PAV+) delivers airway pressure (P_{aw}) in proportion to patient effort (P_{mus}) by using the equation of motion of the respiratory system. PAV+ calculates automatically respiratory mechanics (elastance and resistance); the work of breathing (WOB) is estimated by the ventilator. The accuracy of P_{mus} estimation and hence accuracy of the delivered P_{aw} and WOB calculation have not been assessed. This study aimed at assessing the accuracy of delivered P_{aw} and calculated WOB by PAV+ and examining the factors influencing this accuracy.

Methods: Using an active lung model with different respiratory mechanics, we compared (1) the actual delivered P_{aw} by the ventilator to the theoretical P_{aw} as defined by the equation of motion and (2) the WOB value displayed by the ventilator to the WOB measured from a Campbell diagram.

Results: Irrespective of respiratory mechanics and gain, the ventilator provided a P_{aw} approximately 25 % lower than expected. This underassistance was greatest at the beginning of the inspiration. Intrinsic PEEP (PEEPi), associated with an increase in trigger delay, was a major factor affecting PAV+ accuracy. The absolute value of total WOB displayed by the ventilator was underestimated, but the changes in WOB were accurately detected by the ventilator.

Conclusion: The assistance provided by PAV+ well follows P_{mus} but with a constant underassistance. This is associated with an underestimation by the ventilator of the WOB. PEEPi can be a major factor contributing to PAV+ inaccuracy. Clinical recommendations should include using a high trigger sensitivity and a careful PEEP titration.

Background

Proportional assist ventilation (PAV), described by Younes [1], was the first ventilator mode that introduced the concept of 'patient-driven' ventilation: a patient's effort could influence not only the timing but also the magnitude of the ventilator assistance. This two-way interaction aimed to bypass numerous disadvantages linked to conventional assisted ventilation: patient–ventilator asynchrony, lack of adaptability to changing ventilator demands and loss of normal breathing variability. In critically ill mechanically ventilated patients, PAV has been shown to preserve breathing variability, improve comfort, decrease work of breathing (WOB) and patient–ventilator interaction with the potential to reduce the duration of controlled mechanical ventilation [2–6].

Through automatic calculation of the respiratory system elastance and resistance and using the respiratory system equation of motion, PAV with load adjustable gain factors (PAV+) is able to partition the ventilator (P_{aw}) and the patient (P_{mus}) contribution to total pressure of the respiratory system (P_{tot}) [7–9]. PAV gain, selected by the physician, determines the partition between P_{mus} and P_{tot}. Thus, PAV+ is the only ventilator mode that calculates noninvasively, respiratory mechanics and WOB. This information would be extremely useful to evaluate the efficacy of assistance, to adjust ventilator settings

*Correspondence: brochardl@smh.ca
[1] Keenan Research Centre and Li Ka Shing Knowledge Institute, St. Michael's Hospital, 30 Bond St, Toronto, ON M5B 1W8, Canada
Full list of author information is available at the end of the article

and to assess patient's respiratory status and take therapeutic decisions [10]. Carteaux et al. recently published a study where they used their own calculations of P_{mus} [10]. It was based on the assumption that P_{aw} and P_{mus} were complementary according to the equation of motion and therefore that the ventilator accurately delivered PAV. Second, whether the values of WOB displayed by the ventilator could be used, instead of calculating P_{mus}, was not known. Third, we wanted to assess the effect of intrinsic PEEP in case of obstructive lung disorders.

PAV+ estimations of respiratory system mechanics are indirect and hence, based on a number of assumptions which, if not entirely fulfilled, could affect the accuracy and the reliability of P_{mus} and WOB calculation and, eventually, the delivered P_{aw}. The aim of this study was to assess the accuracy of delivered P_{aw} and calculated WOB by PAV+ under different conditions in terms of respiratory system mechanics and patient breathing pattern and to examine the factors influencing this accuracy. In the first step, we assessed the accuracy of PAV+ by comparing the actual delivered P_{aw} by the ventilator ($P_{aw_{meas}}$) to the theoretical P_{aw} as defined by the equation of motion ($P_{aw_{th}}$). Since P_{aw} provided by the ventilator is always a proportion of P_{mus}, errors in P_{aw} would reflect errors in P_{mus} and, hence, errors in WOB calculation. Therefore, in the second step, we assessed the accuracy of PAV+ WOB calculation by comparing the value displayed by the ventilator to the WOB, estimated by the Campbell diagram.

Methods

A PB840 ventilator (Puritan-Bennett 840; Covidien, Boulder, USA), which is currently the only ventilator able to deliver PAV+, was used. The ventilator was connected to the lung simulator by a conventional circuit with separate inspiratory and expiratory limbs. The circuit was connected to the lung simulator with the use of a heat–moisture exchanger (HME). Prior to each experiment, the ventilator was calibrated and tested for leaks. All experiments took place using room air [fraction of inspired oxygen (FiO_2) 21 %].

Lung model

An Active Servo Lung 5000 (ASL 5000; Ingmar Medical, Pittsburg, PA, USA) was used as described in previous studies [11, 12]. The ASL 5000 is a digitally controlled real-time breathing computerized simulator consisting of a piston moving inside a cylinder. To control the piston's movement, a microprocessor is programmed with a script driver, which uses a mathematical model of the equation of motion. Instantaneous flow (V') and P_{aw} were measured by flow and pressure sensors at the entrance of the piston, and volume (V) is obtained by the integration of V' over time. The spontaneous breathing pattern of the lung simulator was determined by the lung model parameters and the inspiratory effort (P_{mus}). The two main lung model parameters were the compliance C_{RS} and the resistance R_{RS}. The inspiratory effort embodied the breathing rate, effort amplitude, effort slope and inhaled percentage. Thus, a range of respiratory mechanics and inspiratory efforts could be simulated.

Formulas

Equation of motion of the respiratory system

$$P_{tot} = P_{aw} + P_{mus} = V' \times R_{RS} + V \times E_{RS} + \text{PEEPt}$$

where P_{tot} is the total pressure applied to the respiratory system, R_{RS} and E_{RS} the respiratory system resistance and elastance, respectively, V' and V the instantaneous flow and volume and PEEPt the total positive end-expiratory pressure.

PAV gain represents the proportion which balances the ventilator (P_{aw}) and the patient (P_{mus}) contribution to total pressure of the respiratory system (P_{tot}):

$$P_{aw}/P_{mus} = \%\text{Gain}/(100 - \%\text{Gain}).$$

Design of the experiment

Accuracy of P_{aw} delivered during PAV+

The ASL 5000 was set at single-compartment model to resemble four respiratory mechanics conditions: normal (R_{RS} = 10 cmH_2O/L/s and C_{RS} = 60 mL/cmH_2O), obstructive (R_{RS} = 20 cmH_2O/L/s and C_{RS} = 60 mL/cmH_2O), restrictive (R_{RS} = 10 cmH_2O/L/s and C_{RS} = 30 mL/cmH_2O) and mixed obstructive and restrictive (R_{RS} = 20 cmH_2O/L/s and C_{RS} = 30 mL/cmH_2O). A semi-sinusoidal inspiratory waveform was selected. The inspiratory waveform had a rise time of 30 %, inspiratory holding time of 0 % and releasing time of 15 %. PAV+ was tested under different respiratory mechanics (as described above), gains (30 and 60 %), inspiratory trigger (0.8, 5, and 15 L/min), P_{mus} (10 and 15 cmH_2O) and PEEP levels (0 and 5 cmH_2O). Various respiratory rates (RR) (10, 15, 20, 25 and 30 breath/min) were examined during obstructive respiratory mechanics to assess the impact of intrinsic PEEP (PEEPi) on delivered P_{aw}. In total, 24 different conditions were tested.

Accuracy of WOB calculation

The ASL 5000 was set as a single-compartment model to resemble three respiratory mechanics: normal (R_{RS} = 5 cmH_2O/L/s, C_{RS} = 60 mL/cmH_2O), restrictive (R_{RS} = 5 cmH_2O/L/s, C_{RS} = 20 mL/cmH_2O) and obstructive (R_{RS} = 20 cmH_2O/L/s, C_{RS} = 60 mL/cmH_2O). A semi-sinusoidal inspiratory waveform was selected with a rise time of 25 %, inspiratory holding time of 0 % and releasing time of 15 %. Each condition was tested under

2 RR (20 and 30 breaths/min) and across 2 levels of P_{mus} (5 and 10 cmH_2O). The flow triggering was 0.8 L/min and PEEP was 5 cmH_2O.

Moreover, we also used a real esophageal pressure signal, derived from our patients' database, to drive the simulator and test PAV+. This signal was tested under normal, restrictive and obstructive conditions.

The aforementioned scenarios were examined at two PAV+ gain levels (30 and 60 %). Therefore, 15 scenarios at two levels of Gain were assessed (30 conditions in total).

Data collection

Each test was recorded for 5 min, which was the time period for stabilization of the system. Then the last minute of the recording was selected and analyzed offline.

Data acquisition from ASL 5000 was performed at 128 Hz and stored in a laptop computer for subsequent analysis with AcqKnowledge software (Biopac Systems, Goleta, CA, USA). V', P_{mus} and $P_{aw_{meas}}$ curves over time were provided by the ASL 5000. V was derived from V' integration over time.

PEEPi was estimated as the pressure difference between the P_{mus} at the onset of inspiration (defined as the first point where P_{mus} started to decrease at end-expiration) and P_{mus} at the start of inspiratory V'.

Accuracy of P_{aw} delivered

Inspiratory time (Ti) was defined from the beginning of P_{mus} (drop in P_{mus} curve) to the end of inspiratory V' (Additional file 1: Figure S1). Mean P_{aw} during inspiration and P_{aw} at 25, 50, 75 and 100 % of Ti were measured. For each parameter, we averaged three cycles not including an occlusion breath or a breath immediately after an occlusion.

Compliance (C_{vent}) and resistance (R_{vent}) displayed by the ventilator were recorded, and presented values were the values displayed at the ventilator screen after a stabilization period.

$P_{aw_{th}}$ was calculated from the equation of motion as the following equation:

$$\mathrm{P}_{\mathrm{awTh}} = \left[\left(V/C_{\mathrm{RS}} + V' \times R_{\mathrm{RS}}\right) \times \mathrm{Gain}\right] + \text{total PEEP}.$$

where total PEEP = the sum of PEEPi above external PEEP and measured external PEEP at the end of expiration.

The difference between the instantaneous mean $P_{aw_{meas}}$ (i_{meas}) and the mean $P_{aw_{th}}$ (i_{Th}) were calculated over inspiration (Δi) and at 25, 50, 75 and 100 % of Ti ($\Delta P_{aw_{25}}$, $\Delta P_{aw_{50}}$, $\Delta P_{aw_{75}}$ and $\Delta P_{aw_{100}}$). They were expressed in percentage of differences related to the $P_{aw_{th}}$ ($\%\Delta P_{aw}$ and $\%\Delta i$).

The percentage of error in measurement of compliance or resistance (%error C and %error R) was calculated as follows:

$$\%\text{error } C = (C_{\text{vent}} - C_{\text{RS}})/C_{\text{RS}} \times 100,$$

$$\%\text{error } R = (R_{\text{vent}} - R_{\text{RS}})/R_{\text{RS}} \times 100.$$

Accuracy of WOB calculation

Data from the ventilator were recorded throughout a specific set of tests with the aid of a software provided by Covidien© and were stored. Data included ventilator settings and calculation of mean P_{aw}, peak P_{aw}, V, V', minute-ventilation ($V_{E'}$), RR, Ti, C_{vent}, R_{vent}, PEEPi, total PEEP and total displayed WOB in J/L (WOB_{displ}). These values were recorded every second and breath by breath. Based on the Campbell diagram, the patient and ventilator WOB were estimated on a breath-by-breath basis. Patient WOB and ventilator WOB were derived by integration of the area plotted between the P_{mus}–V and P_{aw}–V curves, respectively. Total WOB (WOB_{real}) was the sum of patient and ventilator WOB. Work of breathing was calculated per liter (WOB per minute divided by $V_{E'}$) and was expressed in joules per liter (J/L).

The values of total and patient WOB displayed on the PB 840 screen ($WOBtot_{displ}$, $WOBpt_{displ}$) were recorded and those resulting from Campbell ($WOBtot_{real}$, $WOBpt_{real}$) were calculated. A semiautomated, noncommercially available research software, previously used [13], was used for WOB measurement (SR program, Barcelona).

Statistical analysis

Variables were expressed as medians (25–75th interquartile range, IQR) or means (±standard deviation, SD). Data were analyzed using nonparametric tests. The relationships between WOB_{displ} and WOB_{real}, between $\%\Delta i$ and PEEPi and between %error C and %error R and PEEPi were evaluated using Pearson's correlation. Bland–Altman analysis was used to compare the absolute values of WOB_{displ} with those of WOB_{real} which was regarded as the gold standard.

Statistical significance was defined at p value <0.05. The statistical analysis was performed using Prism (GraphPad Software, La Jolla, CA, USA).

Results

Accuracy of P_{aw} delivered during PAV+

Effect of different respiratory mechanics and gains

Irrespective of respiratory mechanics and gain, i_{meas} was always lower than i_{Th} (Δi and $\%\Delta i$ were -2.9 ± 0.9 cmH_2O and -25.4 ± 4.6 %, respectively), indicating a lower assistance provided by the ventilator than expected from the equation of motion (Table 1). The magnitude of underassistance was greater at the beginning of the inspiratory cycle and decreased toward the end of inspiration (Fig. 1).

Effect of different triggers, P_{mus} and PEEP

The underassistance of PAV+ was also highlighted under different trigger, P_{mus} or PEEP settings in normal respiratory mechanics (Fig. 2; Additional file 2: Tables S1, Additional

Table 1 Measured and theoretical mean airway pressure during inspiration (i_{meas} and i_{Th}) in different respiratory mechanics

Gain (%)	Mechanics	i_{meas} (cmH$_2$O)	i_{Th} (cmH$_2$O)	Δi (cmH$_2$O)	%Δi (%)
30	Normal	6.6	9.4	−2.8	−29.8
	Obstructive	8.4	10.8	−2.4	−22.2
	Restrictive	7.0	8.5	−1.5	−17.6
	Mixed	6.7	8.8	−2.1	−23.9
60	Normal	9.6	13.7	−4.2	−29.9
	Obstructive	9.5	13.6	−4.1	−30.1
	Restrictive	10.2	13.0	−2.8	−21.5
	Mixed	10.3	13.5	−3.2	−23.7
All conditions		8.5 ± 1.6	11.4 ± 2.3	−2.9 ± 0.9	−25.4 ± 4.6

Difference and percentage of difference between i_{meas} and i_{Th} were calculated as follows: $\Delta i = i_{meas} - i_{Th}$ and $\%\Delta i = (i_{meas} - i_{Th})/i_{Th} \times 100$. Inspiratory trigger = 5 L/min; muscular pressure = 10 cmH$_2$O; PEEP = 5 cmH$_2$O; respiratory rate = 20/min. Respiratory system mechanics, normal: resistance (R) = 10 cmH$_2$O/L/s and compliance (C) = 60 mL/cmH$_2$O; obstructive: R = 20 cmH$_2$O/L/s and C = 60 mL/cmH$_2$O; restrictive: R = 10 cmH$_2$O/L/s and C = 30 mL/cmH$_2$O; and mixed: R = 20 cmH$_2$O/L/s and C = 30 mL/cmH$_2$O

file 3: Table S2, Additional file 4: Table S3). A higher trigger value (lower sensitivity) led to greater underassistance at the end of inspiration versus a lower trigger (Fig. 2a). A high P_{mus} was associated with a greater underassistance during the entire inspiration versus a low P_{mus} (Fig. 2b). A decrease in PEEP was associated with a major underassistance at the start of the inspiration (Fig. 2c). These findings were replicated under different trigger, P_{mus} or PEEP settings in obstructive and restrictive respiratory mechanics (Additional file 5: Figure S2). Of note, with obstructive respiratory mechanics and trigger = 15 L/min, the ventilator was unable to estimate initial values for R_{vent} and R_{vent} and the PAV+ mode did not operate.

Effect of PEEPi

To assess the effect of PEEPi on the accuracy of P_{aw} delivered by PAV+, the same experiments were replicated under obstructive respiratory mechanics with increasing RR. An increase in RR leading to an increase in PEEPi resulted in a higher $\%\Delta P_{aw}$ during the entire cycle, showing that PEEPi which is associated with an increase in trigger delay affected PAV+ accuracy (Fig. 3; Additional file 6: Table S4). Combining the data from all conditions, PEEPi was correlated with $\%\Delta i$ (Additional file 7: Figure S3). The higher the PEEPi, the lower the pressure assistance the ventilator provided.

Measurements of C_{RS} and R_{RS}

In comparison with C_{RS}, C_{vent} was globally slightly overestimated for the low value of compliance (30 mL/cmH$_2$O) [34 (IQR 34–36) mL/cmH$_2$O] and slightly underestimated for the high value of compliance (60 mL/cmH$_2$O) [59 (IQR 63–65) mL/cmH$_2$O] (Additional file 8: Figure S4). In comparison with R_{RS}, R_{vent} was always underestimated, irrespective of R_{RS} [8.8 (IQR 8.2–8.9) and 15 (IQR 15–16) cmH$_2$O/L/s for R_{RS} = 10 and 20 cmH$_2$O/L/s, respectively] (Additional file 8: Figure S4).

We found a strong correlation between the percentage of error in the measurement of compliance (%error C) and PEEPi ($r^2 = 0.68$, $p < 0.001$, Additional file 9: Figure S5). The association between the percentage of error in the measurement of resistance (%error R) and PEEPi was weaker ($r^2 = 0.27$, $p = 0.007$). This underestimation of compliance in case of high PEEPi should lead to an increase in the assistance delivered by the ventilator in comparison with $P_{aw_{th}}$ (calculated with the actual compliance of the simulator) and thus counteract in part the underassistance observed in PAV+ when PEEPi is high.

Accuracy of WOB measurements during PAV+

There was a strong linear correlation between total WOB calculated by the ventilator and total WOB based on the Campbell diagram ($r^2 = 0.93$, $p < 0.001$, Fig. 4). The Bland–Altman plot, performed to evaluate the accuracy of the absolute values of total WOB calculation, revealed a mean bias of 0.27 J/L, indicating an underestimation of the $WOB_{tot_{real}}$, with a limit of agreement of 0.6 to −0.11 J/L (Fig. 5). The changes in total WOB were accurately detected by the ventilator, but the absolute values of total WOB displayed by the ventilator were

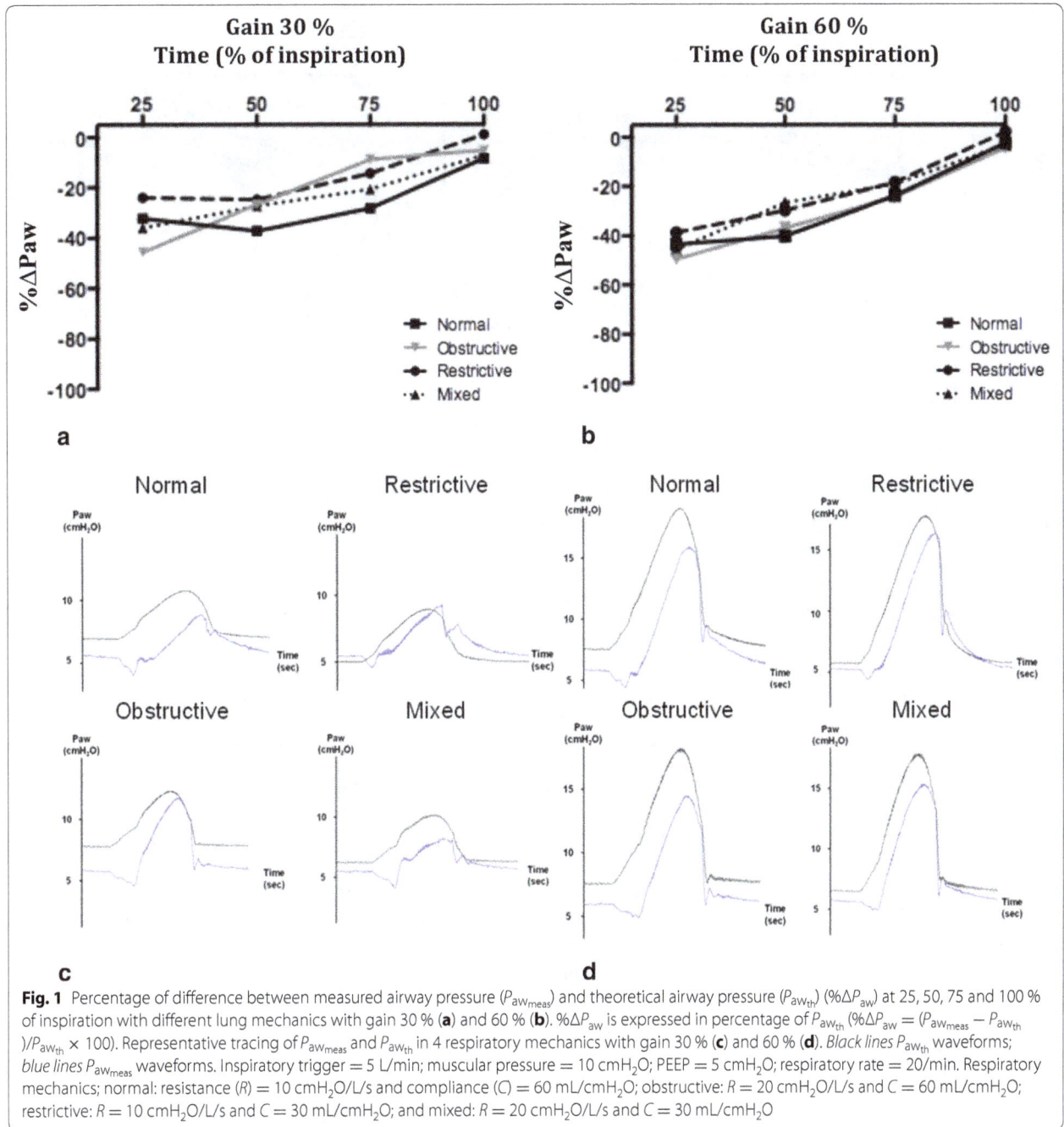

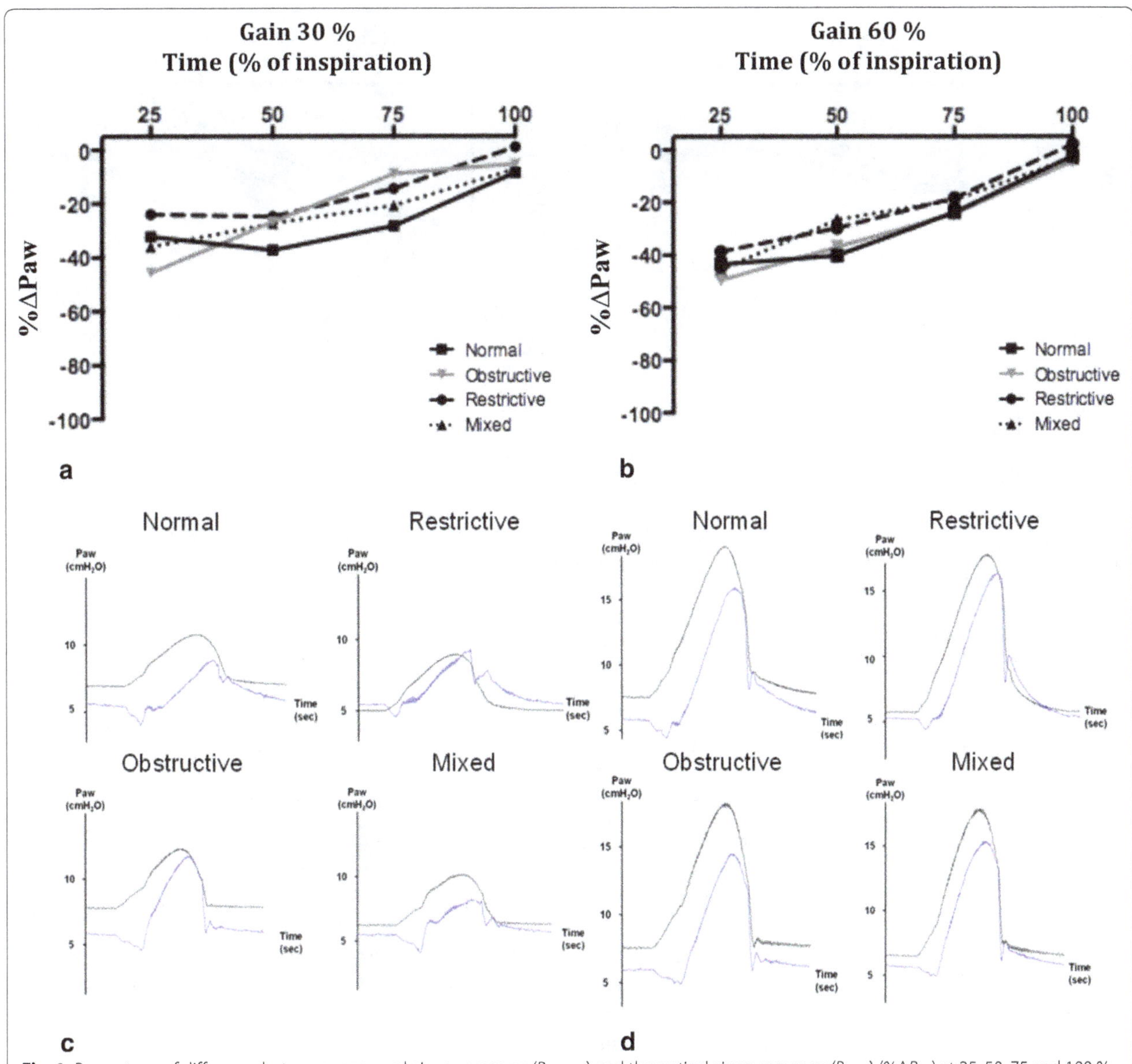

Fig. 1 Percentage of difference between measured airway pressure ($P_{aw_{meas}}$) and theoretical airway pressure ($P_{aw_{th}}$) (%ΔP_{aw}) at 25, 50, 75 and 100 % of inspiration with different lung mechanics with gain 30 % (**a**) and 60 % (**b**). %ΔP_{aw} is expressed in percentage of $P_{aw_{th}}$ (%$\Delta P_{aw} = (P_{aw_{meas}} - P_{aw_{th}})/P_{aw_{th}} \times 100$). Representative tracing of $P_{aw_{meas}}$ and $P_{aw_{th}}$ in 4 respiratory mechanics with gain 30 % (**c**) and 60 % (**d**). *Black lines* $P_{aw_{th}}$ waveforms; *blue lines* $P_{aw_{meas}}$ waveforms. Inspiratory trigger = 5 L/min; muscular pressure = 10 cmH_2O; PEEP = 5 cmH_2O; respiratory rate = 20/min. Respiratory mechanics; normal: resistance (R) = 10 cmH_2O/L/s and compliance (C) = 60 mL/cmH_2O; obstructive: R = 20 cmH_2O/L/s and C = 60 mL/cmH_2O; restrictive: R = 10 cmH_2O/L/s and C = 30 mL/cmH_2O; and mixed: R = 20 cmH_2O/L/s and C = 30 mL/cmH_2O

underestimated. The linear correlation between the patient's WOB as calculated by the ventilator and as computed by the Campbell diagram was significant but much weaker than for WOB_{tot} ($r^2 = 0.63$, $p < 0.001$).

Discussion

This bench study showed that although the P_{aw} delivered by PAV+ reasonably follows the muscular pressure when compared to the theoretical P_{aw} (i.e., the pressure that the

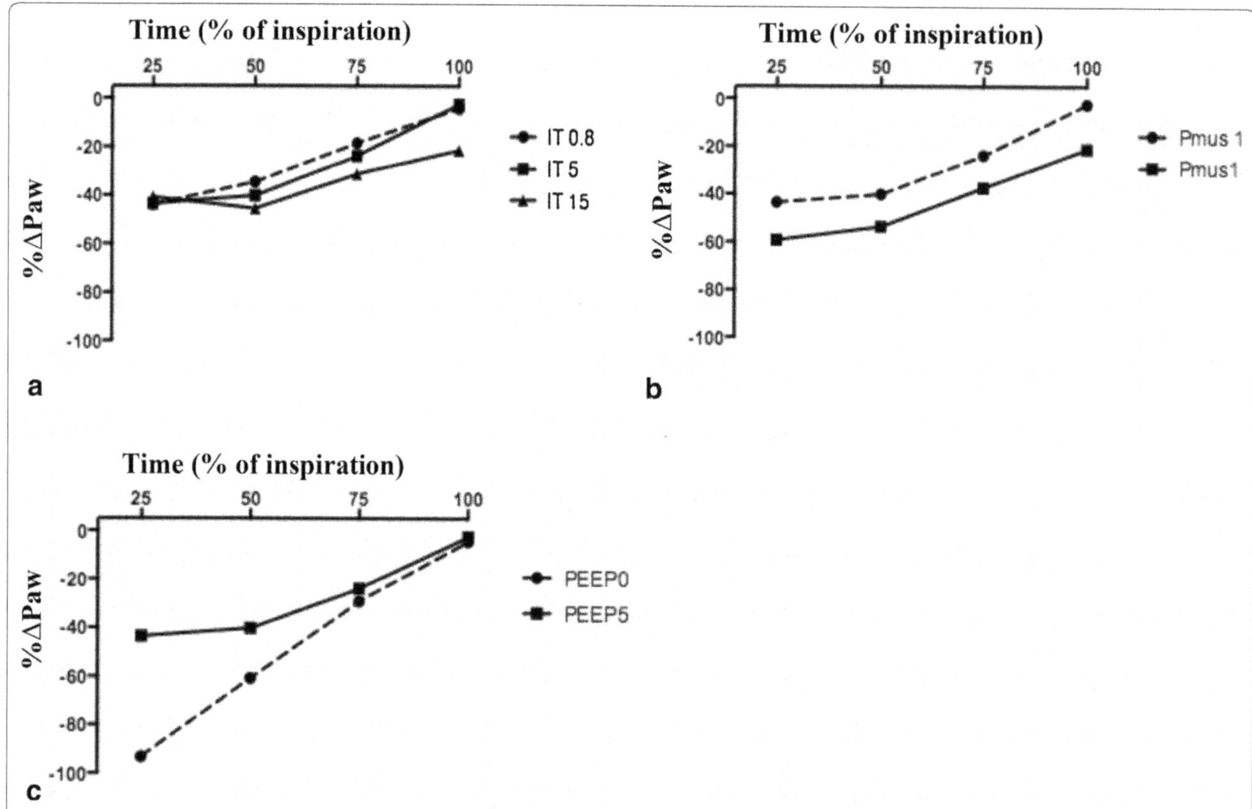

Fig. 2 Percentage of difference between measured airway pressure and theoretical airway pressure (%ΔP_{aw}) at 25, 50, 75 and 100 % of inspiration with different inspiratory trigger (IT) (**a**), muscular pressure (P_{mus}) (**b**) and positive end-expiratory pressure (PEEP) (**c**) under normal respiratory mechanics. Difference between $P_{aw_{meas}}$ and $P_{aw_{th}}$ is expressed in percentage of $P_{aw_{th}}$ (%$\Delta P_{aw} = (P_{aw_{meas}} - P_{aw_{th}})/P_{aw_{th}} \times 100$). Resistance = 10 cmH_2O/L/s; compliance = 60 mL/cmH_2O; gain = 60 %; and respiratory rate = 20/min; **a** different IT at 0.8, 5 and 15 L/min; P_{mus} = 10 cmH_2O; PEEP = 5 cmH_2O. **b** Different P_{mus} at 10 and 15 cmH_2O; IT 5 L/min; PEEP = 5 cmH_2O; **c** different PEEP at 0 and 5 cmH_2O; IT 5 L/min; P_{mus} 10 cmH_2O

ventilator should ideally deliver according to the equation of motion of the respiratory system), the ventilator provides a 25 % underassistance irrespective of the respiratory mechanics or ventilator settings. This underassistance is particularly marked when PEEPi is high. Of note even slight PEEPi values lead to dramatic increases in this underassistance (around 40 % for PEEPi values around 4 cmH_2O).

This inaccuracy in $P_{aw_{meas}}$ compared with $P_{aw_{th}}$ reflects the inaccurate estimation of P_{mus} and is thus associated with an underestimation of WOB. Despite the fact that the absolute values of WOB displayed on the ventilator bar graph underestimated the actual WOB, changes in its values accurately reflect measured changes in WOB.

Trigger delay and PEEPi play a pivotal role in this underassistance and in this relative inaccuracy of WOB measurements in PAV+ mode. PEEPi is associated with an increase in trigger delay. On PAV+ mode, once the ventilator is triggered delivered P_{aw} is continuously proportional to P_{mus}, but during the triggering phase no assistance is provided by the ventilator. A delay in the onset of pressurization by the ventilator reduces the correctly assisted fraction of neural inspiratory time and thus the global assistance by the ventilator. Thus, the further increase in trigger delay due to PEEPi leads to a global underassistance. In critically ill patients ventilated in PAV+ mode, Kondili et al. showed that an increase in PEEPi from 0.8 to 3.2 cmH_2O due to an increase in respiratory workload by chest and abdominal wall compression led to a decrease in the portion of supported inspiratory effort from 86 to 66 % [5]. The conventional pneumatic triggering used in PAV+ ventilation appears as an important limitation especially when compared to the other proportional mode of ventilation (neurally adjusted ventilatory assist), in which the triggering by the electrical activity of the diaphragm (Eadi) is

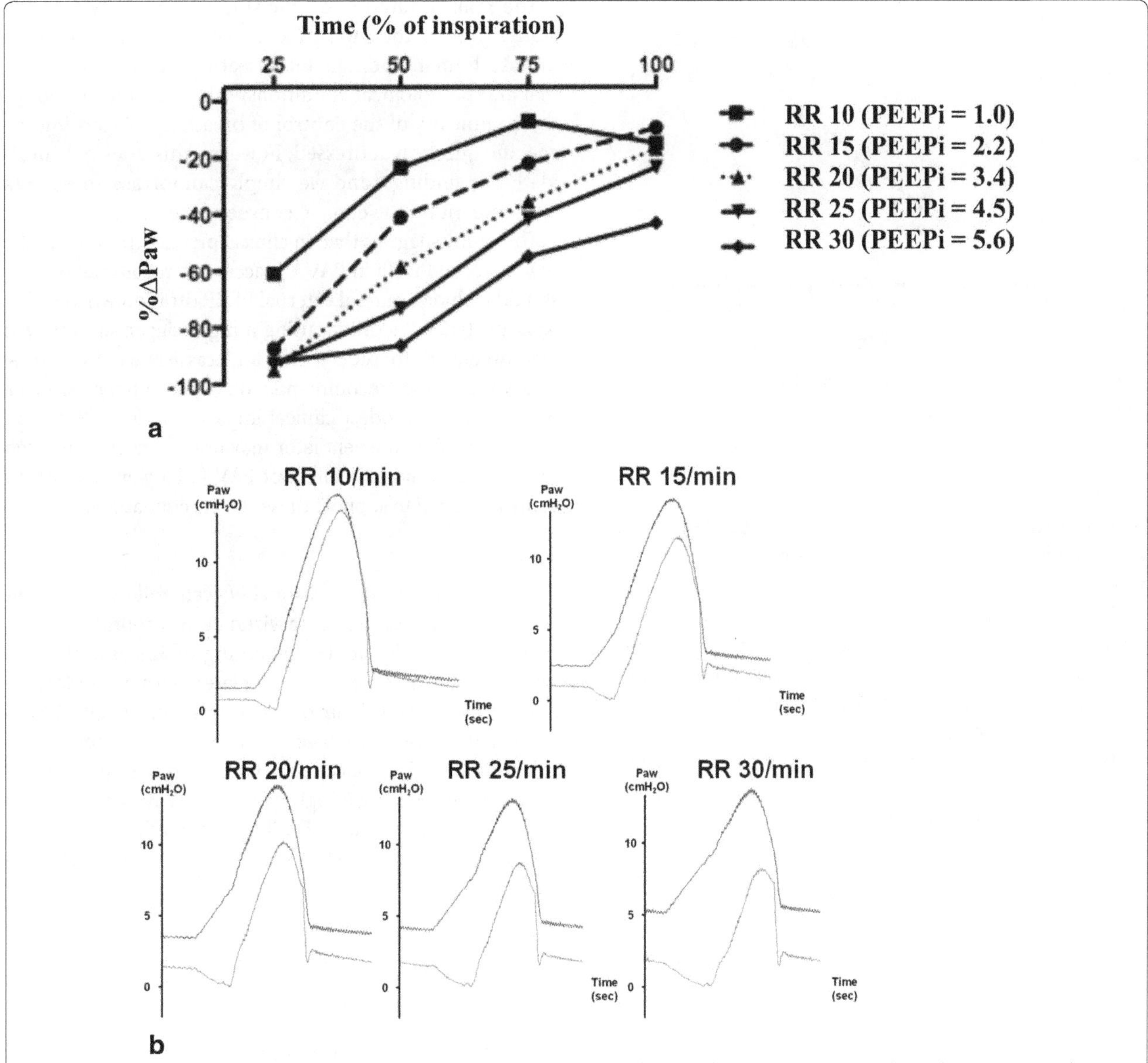

Fig. 3 Percentage of difference between measured airway pressure ($P_{aw_{meas}}$) and theoretical airway pressure ($P_{aw_{th}}$) (%ΔP_{aw}) at 25, 50, 75 and 100 % of inspiration with different respiratory rates in obstructive respiratory mechanics (**a**). Difference between $P_{aw_{meas}}$ and $P_{aw_{th}}$ is expressed in percentage of $P_{aw_{th}}$(% $\Delta P_{aw} = (P_{aw_{meas}} - P_{aw_{th}})/P_{aw_{th}} \times 100$). Representative tracing of $P_{aw_{th}}$ and $P_{aw_{meas}}$ (**b**). *Black lines* $P_{aw_{th}}$ waveforms. *Blue lines* $P_{aw_{meas}}$ waveforms. Resistance = 20 $cmH_2O/L/s$; compliance = 60 mL/cmH_2O; gain = 60 %; inspiratory trigger = 5 L/min; PEEP = 0 cmH_2O; and P_{mus} = 10 cmH_2O

not affected by PEEPi [14, 15]. However, a high PEEPi may also lead to a greater underestimation of C_{RS}. To estimate the compliance, the ventilator applies a 300-ms pause maneuver at the end of inspiration at random intervals of four to 10 breaths [7]. P_{aw} at the end of the occlusion (P_{aw}, occl) is measured and C_{RS} is calculated by the equation of motion ($C = V/(P_{aw}$, occl-totalPEEP)). However, as PB840 cannot detect the actual PEEPi value, this calculated value of C_{RS} may be underestimated in case of dynamic hyperinflation [9]. Thus, the assistance provided by the ventilator calculated by using the equation of motion of the respiratory system is increased as a result of this underestimation of C_{RS}. Overall, PEEPi has two effects on PAV+ accuracy: It is associated with an increase in trigger delay leading to an underassistance, but this effect is in part counterbalanced by the effect

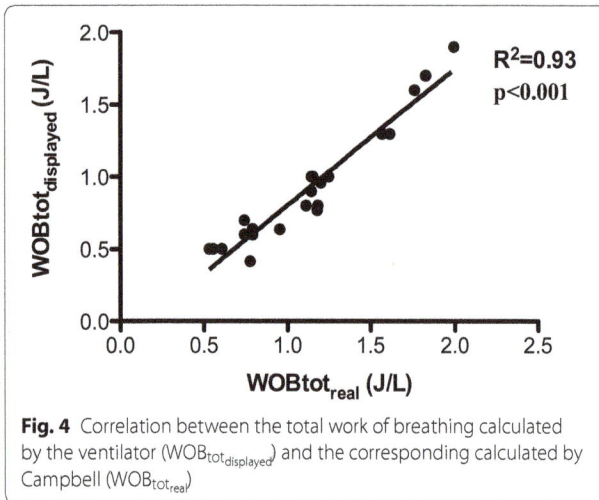

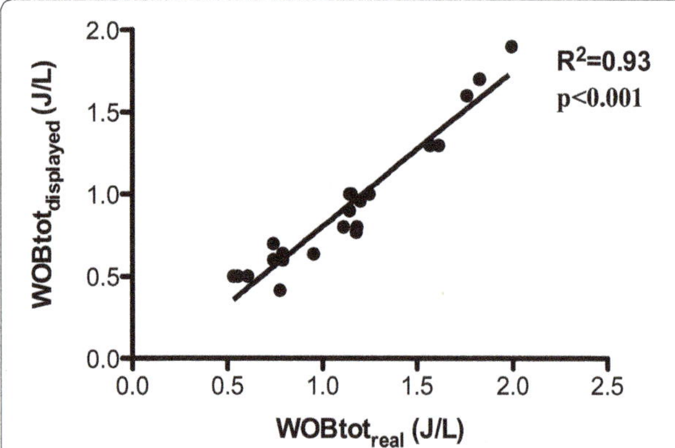

Fig. 4 Correlation between the total work of breathing calculated by the ventilator ($WOB_{tot_{displayed}}$) and the corresponding calculated by Campbell ($WOB_{tot_{real}}$)

on compliance estimation. Of note, this underassistance delivered by PAV+ may prevent the occurrence of runaway phenomena [16].

One of the major advantages of PAV+ is to allow the clinician to assess noninvasively the WOB. We show in this study that the absolute value of total WOB is underestimated by the ventilator. This finding is of particular importance when we consider the way to adjust Gain with a WOB range target [10]. Importantly for clinical practice, the changes in total WOB in a patient are accurately detected by the ventilator.

The main limitation of our study is that it is a bench study. Even if the lung model that we used was set to imitate human spontaneous breathing in different normal and pathological conditions, this does not reproduce the complexity of the control of breathing. Regarding the specific question addressed, however, this does not invalidate our findings, and we simply cannot use these data to comment on the clinical consequences of this.

This study suggests that, in clinical practice, because of the major role of PEEPi in PAV+ inaccuracy, recommendations should include a careful external PEEP titration when PEEPi is suspected. In addition, using a high trigger sensitivity is recommended to reduce the underassistance by PAV+. Following these recommendations, the underassistance has probably a modest clinical impact, whereas WOB values displayed by the ventilator may not be accurate enough to be used to monitor effect of PAV+. However, a clinical study is needed to support these recommendations.

Conclusion

The PAV+ assistance reasonably well follows P_{mus} but provides a constant underassistance of around 25 % on average, especially at the beginning of inspiration. This underassistance is logically associated with an underestimation by the ventilator of the actual total WOB. PEEPi leading to increased trigger delay is a major factor contributing to PAV+ inaccuracy. Clinical recommendations should include using a high trigger sensitivity and a careful PEEP titration when PEEPi is suspected.

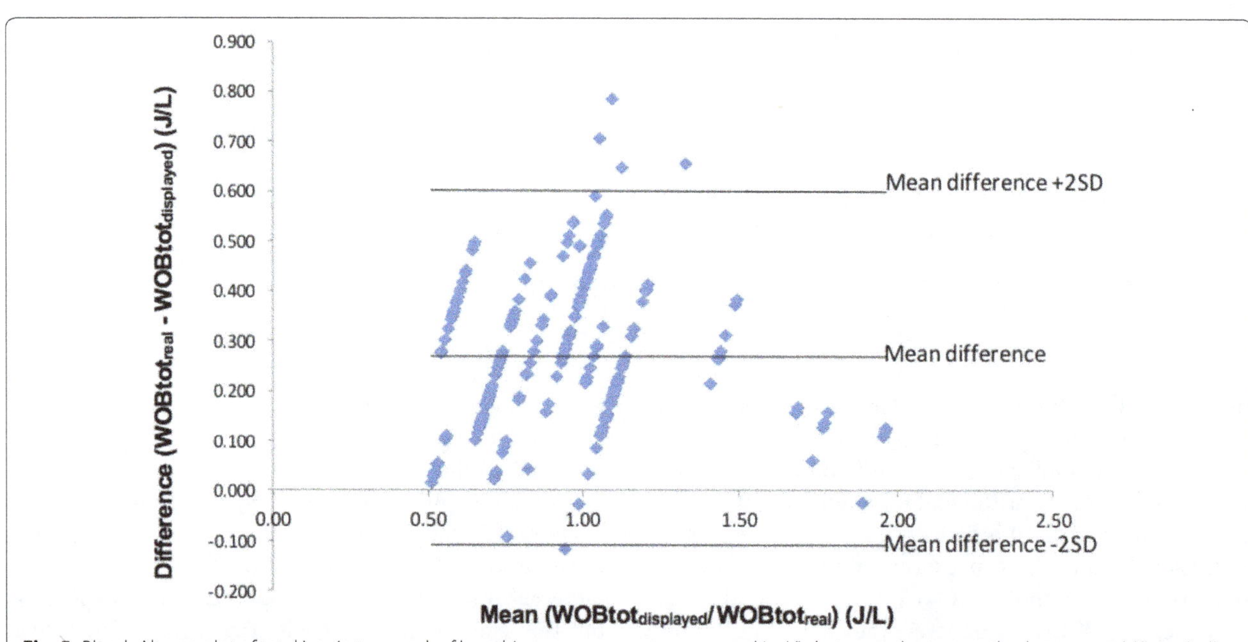

Fig. 5 Bland–Altman plot of total inspiratory work of breathing measurements, expressed in J/L, between the two methods compared (Campbell and Ventilator). $WOB_{tot_{displayed}}$, inspiratory work of breathing calculated by the ventilator; $WOB_{tot_{real}}$, inspiratory work of breathing calculated by the Campbell diagram

Additional files

Additional file 1: Figure S1. Description of measured parameters. (A) Trigger delay time, intrinsic positive end-expiratory pressure (intrinsic PEEP) and inspiratory cycle time (Ti). (B) Theoretical airway pressure (Paw_{Th}) and measured airway pressure (Paw_{meas}) at 25, 50, 75 and 100 % of Ti.

Additional file 2: Table S1. Measured and theoretical mean airway pressure during inspiration (i_{meas} and i_{Th}) with different triggers in different respiratory mechanics.

Additional file 3: Table S2. Measured and theoretical mean airway pressure during inspiration (i_{meas} and i_{Th}) with muscular pressure = 15 cmH_2O in different respiratory mechanics.

Additional file 4: Table S3. Measured and theoretical mean airway pressure during inspiration (i_{meas} and i_{Th}) with PEEP=0 cmH_2O in different respiratory mechanics.

Additional file 5: Figure S2. Percentage of difference between measured airway pressure and theoretical airway pressure (%ΔPaw) at 25, 50, 75 and 100 % of inspiration in obstructive and restrictive respiratory mechanics with different inspiratory triggers (IT) (A, B), muscular pressures (Pmus) (C, D) and positive end-expiratory pressure (PEEP) (E, F). Difference between Paw_{meas} and Paw_{Th} is expressed in percentage of Paw_{Th} (%ΔPaw = (Paw_{meas} − Paw_{Th})/Paw_{Th} × 100). Gain = 60 % and respiratory rate = 20/min; respiratory system mechanics, obstructive: resistance (R) = 20 cmH_2O/L/s and compliance (C) = 60 mL/cmH_2O and restrictive: R = 10 cmH_2O/L/s and C = 30 mL/cmH_2O. (A, B) Different IT at 0.8, 5, and 15 L/min; Pmus = 10 cmH_2O; PEEP = 5 cmH_2O. (C, D) Different Pmus at 10 and 15 cmH_2O. IT 5 L/min; PEEP = 5 cmH_2O. (E, F) Different PEEP at 0 and 5 cmH_2O; IT 5 L/min; Pmus 10 cmH_2O. In obstructive mechanics with IT = 15 L/min, PAV + mode was unable to calculate compliance and resistance and did not operate.

Additional file 6: Table S4. Measured and theoretical mean airway pressure during inspiration (i_{meas} and i_{Th}) with different respiratory rates in obstructive mechanics.

Additional file 7: Figure S3. Correlation between the percentage of difference between measured and theoretical mean airway pressure during inspiration (%Δi) and intrinsic positive end-expiratory pressure (PEEPi). Each point represents each experimental condition.

Additional file 8: Figure S4. Distribution of the values of compliance (A) and resistance (B) measured by the ventilator (C_{vent} and R_{vent}) according to the real values of compliance and resistance (C_{RS} and R_{RS}). Each point represents each experimental condition.

Additional file 9: Figure S5. Correlation between the percentage of error in measurement of compliance (A) or resistance (B) (%error C and %error R) and intrinsic positive end-expiratory pressure (PEEPi). %error C and %error R were calculated as follows: %error C = (C_{vent} - C_{RS})/C_{RS} × 100, %error R = (R_{vent} - R_{RS})/R_{RS} × 100. Each point represents each experimental condition.

Authors' contributions

All authors performed the experiments, interpreted the data, and drafted the manuscript. All authors read and approved the final manuscript.

Author details

[1] Keenan Research Centre and Li Ka Shing Knowledge Institute, St. Michael's Hospital, 30 Bond St, Toronto, ON M5B 1W8, Canada. [2] Medical Intensive Care Unit, Hospital of Angers, University of Angers, Angers, France. [3] Department of Intensive Care Medicine, University Hospital of Heraklion, Crete, Greece. [4] Division of Respiratory Diseases and Tuberculosis, Department of Medicine, Faculty of Medicine Siriraj Hospital, Bangkok, Thailand. [5] Institut Supérieur des Sciences de la Santé, Université Hassan 1er, Settat, Morocco. [6] Interdepartmental Division of Critical Care Medicine, University of Toronto, Toronto, ON, Canada.

Acknowledgements

FB was receiving a Grant from his own institution in France. EA received a Grant from Covidien. NR was receiving a Grant from his own institution in Thailand. LB's laboratory received research Grants from the following companies: Covidien (PAV), General Electric (lung volume measurement), Draeger (SmartCare), Vygon (CPAP), Fisher Paykel (Optiflow).

Competing interests

FB was receiving a Grant from his own institution in France. NR was receiving a Grant from his own institution in Thailand. LB's laboratory has received research Grants from the following companies: Covidien (PAV), General Electric (lung volume measurement), Draeger (SmartCare), Vygon (CPAP), Fisher Paykel (Optiflow). LB has received consultant fees from Covidien and Draeger. St. Michael's Hospital is receiving royalties from Maquet.

References

1. Younes M. Proportional assist ventilation, a new approach to ventilatory support: theory. Am Rev Respir Dis. 1992;145:114–20.
2. Delaere S, Roeseler J, D'hoore W, Matte P, Reynaert M, Jolliet P, Sottiaux T, Liistro G. Respiratory muscle workload in intubated, spontaneously breathing patients without COPD: pressure support vs proportional assist ventilation. Intensive Care Med. 2003;29:949–54.
3. Ranieri VM, Grasso S, Mascia L, Martino S, Fiore T, Brienza A, Giuliani R. Effects of proportional assist ventilation on inspiratory muscle effort in patients with chronic obstructive pulmonary disease and acute respiratory failure. Anesthesiology. 1997;86:79–91.
4. Giannouli E, Webster K, Roberts D, Younes M. Response of ventilator-dependent patients to different levels of pressure support and proportional assist. Am J Respir Crit Care Med. 1999;159:1716–25.
5. Kondili E, Prinianakis G, Alexopoulou C, Vakouti E, Klimathianaki M, Georgopoulos D. Respiratory load compensation during mechanical ventilation—proportional assist ventilation with load-adjustable gain factors versus pressure support. Intensive Care Med. 2006;32:692–9.
6. Xirouchaki N, Kondili E, Vaporidi K, Xirouchakis G, Klimathianaki M, Gavriilidis G, Alexandopoulou E, Plataki M, Alexopoulou C, Georgopoulos D. Proportional assist ventilation with load-adjustable gain factors in critically ill patients: comparison with pressure support. Intensive Care Med. 2008;34:2026–34.
7. Younes M, Webster K, Kun J, Roberts D, Masiowski B. A method for measuring passive elastance during proportional assist ventilation. Am J Respir Crit Care Med. 2001;164:50–60.
8. Younes M, Kun J, Masiowski B, Webster K, Roberts D. A method for noninvasive determination of inspiratory resistance during proportional assist ventilation. Am J Respir Crit Care Med. 2001;163:829–39.
9. Akoumianaki E, Kondili E, Georgopoulos D. Proportional-assist ventilation. Eur Respir Soc Monogr. 2012;55:97–115 **(New developments in Mechanical Ventilation)**.
10. Carteaux G, Mancebo J, Mercat A, Dellamonica J, Richard J-CM, Aguirre-Bermeo H, Kouatchet A, Beduneau G, Thille AW, Brochard L. Bedside adjustment of proportional assist ventilation to target a predefined range of respiratory effort. Crit Care Med. 2013;41:2125–32.
11. Lyazidi A, Thille AW, Carteaux G, Galia F, Brochard L, Richard J-CM. Bench test evaluation of volume delivered by modern ICU ventilators during volume-controlled ventilation. Intensive Care Med. 2010;36:2074–80.
12. Thille AW, Lyazidi A, Richard J-CM, Galia F, Brochard L. A bench study of intensive-care-unit ventilators: new versus old and turbine-based versus compressed gas-based ventilators. Intensive Care Med. 2009;35:1368–76.
13. L'Her E, Deye N, Lellouche F, Taille S, Demoule A, Fraticelli A, Mancebo J, Brochard L. Physiologic effects of noninvasive ventilation during acute lung injury. Am J Respir Crit Care Med. 2005;172:1112–8.

14. Terzi N, Piquilloud L, Rozé H, Mercat A, Lofaso F, Delisle S, Jolliet P, Sottiaux T, Tassaux D, Roesler J, Demoule A, Jaber S, Mancebo J, Brochard L, Richard JC. Clinical review: update on neurally adjusted ventilatory assist-report of a round-table conference. Crit Care Lond Engl. 2012;16:225. doi:10.1186/cc11297.
15. Piquilloud L, Vignaux L, Bialais E, Roeseler J, Sottiaux T, Laterre P-F, Jolliet P, Tassaux D. Neurally adjusted ventilatory assist improves patient–ventilator interaction. Intensive Care Med. 2011;37:263–71.
16. Passam F, Hoing S, Prinianakis G, Siafakas N, Milic-Emili J, Georgopoulos D. Effect of different levels of pressure support and proportional assist ventilation on breathing pattern, work of breathing and gas exchange in mechanically ventilated hypercapnic COPD patients with acute respiratory failure. Respir Int Rev Thorac Dis. 2003;70:355–61.

2

Teamwork enables high level of early mobilization in critically ill patients

Cheryl Elizabeth Hickmann, Diego Castanares-Zapatero, Emilie Bialais, Jonathan Dugernier, Antoine Tordeur, Lise Colmant, Xavier Wittebole, Giuseppe Tirone, Jean Roeseler and Pierre-François Laterre*

Abstract

Background: Early mobilization in critically ill patients has been shown to prevent bed-rest-associated morbidity. Reported reasons for not mobilizing patients, thereby excluding or delaying such intervention, are diverse and comprise safety considerations for high-risk critically ill patients with multiple organ support systems. This study sought to demonstrate that early mobilization performed within the first 24 h of ICU admission proves to be feasible and well tolerated in the vast majority of critically ill patients.

Results: General practice data were collected for 171 consecutive admissions to our ICU over a 2-month period according to a local, standardized, early mobilization protocol. The total period covered 731 patient-days, 22 (3 %) of which met our local exclusion criteria for mobilization. Of the remaining 709 patient-days, early mobilization was achieved on 86 % of them, bed-to-chair transfer on 74 %, and at least one physical therapy session on 59 %. Median time interval from ICU admission to the first early mobilization activity was 19 h (IQR = 15–23). In patients on mechanical ventilation (51 %), accounting for 46 % of patient-days, 35 % were administered vasopressors and 11 % continuous renal replacement therapy. Within this group, bed-to-chair transfer was achieved on 68 % of patient-days and at least one early mobilization activity on 80 %. Limiting factors to start early mobilization included restricted staffing capacities, diagnostic or surgical procedures, patients' refusal, as well as severe hemodynamic instability. Hemodynamic parameters were rarely affected during mobilization, causing interruption in only 0.8 % of all activities, primarily due to reversible hypotension or arrhythmia. In general, all activities were well tolerated, while patients were able to self-regulate their active early mobilization. Patients' subjective perception of physical therapy was reported to be enjoyable.

Conclusions: Mobilization within the first 24 h of ICU admission is achievable in the majority of critical ill patients, in spite of mechanical ventilation, vasopressor administration, or renal replacement therapy.

Keywords: Teamwork, Intensive care unit, Mechanical ventilation, Early mobilization, Physical therapy, Perception

Background

Early mobilization referring to initiating physical exercise or mobilization within the early illness phase is an increasingly common practice in intensive care units (ICU) [1]. Yet the definition of early mobilization is rather vague, as it encompasses a wide range of techniques practiced on different ICU populations [2, 3]. Nevertheless, early mobility interventions in critically ill patients prove to be feasible and safe in preventing bed-rest-associated morbidity [4–6], while improving patients' physical function [7], psychological condition [8], and quality of life [9]. Mobilizing patients at an early time point has been associated with reduced health care costs [10], as such intervention decreases invasive mechanical ventilation (MV) duration, delirium [7, 11], and hospital length of stay [12]. Recent observations suggest that providing mobility as early as possible and extending it to weekends could further improve patient outcomes [13–15].

Reported reasons for not mobilizing patients vary widely and include mechanical ventilation [16],

*Correspondence: pierre-francois.laterre@uclouvain.be
Intensive Care Unit, Cliniques universitaires Saint-Luc, Université catholique de Louvain (UCL), Avenue Hippocrate 10, 1200 Brussels, Belgium

catecholamine infusion [17], impaired consciousness [16], poor functional status [7, 12], safety considerations [9], limited staff capacities, or lack of protocols [18–20]. Safety considerations are indeed crucial in order to prevent additional risks, yet several reported safety issues are instrumental in excluding or delaying intervention in critically ill patients on multiple support systems, whereby this group runs the greatest risk of developing neuromuscular abnormalities.

At the same time, communication [21] and muscular activity [7] remain possible by means of limiting sedation, in line with current recommendations. Nevertheless, there is a lack of data available reporting patients' perceptions in such settings.

In our experience, early mobilization is an integral part of standard care, requiring teamwork combined with either limited sedation or none at all. The primary objective of this study was to demonstrate that early mobilization is feasible in the vast majority of critically ill patients, independently of their severity assessed by the need of MV, high FiO_2, vasopressor doses, or renal replacement therapy (RRT). The secondary objectives included safety of early mobilization, early mobilization rate in MV according to hypoxemia severity and patients' perception. Preliminary data were reported in an Abstract book [22].

Methods

Setting and patients

This was an observational study performed in a tertiary, 14-bed, mixed ICU at Saint-Luc University Hospital. Data were collected from all consecutive patients either already hospitalized in or newly admitted to our ICU between December 1, 2014, and January 31, 2015. The Ethics Committee of the Cliniques universitaires Saint-Luc, Brussels, Belgium, approved the study protocol. A waiver was obtained for written informed consent, given that the described interventions were considered to be part of standard care. Early unwanted effects of mobility, in addition to monitoring data, were anonymously recorded in accordance with Belgian and European law.

Early mobilization and standard care

In accordance with the literature, we define early mobilization as a series of progressive physical activities able to induce acute physiological responses (enhancing ventilation, central and peripheral circulation, muscle metabolism, and alertness) [23] and beginning within 24 h of ICU admission. Our early mobilization protocol includes a few prior contraindications (Fig. 1) [24], such as acute myocardial infarction, active bleeding, increased intracranial pressure with major instability, unstable pelvic fractures, and therapy withdrawal. Moreover, during the morning medical rounds, a multidisciplinary team (physicians, physical therapists, and nurses) evaluates each patient in order to identify limitations to early mobilization. These include low blood pressure despite increasing dose of vasopressors, severe hypoxemia requiring a rapid increase in FiO_2 or prone position, seizures, and patients' refusal.

According to the routine procedure for basic treatment, ICU team first transfers patients out of their beds. The ensuing physical therapy sessions are then designed as passive, active, or manual resistance exercise; cycle ergometer or leg press training; standing; verticalization by means of a tilt table; standing and assisted walking [25]. Activities are selected depending on patients' consciousness; hemodynamic/respiratory stability, as perceived by the team; as well as patients' preferences and physical capabilities. The complete therapeutic regime included getting out of bed together with physical therapy sessions twice a day. The daily mobilization program is otherwise considered to be incomplete.

Physical therapists are present at the ICU from Monday to Friday (7:30 am–5:00 pm), and the senior physical therapist-to-patient ratio is 1:14. The ratio of physical therapy students to senior physical therapists is 2:1. Furthermore, one resident physical therapist is present in the hospital at all times in case of respiratory emergencies. The nurse to patient ratio is 1:1.6 from 7:30 am to 4:00 pm.

Our standard care program consists in limited sedative administration in order to keep patients dozy and calm (RASS score between -1 and $+1$), combined with appropriate analgesia. Our preferred mechanical ventilation mode is pressure support, irrespective of hypoxemia severity or ARDS, provided that the protective volume and pressures guidelines were adhered to [26]. Controlled ventilation modes are mainly restricted to patients undergoing prone position or very severe hypoxemia despite PEEP adjustment.

Data collection

All medical and monitoring data were collected on a routine basis using our software of choice (*Qcare* 4.6 Build 154/2, C3 Critical Care Company NV, Sint-Martens-Latem, Belgium), with subsequent analysis performed by means of a data extraction tool. We extracted from our routine database: demographic characteristics, severity scores, monitoring data, early mobilization activities, reasons for not providing such therapy, as well as any adverse events. Predefined adverse events included death, cardiac or respiratory arrest, falls, medical device removal, and abnormal physiological responses requiring activity interruption [27].

For the first patients' transfer to chair, the nurse monitored hemodynamic and respiratory parameters at

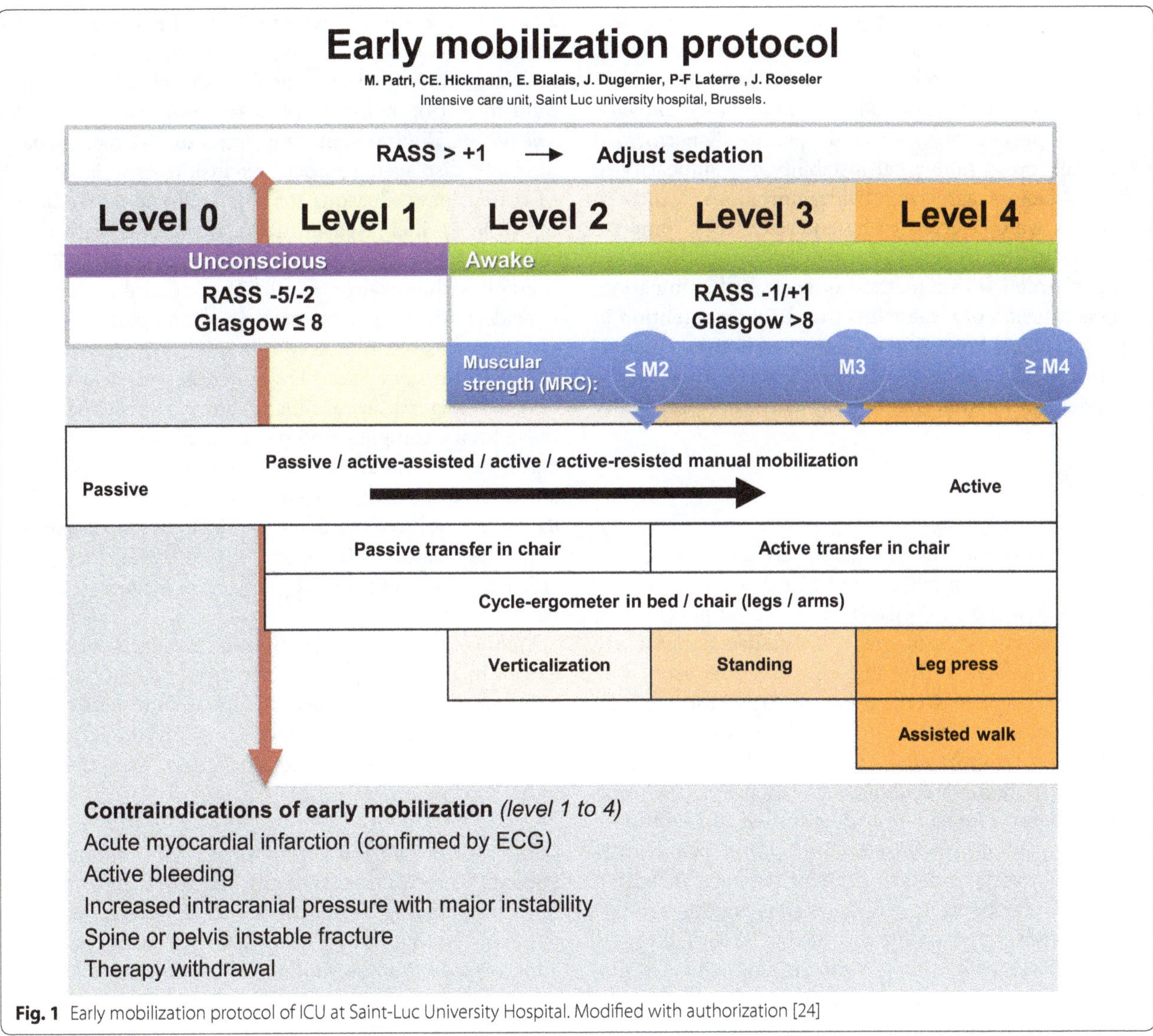

Fig. 1 Early mobilization protocol of ICU at Saint-Luc University Hospital. Modified with authorization [24]

baseline (in bed), and after 5 and 30 min, respectively. Through physical therapy sessions, hemodynamic and respiratory parameters, along with pain scores, were monitored at baseline, as well as at 0 and 15 min afterward, respectively. Pain was assessed in communicative patients on a score of 0 (no pain) to 10 (maximum pain). Patients' perceived exertion was rated from 0 to 10 immediately following physical therapy sessions based on the Borg RPE scale [28], with a similar rating employed to measure perceived enjoyment (0 = no enjoyment, 10 = maximum enjoyment) [29, 30].

Statistical analysis

Analyses were conducted using the software program SPSS software (IBM Corp. Released 2011. IBM SPSS Statistics for Windows, version 20.0. Armonk, NY, USA: IBM Corp). Study periods were expressed in patient-days in terms of performing early mobilization therapy or lack thereof. Descriptive statistics were conducted for demographic, clinical, and activity data and expressed as mean and standard deviation or confidence interval at 95 % (95 % CI) for normally distributed continuous variables, or as median and interquartile range (IQR) for non-normally distributed continuous variables. Categorical data were summarized using numbers or percentages. Characteristics between mobilized and non-mobilized patients were compared using unpaired Student's *t* test or Mann–Whitney *U* test when appropriate. Categorical data were compared with Chi-squared test between groups. One-way repeated measures ANOVA was employed with time as a random factor in order to compare the effect of each activity on hemodynamic and respiratory parameters.

To clearly demonstrate the safety of early mobilization, a multivariate analysis was performed by logistic regression. Adjusted odds ratio (AOR) for 28-day, ICU, and hospital mortality was calculated as follows: Univariate logistic regression analysis was previously performed to identify every numerical instability or collinearity of different factors associated with mortalities. Validated covariates were selected to be entered into a complete multivariate logistic regression model. Variable selection was performed with a method of backward elimination, using a criterion of p value less than 0.20 for retention in the model. Final analysis was performed between covariates reaching a significant p value. Statistical tests were two-sided, and significance was set at the 0.05 probability level.

Results

Population description

In total, 160 consecutive patients were admitted to the ICU over a 2-month period, and 11 others were already being hospitalized at the start of the study period. The overall characteristics of the 171 included patients are presented in Table 1. The mean APACHE II score was 18 ± 7 for the entire ICU population, 20 ± 8 for mechanically ventilated patients, and 22 ± 7 for those affected by severe sepsis or septic shock. Comorbidities were present in 60 % of patients including; active cancer (32 %), end stage cirrhosis (14 %), neurologic disorders (9 %), chronic obstructive pulmonary disease (8 %), and pancreatitis (4 %). MV was provided to 51 % of patients, including 14 % with tracheostomy. Spontaneous modes, principally pressure support, were provided in 96 % of days and controlled modes in only 4 % of the mechanical ventilated population. Remaining patients had oxygenation by mask (13 %), high-flow oxygen therapy (6 %), noninvasive mechanical ventilation (1 %), or nasal cannula (21 %). The mean inspired oxygen fraction (FiO_2) in mechanically ventilated patients was 0.46 ± 0.17. Noradrenaline was the only vasopressor administered, with a mean dose of 0.16 ± 0.23 μg kg^{-1} min^{-1}. The primary sedatives employed were propofol (93 %) and clonidine (23 %). Neuromuscular blocking agents were only administered during tracheal intubation maneuvers, as necessary. Sedatives were administered to 84 % of mechanically ventilated patients. The main analgesic medications, namely opioids and paracetamol, were administrated by means of intravenous bolus, patient-controlled analgesia systems, epidural, or oral route.

Early mobilization therapy

Overall, 139 (81 %) patients underwent early mobilization therapy. The median (IQR) delay from ICU admission to patients' first activity was 19 h [15–23]. Seating in a chair was the first activity for 79 % of patients. In these patients, proportion of hypoxemia according to Berlin classification [31] was as follows: without ($n = 33$), mild ($n = 19$), moderate ($n = 40$), and severe ($n = 19$). The 171 ICU admissions translated to 731 patient-days. Subjects displayed protocol exclusion criteria on 3 % of patient-days. Reasons for this included active bleeding ($n = 7$), increased intracranial pressure with major instability ($n = 3$), unstable pelvic fractures ($n = 2$), and therapy withdrawal ($n = 10$). The remaining 709 were considered to be patient-days on which early mobilization was possible, thus accounting for 709 potential bed-to-chair transfers and 1418 potential physical therapy sessions (Fig. 2), according to our protocol. Based on these totals, complete and partial mobility regimes were carried out on 48 and 86 % of patient-days, respectively, and therefore incorporated into the treatment plan of 81 % of admitted patients. Subjects were transferred from their beds to chairs on 74 % of patient-days, with at least one physical therapy session provided on 59 % of patient-days.

Mobilized and non-mobilized patients' characteristics are described in Table 2. MV, vasopressors, and RRT were provided on 46, 30, and 16 % of patient-days, respectively. Patients treated using all the aforementioned support systems were transferred out of their beds on 60 % of patient-days.

Description of early mobilization

Patients were transferred from bed to chair with assistance in standing upright in 60 % of cases. They were manually lifted up by an ICU team in 36 % of cases, with a motorized lift employed in the remaining 4 %. Patients remained in their chairs for a median (IQR) duration of 300 (152–300) min. Hemodynamic variations during the first sitting session did not differ between patients on mechanical ventilation and those without it (Additional file 1).

Active physical therapy sessions were provided to 61 % of cases. Median (IQR) potency during active leg cycle ergometer sessions in seated and lying positions was recorded at 4 [3–5] watts and 3 [3–5] watts, respectively. Median (IQR) durations and RASS scores recorded during each activity are documented in Table 3.

The subjective perceptions of communicative patients were recorded on each physical therapy session (Table 3). Overall exertion ratings were moderate (5 ± 3); however, patients' enjoyment scores following physical therapy sessions were higher, indicating pleasant perceptions of their activity (8 ± 3), with even better values observed after more demanding activities, such as walking or active cycling. It is worth noting that pain was not significantly affected by physical activity.

Table 1 Descriptive patient characteristics

All admissions ($n = 171$)	Mobilized $n = 139$	Never mobilized $n = 32$	p value
Age[a]	59 ± 17	62 ± 17	0.36
Male[b]	80 (58 %)	18 (56 %)	0.99
SOFA score[a]	5 ± 3	8 ± 5	0.01
APACHE II score[a]	17 ± 7	22 ± 9	<0.001
Predicted mortality (APACHE II)	29 %	44 %	0.017
In-hospital mortality[b]	26 (19 %)	16 (50 %)	<0.001
In ICU mortality[b]	11 (8 %)	13 (41 %)	<0.001
28-day mortality[b]	15 (11 %)	15 (47 %)	<0.001
ICU length of stay[a]	6.4 ± 11.7	1.4 ± 2.1	0.017
Vasoactive drug use[b]	47 (34 %)	11 (34 %)	0.99
Sedative drug use[b]	68 (49 %)	13 (41 %)	0.43
Opioids use[b]	86 (62 %)	15 (47 %)	0.16
Renal replacement therapy[b]	12 (9 %)	5 (16 %)	0.32
Admission cause			
Medical[b]	74 (53 %)	15 (47 %)	0.56
Elective surgery[b]	49 (35 %)	9 (28 %)	0.54
Urgent surgery[b]	16 (12 %)	8 (25 %)	0.08
Mechanically ventilated patients ($n = 88$)	**Mobilized $n = 69$**	**Never mobilized $n = 19$**	**p value**
Age[a]	61 ± 16	66 ± 14	0.24
Male[b]	40 (58 %)	12 (63 %)	0.79
SOFA score[a]	7 ± 4	10 ± 5	0.01
APACHE II score[a]	19 ± 7	25 ± 9	0.005
Predicted mortality (APACHE II)	36 %	60 %	0.003
In-hospital mortality[b]	20 (29 %)	13 (68 %)	0.002
In ICU mortality[b]	11 (16 %)	12 (63 %)	<0.001
28-day mortality[b]	10 (14 %)	13 (68 %)	<0.001
ICU length of stay (days)[a]	10.7 ± 15.5	1.7 ± 2.6	<0.001
MV duration (days)[a]	4.9 ± 7.7	1.3 ± 1.1	0.04
Vasoactive drug use[b]	39 (57 %)	10 (53 %)	0.79
Sedative drug use[b]	58 (84 %)	13 (68 %)	0.18
Opioids use[b]	47 (68 %)	9 (47 %)	0.18
Renal replacement therapy[b]	10 (14 %)	5 (26 %)	0.30
PaO_2/FiO_2 ratio[b]			
>300 ($n = 11$)	10 (91 %)	1 (9 %)	0.44
201–300 (mild) ($n = 13$)	9 (69 %)	4 (31 %)	0.46
101–200 (moderate) ($n = 42$)	34 (81 %)	8 (19 %)	0.61
≤100 (severe) ($n = 22$)	16 (73 %)	6 (27 %)	0.55
Non-mechanically ventilated ($n = 83$)	**Mobilized $n = 70$**	**Never mobilized $n = 13$**	**p value**
Age[a]	56 ± 17	56 ± 20	0.96
Male[b]	40 (57 %)	6 (46 %)	0.54
SOFA score[a]	4 ± 3	5 ± 5	0.56
APACHE II score[a]	15 ± 6	16 ± 8	0.67
Predicted mortality (APACHE II)	22 %	19 %	0.69

Table 1 continued

Non-mechanically ventilated ($n = 83$)	Mobilized $n = 70$	Never mobilized $n = 13$	p value
In-hospital mortality[b]	6 (8 %)	3 (23 %)	0.14
In ICU mortality[b]	0 (0 %)	1 (8 %)	0.15
28-day mortality[b]	5 (7 %)	2 (15 %)	0.30
ICU length of stay[a]	2.2 ± 1.6	0.8 ± 0.5	<0.001
Vasoactive drug use[b]	8 (11 %)	1 (8 %)	0.99
Sedative drug use[b]	10 (14 %)	0 (0 %)	0.34
Opioids use[b]	39 (56 %)	6 (46 %)	0.55
Renal replacement therapy[b]	2 (3 %)	0 (0 %)	0.99
PaO_2/FiO_2 ratio[b]			
> 300 ($n = 37$)	29 (78 %)	8 (22 %)	0.22
201–300 (mild) ($n = 22$)	19 (86 %)	3 (14 %)	0.99
101–200 (moderate) ($n = 16$)	15 (94 %)	1 (6 %)	0.44
≤100 (severe) ($n = 8$)	7 (88 %)	1 (13 %)	0.99

APACHE II acute physiology and chronic health evaluation II score, *SOFA* sequential organ failure assessment score

[a] Values expressed as mean ± SD

[b] Values expressed as number (percentage)

Hemodynamic parameters were recorded for 242 activities, 95 of which carried out by patients on MV while 147 involved no MV (Additional file 2). Heart rate, respiratory rate, or arterial pressure variations observed immediately after active exercises like walking, cycling, or manual mobilization were not clinically significant, returning to baseline values after 15 min. Hemodynamic variations on active mobilization were similar for MV and non-MV patients.

Limiting factors for mobilization activities

Table 4 summarizes the limiting factors for early mobilization. ICU procedures (surgery, medical/nursing intervention, and imaging) were the most common reasons for patients not to perform mobilization activities, followed by physiological instability as perceived by the team, and then patients' refusal. The failure to provide any given physical therapy session was primarily accounted for by staff limitations on weekends, and the same applies to several physical therapist consultations during the week. To a lesser extent, mobilization activities were limited due to patients' refusal, ICU procedures, or physiological instability.

Hemodynamic instability was the most commonly reported physiological limitation to mobility, in patients receiving a mean dose of noradrenaline at 0.31 (95 % CI 0.15–0.47) $\mu g\,kg^{-1}\,min^{-1}$. Noradrenaline was administered during 361 mobilization activities at a mean dose of 0.10 (95 % CI 0.09–0.11) $\mu g\,kg^{-1}\,min^{-1}$. Active physical therapy was successfully performed for eight sessions, while the patients were on noradrenaline >0.2 $\mu g\,kg^{-1}\,min^{-1}$ [mean

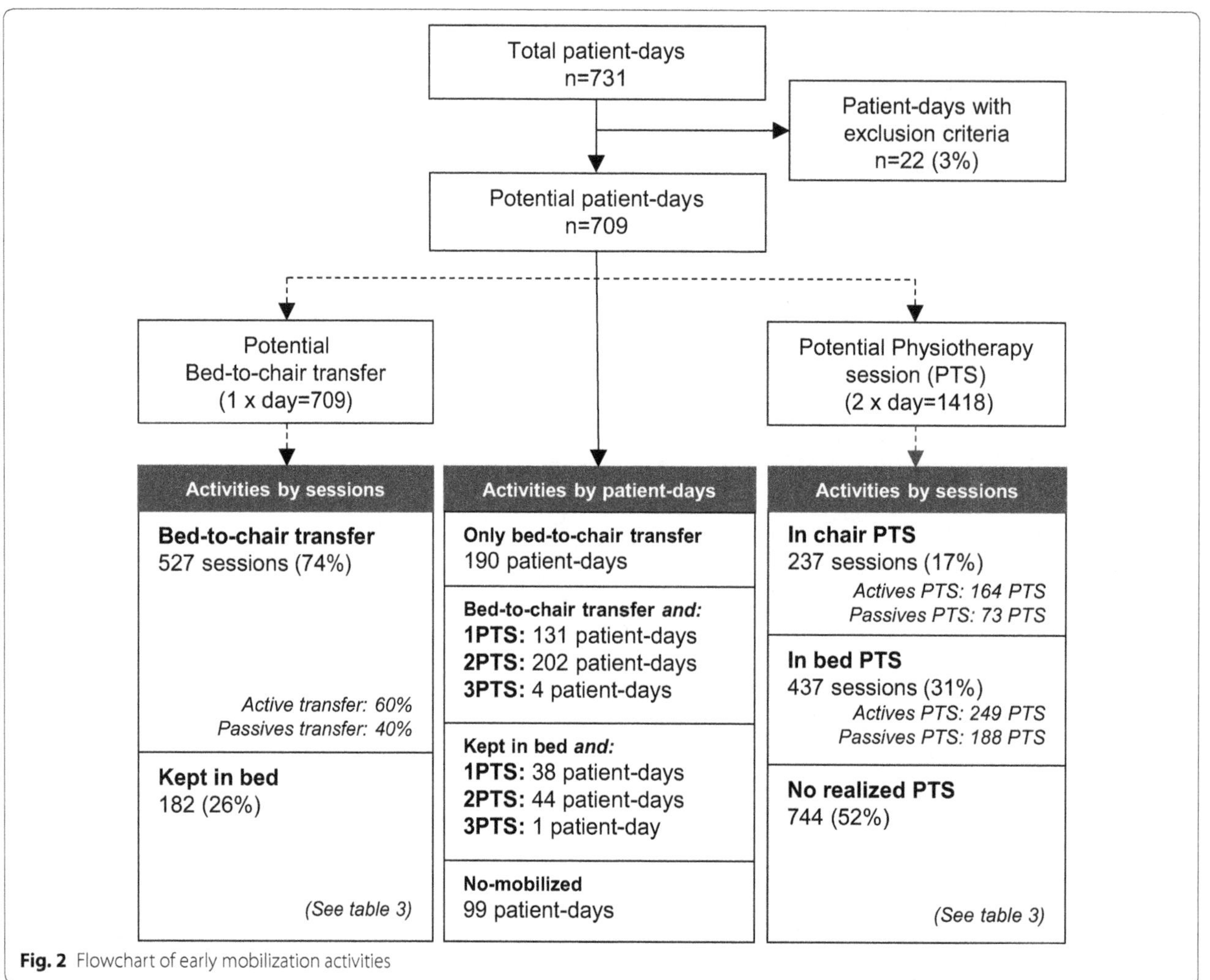

Fig. 2 Flowchart of early mobilization activities

dose: 0.34 (95 % CI 0.11–0.44)] and transfer from bed to chair was performed for 11 sessions in the same condition [mean dose: 0.30 (95 % CI 0.22–0.37)].

The second limiting factor was related to respiratory dysfunction on account of recent intubation/extubation ($n = 12$), prone position ($n = 2$), or occurrence of severe hypoxemia ($n = 19$). In these patients, mean FiO_2 was 0.62 (95 % CI 0.51–0.73). Nevertheless, 78 % of MV patients were successfully mobilized with a mean FiO_2 at 0.47 (95 %CI 0.46–0.49). We carried out 23 active and 49 passive physical therapy sessions with $FiO_2 \geq 0.60$ (mean FiO_2 at 0.83 (95 %CI 0.77–0.88) and 0.71 (95 %CI 0.67–0.76), respectively), as well as 50 bed-to-chair transfers with mean FiO_2 of 0.78 (95 %CI 0.74–0.82). Maximum FiO_2 at 1.0 was observed during 18 mobility activities: nine chair sittings and nine physiotherapy activities.

Adverse events

Activities were discontinued due to medical/nursing procedures in 11 cases and at patient request (pain, high perceived exertion, or digestive transit acceleration) in eight cases. Adverse events occurred in 10 interventions, representing 0.8 % of total mobilizations; hypotension occurred in two patients receiving low-dose vasopressors, hypertension in two, and tachycardia in three. In the sitting position, one patient experienced faintness and was subsequently diagnosed with pulmonary embolism, while another epileptic patient experienced seizures. Moreover, one patient's operative wound exhibited slight oozing after a walking session. All events were reversible following activity interruption, displaying no impact on clinical outcome. There was no evidence of induced tissue hypoxia, as confirmed by means of steady lactate levels after mobilization available for 370 patients-days.

Table 2 Characteristics of mobilized and non-mobilized patients

	ICU patient-days	EM performed				No EM performed
		Sitting in chair			In bed PTS+	
		All sitting in chair	PTS+	PTS-		
Total	709	527	337	190	83	99
Invasive mechanical ventilation (MV)	327	223 (68 %)	142 (43 %)	81 (25 %)	40 (12 %)	64 (20 %)
Severe sepsis/sepsis shock	241	166 (69 %)	102 (42 %)	64 (27 %)	28 (12 %)	47 (20 %)
Vasoactive drugs (VAD)	211	149 (71 %)	99 (47 %)	50 (24 %)	25 (12 %)	37 (18 %)
Renal replacement therapy (RRT)	115	76 (66 %)	59 (51 %)	17 (15 %)	11 (10 %)	28 (24 %)
Sedatives (SD)	260	193 (74 %)	122 (47 %)	71 (27 %)	22 (8 %)	45 (17 %)
MV + VAD	158	104 (66 %)	72 (46 %)	32 (20 %)	21 (13 %)	33 (21 %)
MV + VAD + RRT	77	46 (60 %)	38 (49 %)	8 (10 %)	8 (10 %)	23 (30 %)
MV + without SD	122	77 (63 %)	49 (40 %)	28 (23 %)	22 (18 %)	23 (19 %)
RASS −1 to +1	576	454 (79 %)	284 (49 %)	170 (30 %)	58 (10 %)	64 (11 %)
RASS >+1	25	21 (84 %)	18 (72 %)	3 (12 %)	1 (0.4 %)	3 (12 %)
RASS <−1	108	50 (46 %)	33 (31 %)	17 (16 %)	22 (20 %)	36 (33 %)

Values expressed as number (percentage)

MV mechanical ventilation, *VAD* vasoactive drugs, *RRT* renal replacement therapy, *SD* sedatives drug, *RASS* Richmond agitation-sedation scale, *PTS+* physical therapy session carried out, *PTS−* no physical therapy session carried out, *EM* early mobilization

Table 3 Early mobilization activities and patients' perception

	Total	Duration[a]	RASS[a]	Patient perception (0–10)[b]						
				Pain				*n*	Fatigue	Enjoyment
	n	min	(−5 to +4)	*n*	Before	0 min	15 min		0 min	0 min
In-bed passive mobilization	151	17 [15–20]	−2 [−4 to 0]	11	4 ± 3	3 ± 3	3 ± 3	11	6 ± 3	8 ± 1
In-bed active mobilization	177	18 [15–22]	0 [0 to 0]	121	4 ± 3	4 ± 3	4 ± 3	108	6 ± 3	7 ± 3
In-bed passive cycling (legs/arms)	37	20 [15–21]	−1 [−4 to 0]	7	2 ± 3	2 ± 3	2 ± 3	7	5 ± 3	8 ± 2
In-bed active cycling (legs/arms)	69	20 [15–22]	0 [0 to 0]	64	2 ± 2	2 ± 2	3 ± 2	65	5 ± 3	9 ± 2
In-bed leg press	3	16 [10–20]	0 [0 to 0]	3	3 ± 1	3 ± 1	3 ± 1	3	5 ± 1	9 ± 1
In-chair sitting	526	300 [152–300]	0 [0 to 0]	–	–	–	–	–	–	–
In-chair passive mobilization	14	15 [12–18]	−2 [−5 to 0]	3	4 ± 4	4 ± 4	5 ± 5	1	3	5
In-chair active mobilization	41	15 [13–20]	0 [0 to 0]	22	4 ± 3	4 ± 3	4 ± 3	16	6 ± 2	6 ± 3
In-chair passive cycling (legs/arms)	59	20 [15–20]	0 [−1 to 0]	9	3 ± 3	4 ± 3	3 ± 3	4	4 ± 1	5 ± 1
In-chair active cycling (legs/arms)	93	20 [15–20]	0 [0 to 0]	74	4 ± 3	4 ± 3	3 ± 3	65	5 ± 3	7 ± 3
In-chair leg press	1	20	0	1	2	2	2	–	–	–
Standing/walking	29	28 [20–40]	0 [0 to 0]	24	2 ± 2	3 ± 3	3 ± 2	23	3 ± 2	9 ± 2

n Patient-days

[a] Values expressed as median [IQR]

[b] Values expressed as mean ± SD

Safety of early mobilization

By multivariate analyses, we were able to assess several risk factors associated with in ICU, 28-day, and in-hospital mortality (Additional file 3). Interestingly, after adjustment for severity covariates, early mobilization was not associated with increased mortality and was identified as a significant protective factor in all multivariate models (AOR (95 % CI): 0.06 (0.01–0.29), $p = 0.001$; 0.13 (0.04–0.47), $p = 0.002$ and 0.31 (0.11–0.91), $p = 0.03$ for ICU, 28-day, and in-hospital mortalities, respectively). Longer ICU length of stay, advanced age, severity of hypoxemia according to Berlin classification, and higher SOFA score were risk factors for ICU mortality. Vasoactive drug use and higher APACHE II score were risk factors for 28-day

Table 4 Limiting factors to early mobilization

	Limiting factors to	
	Bed-to-chair transfer	Physical therapy sessions
	182 out of 709 (26 %)	744 out of 1418 (52 %)
Patient-dependent limiting factors		
Severe physiological instability	42 (23 %)	42 (6 %)
Hemodynamic instability	21	9
Respiratory instability	5	27
Neurological instability	16	6
Patient refusal	26 (14 %)	62 (8 %)
Patient-independent limiting factor		
ICU interventions	45 (25 %)	49 (7 %)
Surgery (transferred to OR)	16	16
Medical/imaging procedures	17	22
Nurse procedures	12	13
Insufficient staff (weekend)	11 (6 %)	396 (53 %)
Insufficient staff (weekdays)	0 (0 %)	16 (2 %)
No reported physical therapist consultation during week	–	177 (24 %)
Unspecified	58 (32 %)	2 (0 %)

Values expressed as number (%)

OR operative room

mortality. Finally, tracheostomy and higher APACHE II score were identified as risk factors for hospital mortality.

Discussion

This observational study demonstrates the utility of teamwork in successfully carrying out early mobilization, as assessed on 171 consecutive critically ill patients. The study's main observation is that mobility was provided at least once in 81 % of all patients within 24 h of ICU admission. Bed-to-chair transfer was achievable in the vast majority of ICU patient-days. As shown by our study data, a teamwork approach exhibited an excellent safety profile when initiated very early after ICU admission, even in patients on support by vasoactive agents, MV, or RRT. Safety of our early mobilization approach was confirmed through a multivariate analysis taking into account patients' severity. After adjustment, early mobilization was identified not only as safe, but as a significant protective factor.

Despite the growing body of evidence confirming the feasibility, safety, and improved outcome displayed by early mobilization, it still remains a nonstandard and uncommon practice in ICUs. Moreover, initiation times vary significantly in the literature, ranging from 1.5 to 2 days [7, 32] to several days after intubation [9], or even weeks after ICU admission [33, 34]. Furthermore, several reports describe rehabilitation initiation occurring only after ICU discharge due to a lack of physical therapists or mobility teams within the ICU in question [35, 36]. In a large-scale multicenter cohort study on MV patients, mobility was achieved in only 16 % of overall sessions, reporting intubation and sedation as the primary limiting factors. In this report, authors founded a high incidence of muscular weakness and associated with higher mortality [16]. Furthermore, no clear improvement in outcome has been reported when reinforcement of physical activity was provided only after patients' awakening [37].

Recent expert recommendations on safety criteria for early mobilization mentioned that vasopressor use [38, 39], endotracheal intubation, RRT [38], or even life support devices like ECMO [40] should not be considered as contraindications for active mobilization. Despite that, besides the study of Pohlman et al. [32] performing in-bed mobilization with maximal FiO_2 at 1.0 and vasoactive drug, no study has explored the safety of very early mobilization in critically ill patients on multiple support systems. To date, there is no consensus regarding vasoactive doses or maximum FiO_2, but <0.60 was considered safe for initiating active mobilization [38]. Some authors consider a maximum noradrenaline dose of 0.2 $\mu g\ kg^{-1}\ min^{-1}$ and $FiO_2 < 0.55$ or 0.60 to be safe [9, 38]. In the protocol at hand, we made a conscious effort to predefine a few contraindications, in order to assess each patient's potential to undergo early activity. Our results demonstrate that mobilizing patients with higher vasopressor doses and FiO_2 is achievable without increased risks. However, based on our data we are unable to propose theoretical limits to mobilization. Indeed, there is to our view no limiting FiO_2 or vasopressor dose, but rather a stabilized patient's condition with all supports.

Adverse event rates were shown to vary across studies. Pohlman et al. [32] reported the feasibility of early physical therapy and occupational therapy in 90 % of MV patients on life support devices combined with daily sedation interruption. In their study, the mean Apache II score was 20, and mobility was initiated within 1.5 days following intubation, with adverse events occurring in 16 % of overall sessions. In line with other studies, we clearly showed that most patients receiving MV and supportive therapy can be mobilized very early, within the first day of ICU admission. Furthermore, such activities were rarely interrupted due to adverse events like hypotension or arrhythmia, while requiring no additional intervention nor causing adverse outcome. We also demonstrated that mobility activities can be performed by patients following major abdominal surgery, patient that are often excluded of clinical trials.

As previously described, providing early mobilization with a high degree of supportive care requires experienced and coordinated multidisciplinary teams [41]. This is a mandatory aspect to ensure patients' security during early mobilization implementation.

Our principal limiting factor for specific physical therapy activities stemmed from staffing capacities, resulting in 28 % of overall weekend and 12 % of weekday physical therapy activities not being performed. This likewise accounted for the low rate of walks, since emphasis was placed on less time-consuming therapies, such as ergometer cycling, in an attempt to mobilize every patient. Based on our data, we estimated the ideal ratio of senior physiotherapists to patients to be 1:7 (including on weekends) in order to achieve the optimal number of daily physical therapy activities. Furthermore, the vast majority of patients were able to be moved out of bed by the nursing team on weekends. This observation confirms that a teamwork- and protocol-driven approach is recommended in order to ensure maximum mobilization, even in the presence of a limited number of physical therapists [19]. Moreover, even if more staff is required to mobilize patients out of bed, seating patients in a chair seems to be more advantageous in the ability to achieve a greater angle of inclination and to remain in a more stable position, compared with semi-recumbent position on bed, with non-additional risks [42].

Deep sedation is usually associated with limited mobility [43]. In our study, it was therefore unsurprising to observe a lower rate of bed-to-chair transfers for patients with a RASS score <-1. Current guidelines on sedation recommend maintaining consciousness with adequate analgesia, which results in a reduction in MV duration [44], vasopressor dosage, and in-hospital mortality [45]. In line with this recommendation, RASS scores in our study primarily ranged between -1 and $+1$, allowing patients to communicate and self-regulate both exercise intensity and duration. In addition, patients were also allowed to refuse mobilization initiation, when expressing their inability to leave their beds or perform any physical activity. This overall approach therefore represents our optimal strategy to individually dose activity intensity and duration, coupled with vital parameter monitoring. In terms of severely ill unconscious patients, passive mobility has previously been reported to be associated with negligible variation in oxygen consumption and hemodynamic parameters [46–48].

Emerging clinical research now takes into consideration the subjective feelings of critically ill patients undergoing physical therapy in order to better dose their activities' intensity [49]. In accordance with such methods, overall exertion values in our population were moderate, coupled with higher perceptions of enjoyment post-exercise. These observations are highly relevant for this new approach of patient-centered outcomes in critical care. Surprisingly, even during the more demanding physical activities, patients reported high enjoyment ratings.

Our study has some limitations. Firstly, this was a single-center study conducted in an ICU with a strong culture of both mobilization and minimal sedation. It may thus prove difficult to extrapolate our results to other centers. Secondly, in line with our observational study design, muscle strength or other functional outcomes were not assessed. Moreover, the protective effect of early mobilization has to be considered as an observation in our study cohort and must be confirmed by a randomized controlled trial. At last, due to the layout of the critical care units in our hospital, we did not include ischemic or heart failure patients in our study.

In conclusion, we observed that early mobilization is achievable and well tolerated in the vast majority of critically ill patients, despite commonly described contraindications such as MV, vasopressor administration, and RRT. It is of great interest to note that patients reported very positive experiences and feelings of well-being following various modalities of physical therapy sessions.

Abbreviations

ICU: intensive care unit; MV: mechanical ventilation; RRT: renal replacement therapy; ECMO: extracorporeal membrane oxygenation; FiO_2: fraction of inspired oxygen; PTS: physiotherapy session; EM: early mobilization; AOR: adjusted odds ratio.

Authors' contributions

CEH, CD, EB, JD, XW, JR, and PFL contributed to the conception and design of the research; AT, LC, GT, EB, JD, and JR contributed to data collection; all authors contributed to data analysis and interpretation and drafting of the manuscript. Furthermore, they all were involved in critically revising the manuscript and agree to be held fully accountable for ensuring the integrity and accuracy of their work. All authors read and approved the final manuscript.

Acknowledgements

The authors would like to thank Dr. Jean-Louis Bachy for his fundamental IT support and Professor Annie Robert for her assistance in statistical analyses.

Competing interests

The authors declare that they have no competing interests.

References

1. Burns JR. Letter: early ambulation of patients requiring ventilatory assistance. CHEST J. 1975;68(4):608a.
2. Bailey PP, Miller RR 3rd, Clemmer TP. Culture of early mobility in mechanically ventilated patients. Crit Care Med. 2009;37(10 Suppl):S429–35.
3. Stiller K. Physiotherapy in intensive care: an updated systematic review. Chest. 2013;144(3):825–47.
4. Chambers MA, Moylan JS, Reid MB. Physical inactivity and muscle weakness in the critically ill. Crit Care Med. 2009;37(10 Suppl):S337–46.
5. Griffiths RD, Palmer TE, Helliwell T, et al. Effect of passive stretching on the wasting of muscle in the critically ill. Nutrition. 1995;11(5):428–32.
6. Weber-Carstens S, Schneider J, Wollersheim T, et al. Critical illness myopathy and GLUT4: significance of insulin and muscle contraction. Am J Respir Crit Care Med. 2013;187(4):387–96.
7. Schweickert WD, Pohlman MC, Pohlman AS, et al. Early physical and occupational therapy in mechanically ventilated, critically ill patients: a randomised controlled trial. Lancet. 2009;373(9678):1874–82.
8. Hopkins RO, Suchyta MR, Farrer TJ, et al. Improving post-intensive care unit neuropsychiatric outcomes: understanding cognitive effects of physical activity. Am J Respir Crit Care Med. 2012;186(12):1220–8.
9. Burtin C, Clerckx B, Robbeets C, et al. Early exercise in critically ill patients enhances short-term functional recovery. Crit Care Med. 2009;37(9):2499–505.
10. Lord RK, Mayhew CR, Korupolu R, et al. ICU early physical rehabilitation programs: financial modeling of cost savings. Crit Care Med. 2013;41(3):717–24.
11. Skrobik Y, Chanques G. The pain, agitation, and delirium practice guidelines for adult critically ill patients: a post-publication perspective. Ann Intensive Care. 2013;3(1):9.
12. Morris PE, Goad A, Thompson C, et al. Early intensive care unit mobility therapy in the treatment of acute respiratory failure. Crit Care Med. 2008;36(8):2238–43.
13. Calvo-Ayala E, Khan BA, Farber MO, et al. Interventions to improve the physical function of ICU survivors: a systematic review. Chest. 2013;144(5):1469–80.
14. Peiris C, Shields N, Brusco N, et al. Additional Saturday rehabilitation improves functional independence and quality of life and reduces length of stay: a randomized controlled trial. BMC Med. 2013;11(1):198.
15. Hakkennes S, Lindner C, Reid J. Implementing an inpatient rehabilitation Saturday service is associated with improved patient outcomes and facilitates patient flow across the health care continuum. Disabil Rehabil. 2015;37(8):721–7.
16. TEAM Study Investigators. Early mobilization and recovery in mechanically ventilated patients in the ICU: a bi-national, multi-centre, prospective cohort study. *Crit Care* 2015;19(1):81.
17. Bailey P, Thomsen GE, Spuhler VJ, et al. Early activity is feasible and safe in respiratory failure patients. Crit Care Med. 2007;35(1):139–45.
18. Barber EA, Everard T, Holland AE, et al. Barriers and facilitators to early mobilisation in Intensive Care: a qualitative study. Aust Crit Care. 2015;28(4):177–82 **(quiz 83)**.
19. Jolley SE, Regan-Baggs J, Dickson RP, et al. Medical intensive care unit clinician attitudes and perceived barriers towards early mobilization of critically ill patients: a cross-sectional survey study. BMC Anesthesiol. 2014;14:84.
20. Bakhru RN, Wiebe DJ, McWilliams DJ, et al. An environmental scan for early mobilization practices in U.S. ICUs. Crit Care Med. 2015;43(11):2360–9.
21. Egerod I, Bergbom I, Lindahl B, et al. The patient experience of intensive care: a meta-synthesis of Nordic studies. Int J Nurs Stud. 2015;52(8):1354–61.
22. Jaillette E, Girault C, Brunin G, et al. French Intensive Care Society, International congress—Réanimation 2016. Ann Intensive Care. 2016;6(1):1–236.
23. Gosselink R, Bott J, Johnson M, et al. Physiotherapy for adult patients with critical illness: recommendations of the European Respiratory Society and European Society of Intensive Care Medicine Task Force on Physiotherapy for Critically Ill Patients. Intensive Care Med. 2008;34(7):1188–99.
24. Offenstadt G. *Réanimation - Traité de référence en Médecine Intensive et Réanimation*. 3ème édition ed. Paris: Elsevier; 2016.
25. Choi J, Tasota FJ, Hoffman LA. Mobility interventions to improve outcomes in patients undergoing prolonged mechanical ventilation: a review of the literature. Biol Res Nurs. 2008;10(1):21–33.
26. Ventilation with lower tidal volumes as compared with traditional tidal volumes for acute lung injury and the acute respiratory distress syndrome The acute respiratory distress syndrome network. *N* Engl J Med 2000;342(18):1301–8.
27. Lee H, Ko YJ, Suh GY, et al. Safety profile and feasibility of early physical therapy and mobility for critically ill patients in the medical intensive care unit: beginning experiences in Korea. J Crit Care. 2015;30(4):673–7.
28. Borg G, Ljunggren G, Ceci R. The increase of perceived exertion, aches and pain in the legs, heart rate and blood lactate during exercise on a bicycle ergometer. Eur J Appl Physiol Occup Physiol. 1985;54(4):343–9.
29. Baron B, Moullan F, Deruelle F, et al. The role of emotions on pacing strategies and performance in middle and long duration sport events. Br J Sports Med. 2011;45(6):511–7.
30. Kilpatrick M, Kraemer R, Bartholomew J, et al. Affective responses to exercise are dependent on intensity rather than total work. Med Sci Sports Exerc. 2007;39(8):1417–22.
31. Ranieri VM, Rubenfeld GD, Thompson BT, et al. Acute respiratory distress syndrome: the Berlin definition. JAMA. 2012;307(23):2526–33.
32. Pohlman MC, Schweickert WD, Pohlman AS, et al. Feasibility of physical and occupational therapy beginning from initiation of mechanical ventilation. Crit Care Med. 2010;38(11):2089–94.
33. Chiang LL, Wang LY, Wu CP, et al. Effects of physical training on functional status in patients with prolonged mechanical ventilation. Phys Ther. 2006;86(9):1271–81.
34. Martin UJ, Hincapie L, Nimchuk M, et al. Impact of whole-body rehabilitation in patients receiving chronic mechanical ventilation. Crit Care Med. 2005;33(10):2259–65.
35. Thomsen GE, Snow GL, Rodriguez L, et al. Patients with respiratory failure increase ambulation after transfer to an intensive care unit where early activity is a priority. Crit Care Med. 2008;36(4):1119–24.
36. O'Connor ED, Walsham J. Should we mobilise critically ill patients? A review. Crit Care Resusc. 2009;11(4):290–300.
37. Moss M, Nordon-Craft A, Malone D, et al. A randomized trial of an intensive physical therapy program for patients with acute respiratory failure. Am J Respir Crit Care Med. 2016;193(10):1101–10.
38. Hodgson CL, Stiller K, Needham DM, et al. Expert consensus and recommendations on safety criteria for active mobilization of mechanically ventilated critically ill adults. Crit Care. 2014;18(6):658.
39. Roeseler J, Sottiaux T, Lemiale V, et al. Management of early mobilisation (including electrostimulation) in adult and pediatric patients in the intensive care unit. Réanimation. 2013;22(2):207–18.
40. Ko Y, Cho YH, Park YH, et al. Feasibility and safety of early physical therapy and active mobilization for patients on extracorporeal membrane oxygenation. ASAIO J. 2015;61(5):564–8.

41. Bassett RD, Vollman KM, Brandwene L, et al. Integrating a multidisciplinary mobility programme into intensive care practice (IMMPTP): a multicentre collaborative. Intensive Crit Care Nurs. 2012;28(2):88–97.
42. Thomas P, Paratz J, Lipman J. Seated and semi-recumbent positioning of the ventilated intensive care patient—effect on gas exchange, respiratory mechanics and hemodynamics. Heart Lung. 2014;43(2):105–11.
43. Leditschke IA, Green M, Irvine J, et al. What are the barriers to mobilizing intensive care patients? Cardiopulm Phys Ther J. 2012;23(1):26–9.
44. De Jonghe B, Bastuji-Garin S, Fangio P, et al. Sedation algorithm in critically ill patients without acute brain injury. Crit Care Med. 2005;33(1):120–7.
45. Tanaka LM, Azevedo LC, Park M, et al. Early sedation and clinical outcomes of mechanically ventilated patients: a prospective multicenter cohort study. Crit Care. 2014;18(4):R156.
46. Hickmann CE, Roeseler J, Castanares-Zapatero D, et al. Energy expenditure in the critically ill performing early physical therapy. Intensive Care Med. 2014;40(4):548–55.
47. Pires-Neto RC, Kawaguchi YMF, Hirota AS, et al. Very early passive cycling exercise in mechanically ventilated critically ill patients: physiological and safety aspects—a case series. PLoS One. 2013;8(9):e74182.
48. Koch SM, Fogarty S, Signorino C, et al. Effect of passive range of motion on intracranial pressure in neurosurgical patients. J Crit Care. 1996;11(4):176–9.
49. Sottile PD, Nordon-Craft A, Malone D, et al. Patient and family perceptions of physical therapy in the medical intensive care unit. J Crit Care. 2015;30(5):891–5.

3

External validation of the APPS, a new and simple outcome prediction score in patients with the acute respiratory distress syndrome

Lieuwe D. Bos[1*], Laura R. Schouten[1], Olaf L. Cremer[2], David S. Y. Ong[2,3], Marcus J. Schultz[1]
and MARS consortium

Abstract

Background: A recently developed prediction score based on age, arterial oxygen partial pressure to fractional inspired oxygen ratio (PaO_2/FiO_2) and plateau pressure (abbreviated as 'APPS') was shown to accurately predict mortality in patients diagnosed with the acute respiratory distress syndrome (ARDS). After thorough temporal external validation of the APPS, we tested the spatial external validity in a cohort of ARDS patients recruited during 3 years in two hospitals in the Netherlands.

Methods: Consecutive patients with moderate or severe ARDS according to the Berlin definition were included in this observational multicenter cohort study from the mixed medical-surgical ICUs of two university hospitals. The APPS was calculated per patient with the maximal airway pressure instead of the plateau pressure as all patients were ventilated in pressure-controlled mode. The predictive accuracy for hospital mortality was evaluated by calculating the area under the receiver operating characteristics curve (AUC-ROC). Additionally, the score was recalibrated and reassessed.

Results: In total, 439 patients with moderate or severe ARDS were analyzed. All-cause hospital mortality was 43 %. The APPS predicted all-cause hospital mortality with moderate accuracy, with an AUC-ROC of 0.62 [95 % confidence interval (CI) 0.56–0.67]. Calibration was moderate using the original cutoff values (Hosmer–Lemeshow goodness of fit $P < 0.001$), and recalibration was performed for the cutoff value for age and plateau pressure. This resulted in good calibration ($P = 1.0$), but predictive accuracy did not improve (AUC-ROC 0.63, 95 % CI 0.58–0.68).

Conclusions: The predictive accuracy for all-cause hospital mortality of the APPS was moderate, also after recalibration of the score, and thus the APPS does not seem to be fitted for that purpose. The APPS might serve as simple tool for stratification of mortality in patients with moderate or severe ARDS. Without recalibrations, the performance of the APPS was moderate and we should therefore hesitate to blindly apply the score to other cohorts of ARDS patients.

Keywords: ARDS, Prediction, Mortality, Sensitivity, Specificity, APPS

Background

Outcome prediction in critically ill patients is commonly performed using general-purpose scoring systems such as the Acute Physiology and Chronic Health Evaluation (APACHE) score [1] and the Simplified Acute Physiology Score (SAPS) [2], which have been developed in unselected series of ICU patients. Other scoring systems have been developed for selective patient groups in the intensive care unit (ICU), e.g., for patients who develop acute kidney injury [3, 4] and liver failure [5].

Unfortunately, no such prediction system has been developed for patients with the acute respiratory distress syndrome (ARDS). Outcome prediction in patients with ARDS based on PaO_2/FiO_2, as proposed in the American-European Consensus Conference (AECC) criteria [6]

*Correspondence: l.d.bos@amc.nl
[1] Department of Intensive Care, Academic Medical Center, Meibergdreef 9, 1105 AZ Amsterdam, The Netherlands
Full list of author information is available at the end of the article

and the Berlin definition for ARDS [7], does neither show good predictive accuracy nor show calibration [7–9]. Very recently, a scoring system was developed that predicts hospital mortality with good accuracy in patients with ARDS [10]. This score is based on three routinely available variables: age, the arterial oxygen partial pressure to fractional inspired oxygen ratio (PaO_2/FiO_2) and plateau pressure measured 24 h after the initial diagnosis of ARDS, and was thus coined the APPS. However, after excellent results of temporal external validation of this so-called APPS by the original authors, spatial external validation (e.g., the accuracy of prediction in another location) is highly needed.

Therefore, we tested the predictive accuracy and calibration of the APPS in a cohort of consecutive prospectively identified ARDS patients in two university hospitals in the Netherlands and recalibrated the score for our population of patients. We hypothesized that the ability of the APPS to predict hospital mortality remains excellent after spatial external validation.

Methods

Study design

The patient cohort was previously described by Gebobers et al. [11]. Patients with ARDS, according to the Berlin definition, were selected from the parent 'Molecular Diagnosis and Risk Stratification' (MARS) study, performed in the ICUs of two tertiary care hospitals in the Netherlands (Academic Medical Center, Amsterdam, The Netherlands; University Medical Center, Utrecht, The Netherlands). The Medical Ethics Committees of both hospitals approved the study protocol and opt-out consent method. The patient or their legal representative was presented with a brochure and opt-out form, to be completed in case of unwillingness to participate.

Setting

ICUs are closed-format units, with a team of board-certified critical care physicians, fellows in critical care medicine and board-certified ICU nurses caring for a mixed medical-surgical population of patients. The nurse-to-patient ratio was from 1:1 to 1:2. Patients received lung-protective mechanical ventilation per protocol, which mandated the use of low tidal volumes (6–8 mL/kg predicted body weight), a minimum level of positive end-expiratory pressure of 5 cmH_2O, which together with FiO_2 was titrated based on frequent PaO_2 measurements. As part of standard care, nurses and attending physicians checked hourly whether there were signs of spontaneous breathing activity by comparing the set and measured respiratory rate and by observing flow curves at the ventilator. In case this was seen, the ventilator could be switched to an assisted ventilation mode, or additional sedation was given. Recruitment maneuvers and prone ventilation were used early and frequently if hypoxemia did not respond to higher levels of PEEP and FiO_2. Details of the ventilation protocol were reported before [12]. A conservative fluid strategy was followed according to the ARDSnet protocol [13], and analgo-sedation was applied using sedation scales and bolus sedation with midazolam or continuous sedation with propofol. Details of the analgo-sedation protocol were also reported before [14]. Neuromuscular blocking agents were not routinely used, and if used only as a bolus.

Inclusion and exclusion criteria

Consecutive adult patients admitted to the ICU with an expected length of stay of more than 24 h from January 2011 to December 2013 were eligible for participation in the MARS study. ARDS was defined according to the criteria stated by the American-European Consensus Conference on ARDS: i.e., the diagnosis required an acute onset of symptoms, the presence of bilateral infiltrates on chest radiography, a pulmonary-artery wedge pressure <18 mmHg and/or the absence of signs of left ventricular dysfunction, and a $PaO_2/FiO_2 \leq 200$. Although our study started in 2011, before the recent 'Berlin definition for ARDS', we found that 100 % patients would have fulfilled the criteria of the new definition. Patients that were discharged or transferred to another ICU within 24 h after the diagnosis of ARDS were excluded from the present analysis, as they could not be used to validate the results reported by the ALIEN Network investigators. There were no additional inclusion or exclusion criteria for the present analysis. ARDS was diagnosed by a dedicated team of researchers who were trained in the proper use of the AECC criteria for ARDS [12]. The cause for ARDS was determined and scored in the following categories: pneumonia, aspiration, other pulmonary (i.e., inhalation trauma, near drowning), sepsis, trauma or major surgery, pancreatitis or other non-pulmonary (i.e., blood transfusion, toxic medication). In the event of multiple causes for ARDS, each cause was scored separately.

APPS

The APPS was calculated as proposed in the original publication [10]. However, instead of plateau pressure, maximal airway pressure was used since pressure-controlled ventilation was used exclusively in our setting. The maximal airway pressure during pressure-controlled ventilation is equal to the plateau pressure during volume-controlled ventilation under most circumstances. As described above, nurses and physicians screened whether the ventilator could be switched to an assisted ventilation mode.

Outcomes

All-cause in-hospital mortality was used as the primary endpoint. The data collectors were blind for this outcome at the moment of data collection as the all parameters were collected prospectively. If a patient was transferred to another hospital, that hospital was contacted to obtain the date of hospital discharge. Follow-up was complete for all patients.

Statistical analysis

Data were expressed as mean ± SD, median with interquartile range or number with percentage, as appropriate. Differences between groups were tested with the Pearson Chi-square or Fisher exact test for categorical variables and with *T* test, one-way ANOVA, Mann–Whitney or Kruskal–Wallis test for numerical variables. A *P* value below 0.05 was considered significant. All analyses were performed in R via the R-studio interface.

The predictive performance of the APPS was assessed by quantifying the calibration and the accuracy of the score [15]. The predictive accuracy was expressed in the area under the receiver operating characteristics curve (AUC-ROC), and the predictive accuracy of the APPS was compared to the APACHE IV score. Sensitivity, specificity and likelihood ratios were calculated for the optimal cutoff obtained by the Youden index. A Kaplan–Meier curve was constructed for the APPS categories 3–4, 5–7, 8–9, as in the original report on the APPS [10]. Calibration was visualized by plotting the APPS against the percentage of non-survivors at that score and quantified by the Hosmer–Lemeshow goodness-of-fit test. Recalibration was performed manually, and measures of calibration and predictive accuracy were reassessed. A sensitivity analysis was performed in patients that received mechanical ventilation according to the ventilation protocol in the derivation study for the APPS (i.e., patients were ventilated using the following settings: PEEP $\geq$ 10 cmH_2O and $FiO_2 \geq 50$ %). A *P* value below 0.05 was considered significant. All analyses were performed in R via the R-studio interface.

Results

The cohort consisted of 439 patients with moderate or severe ARDS. Baseline characteristics are described in Table 1. Pressure-controlled ventilation was exclusively used; indeed, volume-controlled ventilation and assisted ventilation modes were not used at the moments data were collected for the present investigation. All-cause hospital mortality was 43 %. The mean APPS was 5 in surviving patients and 6 in non-surviving patients (Additional file 1: Figure E1; $P < 0.001$). The APPS predicted all-cause hospital mortality with moderate accuracy with an AUC-ROC of 0.62 (95 % confidence interval 0.56–0.67, see Fig. 1; Table 2), which was not significantly different from the predictive value of the APACHE IV score (AUC-ROC 0.66, 95 % CI 0.61–0.71; $P = 0.22$). The APPS showed a disturbed calibration at a score of 4–5 (Fig. 1; $P < 0.001$). This was mainly due to the categorization of the variables age and Pmax (Table 3, Additional file 1: Figure E2). This was translated into overlapping Kaplan–Meier curves for the APPS categories 3–4 and 5–7 (Additional file 1: Figure E3).

Recalibration was performed for two of the three facets of the APPS. The age limit for 2 points was set to 47 and for 3 points to above 59 years (see Table 4). A maximum airway pressure above 30 resulted in 2 points and above 33 in 3 points. This resulted in good calibration (Fig. 1; Table 4; Additional file 1: Figure E4, E5, $P = 1.0$), but predictive accuracy remained moderate (AUC-ROC 0.63, 95 % CI 0.58–0.68, Fig. 1). Survival was significantly different when the APPS categories were changed to 3, 4–7 and 8–9 ($P < 0.001$, Additional file 1: Figure E6).

A sensitivity analysis was limited to patients that were ventilated following the protocol that was used in the derivation cohort ($N = 151$), where the ventilation data were collected under the following standardized ventilatory settings: PEEP $\geq$ 10 cmH_2O and $FiO_2 \geq 50$ %. This analysis confirmed a moderate predictive accuracy for the original (AUC-ROC 0.62, 95 % CI 0.54–0.71) and the recalibrated APPS (AUC-ROC 0.64, 95 % CI 0.55–0.73).

Discussion

Spatial external validation of the APPS in two university hospitals in the Netherlands showed a considerable lower predictive accuracy for all-cause hospital mortality than in the derivation and temporal validation population in the Spanish hospitals. Calibration was also disturbed, but this was resolved after minor modification of the score.

Patient characteristics were strikingly similar in both studies. For example, hospital mortality was comparable between the cohorts (46 % in the derivation cohort, 42 % in temporal validation cohort and 43 % in spatial validation cohort). Furthermore, ventilator parameters were also comparable, with the exception of FiO_2 (80 % in derivation and temporal validation cohorts, 60 % in spatial validation cohort). Additionally, the strength of the association between aspects of the APPS and mortality, as exemplified by the odds ratio (Tables 2, 3), was similar between the cohorts. Importantly, the odds ratio is a measure of effect size and not of discrimination. This implies that the association between hospital mortality and age, PaO_2/FiO_2 and plateau pressure was very similar between the cohorts, but that this did not result in sufficient discrimination in the population we included.

Any difference in patient selection, practice or data collection between the temporal validation and spatial

Table 1 Baseline characteristics of 439 survivors and non-survivors with the acute respiratory distress syndrome in the Netherlands

	Survivors ($N = 252$)	Non-survivors ($N = 187$; 43 %)	P
Gender, male, N (%)	163 (64.7)	120 (64.2)	0.92
Age, mean ± SD	58.5 ± 15.4	63.1 ± 12.7	0.001
Cause of ARDS, N (%)			
Pneumonia	154 (61.1)	115 (61.5)	1.0
Aspiration	25 (9.9)	16 (8.6)	0.76
Other pulmonary	2 (0.8)	1 (0.5)	1.0
Sepsis	144 (57.1)	132 (70.6)	0.003
Trauma	38 (15.1)	15 (8.0)	0.029
Pancreatitis	2 (0.8)	6 (3.2)	0.069
Other non-pulmonary	29 (11.5)	17 (9.1)	0.43
Disease severity, mean ± SD			
APACHE IV	85.5 ± 27	102.7 ± 30.7	<0.001
SOFA score	8.6 ± 3.2	10.1 ± 4.1	<0.001
Physiological parameters, mean ± SD			
pH, median ± IQR	7.4, 7.4–7.5	7.4, 7.3–7.4	0.001
$PaCO_2$	42.1 ± 9	44.4 ± 12.1	0.039
PaO_2/FiO_2	126.8 ± 38.3	127.7 ± 43.1	0.81
Respiratory system compliance	28.9 ± 15.6	37.4 ± 20.9	<0.001
Ventilation parameters, mean ± SD			
Tidal volume (ml/kg PBW)	7.7 ± 2	7.5 ± 1.7	0.38
FiO_2	53.2 ± 12.9	56.7 ± 16.7	0.017
Respiratory rate	22 ± 7	25 ± 8	<0.001
PEEP (cmH_2O)	10.4 ± 3.6	10.9 ± 4	0.2
P_{max} (cmH_2O)	26.2 ± 7.9	28.2 ± 9.4	0.018

validation cohorts may explain the differences in discrimination. First, it could be argued that differences arose because we used the maximal airway pressure instead of the plateau pressure. Although the maximal airway pressure can be used to approximate the plateau pressure in theory [16], it could be that, for example, during undetected spontaneous breathing effort these values were influenced [17]. In our setting, however, nurses and physicians carefully and hourly check whether a patient is breathing spontaneously. If so, the local ventilation protocol dictates the use of an assisted ventilation mode, and this was not seen at the moments of data collection for this study. The maximal airway pressure and the plateau pressure are both surrogate measures for alveolar distending pressure, and the accuracy of the score may improve if that pressure would be measured directly. PaO_2/FiO_2 may be influenced by ventilator settings [8], and therefore we performed a sensitivity analyses for patients that were using the standardized ventilator settings (PEEP $\geq$ 10 cmH_2O and $FiO_2 \geq 50$ %) that were used in the original study. However, this did not change the results. This implies that differences in ventilation strategies are not likely to have caused the lower predictive accuracy. Thus, the APPS may have been over-fitted to the setting in which it is developed and validation. This observation is further supported by the observation that not only maximal airway pressure and PaO_2/FiO_2 discriminated differently between the cohorts, but that this lower accuracy was also found for age. In contrast to the former, data collection will not influence the age of the patient. Thereby, we can establish that the lower accuracy may partly be due to differences in data collection, but also that the APPS cannot be generalized to other populations due to over-fitting to the derivation population.

The presented data suggest that calibration of the APPS is sufficiently good after slight modification of the original score. Calibration may be more important than predictive accuracy for some purposes. For example, for inclusion into clinical trials the added value of discrimination is limited, while calibration is pivotal. A well-calibrated score could lead to the inclusion of a patient population with the mortality to which the study is powered (prognostic enrichment), something that has been an issue in many investigational trials [18–20]. However, it is worrisome that recalibration of the cutoffs for age and pressure was needed as this limits the implementation of the score in new clinical environments. Additional

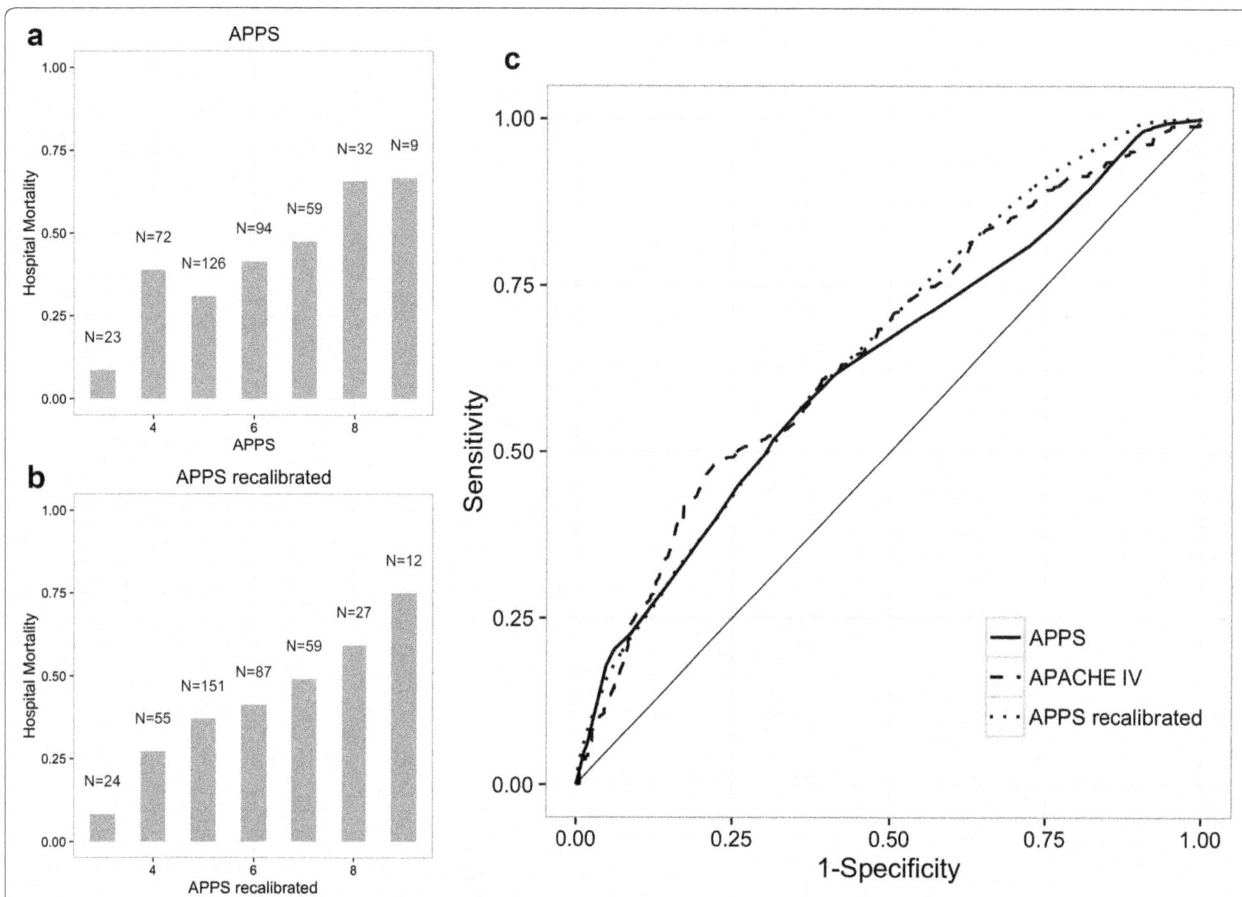

Fig. 1 Calibration and predictive accuracy of the APPS for hospital mortality. **a** Original APPS. **b** Recalibrated APPS. **c** ROC curves. Each *bar* represents the percentage of patients that did not survive that hospital admission. The *number* indicates the total number of patients with that APPS

Table 2 Test characteristics

	ROC	CI	Cutoff	Sens	Spec	LR+	LR−
Complete cohort ($N = 439$)							
APPS	0.62	0.56–0.67	5.5	0.63	0.56	1.43	0.66
Recalibrated APPS	0.63	0.58–0.68	5.5	0.63	0.56	1.43	0.66
Sensitivity analysis ($N = 151$)							
APPS	0.62	0.54–0.71	5.5	0.38	0.85	2.53	0.73
Recalibrated APPS	0.64	0.55–0.73	5.5	0.48	0.78	2.18	0.37

ROC receiver operating characteristics curve, *CI* 95 % confidence interval of area under the ROC curve, *Sens* sensitivity, *Spec* specificity, *LR* likelihood ratio

validation attempts could further clarify the optimal cutoffs for the score and may allow for stratification of newly recruited ARDS patients.

Based on our data, the validity of the APPS as a prediction score for mortality in ARDS is disputable. But what purpose would a prediction score for mortality serve? The authors that proposed the APPS suggest that the score may be used to identify patients in whom benefit from the treatment may be limited. However, here the same point can be made as in the previous paragraph; it may be sufficient to identify groups of patients that have a higher or lower mortality and treat those groups differently. A well-calibrated score will serve this point, and for that purpose, the APPS may still qualify. It could be argued that we should have improved the prediction score. However, this was not the aim of this study. Thorough validation of well-developed scores is more important than development of multiple prediction tools [21].

Table 3 Odds ratios per category APPS

Variable	Range	Category	*N*	Hospital mortality (%)	OR	OR 2.5 %	OR 97.5 %	*P* for trend
Age	<47	1	72	26.4	1			0.0046
	47–66	2	196	43.9	2.18	1.2	3.95	
	>66	3	171	48	2.57	1.41	4.7	
PaO_2/FiO_2	>158	1	239	36.4	1			0.0015
	105–158	2	135	46.7	1.53	1	2.35	
	<105	3	65	56.9	2.31	1.32	4.03	
P_{max}	<27	1	233	34.8	1			0.0021
	27–30	2	48	25	0.63	0.31	1.27	
	>33	3	134	52.2	2.05	1.33	3.17	

Table 4 Odds ratios per category recalibrated APPS

Variable	Range	Category	*N*	Hospital mortality (%)	OR	OR 2.5 %	OR 97.5 %	*P* for trend
Age	<47	1	72	26.4	1			0.0021
	47–59	2	96	41.7	1.99	1.03	3.87	
	>59	3	271	47.2	2.5	1.4	4.44	
PaO_2/FiO_2	>158	1	239	36.4	1			0.0015
	105–158	2	135	46.7	1.53	1.00	2.35	
	<105	3	65	56.9	2.31	1.32	4.03	
P_{max}	<30	1	281	33.1	1			0.0001
	30–33	2	40	45	1.65	0.85	3.23	
	>33	3	94	55.3	2.5	1.55	4.03	

The two-center, single national design is another limitation of the present study as ideally the accuracy of a predictive test such as the APPS is validated in a prospective, international observational cohort study.

To conclude, our data suggest the APPS could serve as simple tool for stratification of mortality in patients with moderate or severe ARDS. Importantly, without recalibrations the performance of the APPS was moderate and we should therefore hesitate to blindly apply the score to new series of patients. The predictive accuracy for all-cause hospital mortality was moderate, also after recalibration of the score, and thus the APPS does not seem to be fitted for that purpose.

Authors' contributions

All authors were involved in conception and design. LDB, LRS, MJS analyzed and interpreted the data. LDB, MJS drafted the manuscript. All authors revised and approved the manuscript. All authors read and approved the final manuscript.

Author details

[1] Department of Intensive Care, Academic Medical Center, Meibergdreef 9, 1105 AZ Amsterdam, The Netherlands. [2] Department of Intensive Care Medicine, University Medical Center Utrecht, Utrecht, The Netherlands. [3] Department of Medical Microbiology, University Medical Center Utrecht, Utrecht, The Netherlands.

Competing interests

The authors declare that they have no competing interests.

Funding

This study was supported by a grant from the Center of Translational Molecular Medicine.

A complete list of members of the MARS Consortium is given in the "Appendix".

Appendix: Members of the MARS consortium

Jos F. Frencken (Department of Intensive Care Medicine and Julius Center for Health Sciences and Primary Care, University Medical Center Utrecht, Utrecht, the Netherlands); Marc Bonten, Peter M. C. Klein Klouwenberg, David Ong (Department of Medical Microbiology, University Medical Center Utrecht, Utrecht, the Netherlands); and Roosmarijn T. M. van Hooijdonk, Mischa A. Huson, Laura R. A. Schouten, Marleen Straat, Lonneke A. van Vught, Maryse A. Wiewel, Esther Witteveen,

Gerie J. Glas, and Luuk Wieske (Department of Intensive Care Medicine, Academic Medical Center, University of Amsterdam); Tom van der Poll (Center of Experimental Molecular Medicine; CEMM, Academic Medical Center, University of Amsterdam).

References

1. Knaus WA, Draper EA, Wagner DP, et al. APACHE II: a severity of disease classification system. Crit Care Med. 1985;13:818–29.
2. Le Gall JR, Lemeshow S, Saulnier F. A new Simplified Acute Physiology Score (SAPS II) based on a European/North American multicenter study [Internet]. JAMA. 1993;270:2957–63. http://jama.jamanetwork.com/article.aspx?articleid=409979.
3. Bellomo R, Ronco C, Kellum JA, et al. Acute renal failure—definition, outcome measures, animal models, fluid therapy and information technology needs: the Second International Consensus Conference of the Acute Dialysis Quality Initiative (ADQI) Group. Crit Care. 2004;8:R204–12.
4. Mehta RL, Kellum JA, Shah SV, et al. Acute Kidney Injury Network: report of an initiative to improve outcomes in acute kidney injury. Crit Care. 2007;11:R31.
5. Campbell J, McPeake J, Shaw M, et al. Validation and analysis of prognostic scoring systems for critically ill patients with cirrhosis admitted to ICU [Internet]. Crit Care. 2015;19:364. http://ccforum.com/content/19/1/364.
6. Bernard GR, Artigas A, Brigham KL, et al. The American-European Consensus Conference on ARDS. Definitions, mechanisms, relevant outcomes, and clinical trial coordination [Internet]. Am J Respir Crit Care Med. 1994;149:818–24. http://www.ncbi.nlm.nih.gov/entrez/query.fcgi?cmd=Retrieve&db=PubMed&dopt=Citation&list_uids=7509706.
7. Ards Definition Task Force T. Acute respiratory distress syndrome: the Berlin definition [Internet]. JAMA. 2012;307:2526–33. http://dx.doi.org/10.1001/jama.2012.5669.
8. Villar J, Blanco J, Del Campo R, et al. Assessment of PaO_2/FiO_2 for stratification of patients with moderate and severe acute respiratory distress syndrome. [Internet]. BMJ Open. 2015;5:e006812 [cited 2015 Apr 3]. http://bmjopen.bmj.com/content/5/3/e006812.short.
9. Hernu R, Wallet F, Thiollière F, et al. An attempt to validate the modification of the American-European consensus definition of acute lung injury/acute respiratory distress syndrome by the Berlin definition in a university hospital. [Internet]. Intensive Care Med. 2013;39:2161–70 [cited 2015 Mar 30]. http://www.ncbi.nlm.nih.gov/pubmed/24114319.
10. Villar J, Ambrós A, Soler J, Martínez D, Ferrando C, Solano R, et al. Age, PaO2 /FIO2, and Plateau pressure score: a proposal for a simple outcome score in patients with the acute respiratory distress syndrome. Crit Care Med. 2016;44:1361–9.
11. Geboers DGPJ, de Beer FM, Boer AMT, et al. Plasma suPAR as a prognostic biological marker for ICU mortality in ARDS patients [Internet]. Intensive Care Med. 2015;41:1281–90 [cited 2015 Jun 26]. http://link.springer.com/10.1007/s00134-015-3924-9.
12. Schultz MJ, De Pont AC. Prone or PEEP, PEEP and prone. Intensive Care Med. 2011;37:366–7.
13. National Heart and Blood Institute Acute Respiratory Distress Syndrome (ARDS) Clinical Trials Network L. Comparison of two fluid-management strategies in acute lung injury. N Engl J Med. 2006;354:2564–75.
14. Veelo DP, Dongelmans DA, Binnekade JM, et al. Tracheotomy does not affect reducing sedation requirements of patients in intensive care—a retrospective study. [Internet]. Crit Care. 2006;10:R99. http://www.pubmedcentral.nih.gov/articlerender.fcgi?artid=1751026&tool=pmcentrez&rendertype=abstract.
15. Steyerberg EW, Vickers AJ, Cook NR, et al. Assessing the performance of prediction models: a framework for Some Traditional and Novel Measures. Epidemiology. 2013;21:128–38.
16. Chatburn RL, Volsko TA, et al. Documentation issues for mechanical ventilation in pressure-control modes. Respir Care. 2010;55:1705–16.
17. Rittayamai N, Katsios CM, Beloncle F, et al. Pressure-controlled vs volume-controlled ventilation in acute respiratory failure: a physiology-based narrative and systematic review. Chest. 2015;148:340–55.
18. ARDS-Network. Ventilation with lower tidal volumes as compared with traditional tidal volumes for acute lung injury and the acute respiratory distress syndrome. The Acute Respiratory Distress Syndrome Network. N Engl J Med. 2000;342:1301–8.
19. Takeda S, Ishizaka A, Fujino Y, et al. Time to change diagnostic criteria of ARDS: toward the disease entity-based subgrouping [Internet]. Pulm Pharmacol Ther. 2005;18:115–9. http://www.sciencedirect.com/science/article/pii/S1094553904001385.
20. Ospina-Tascón GA, Büchele GL, Vincent J-L. Multicenter, randomized, controlled trials evaluating mortality in intensive care: doomed to fail? [Internet]. Crit Care Med. 2008;36:1311–22 [cited 2015 Dec 29]. http://www.ncbi.nlm.nih.gov/pubmed/18379260.
21. Moons KGM, Kengne AP, Grobbee DE, et al. Risk prediction models: II. External validation, model updating, and impact assessment [Internet]. Heart. 2012;98:691–8. http://heart.bmj.com/content/98/9/691.abstract.

4

ICU management based on PiCCO parameters reduces duration of mechanical ventilation and ICU length of stay in patients with severe thoracic trauma and acute respiratory distress syndrome

Zhong Yuanbo, Wang Jin, Shi Fei, Long Liangong, Liu Xunfa, Xu Shihai and Shan Aijun*

Abstract

Background: This study aimed to assess whether a management algorithm using data obtained with a PiCCO system can improve clinical outcomes in critically ill patients with acute respiratory distress syndrome (ARDS).

Results: The PaO_2/FiO_2 ratio increased over time in both groups, with a sharper increase in the PiCCO group. There was no difference in 28-day mortality (3.2 vs. 3.6%, $P = 0.841$). Days on mechanical ventilation (3 vs. 5 days, $P = 0.002$) and ICU length of stay (6 vs. 11 days, $P = 0.004$) were significantly lower in the PiCCO group than in the CVP group. Treatment costs were lower in the PiCCO group than in the CVP group. Multivariate logistic regression model showed that the monitoring method (PiCCO vs. CVP) was independently associated with the length of ICU stay [odds ratio (OR) 3.16, 95% confidence interval (95% CI) 1.55–6.63, $P = 0.001$], as well as shock (OR 3.41, 95% CI 1.74–6.44, $P = 0.002$), shock and ARDS (OR 3.46, 95% CI 1.79–6.87, $P = 0.002$), and APACHE II score (OR 1.17, 95% CI 1.02–1.86, $P = 0.014$).

Conclusions: This study investigated the usefulness of the PiCCO system in improving outcomes for patient with severe thoracic trauma and ARDS and provided new evidence for fluid management in critical care settings.

Keywords: Thoracic trauma, Acute respiratory distress syndrome, PiCCO, PaO_2/FiO_2, ICU stay

Background

Thoracic trauma is directly responsible for 25% of all trauma-related deaths and plays a major role in 25% of the remaining trauma deaths [1]. Among patients with severe thoracic trauma and acute respiratory distress syndrome (ARDS), which is usually accompanied by hypotensive shock, mortality would significantly increase if the patients receive massive blood or fluid transfusion [2]. Therefore, optimizing the management of fluid status is still a challenge in critical care. Indeed, severe pulmonary edema may result from fluid overload, which will lead to increased mortality [3, 4]. On the other hand, inadequate fluid volume will result in insufficient oxygen delivery due to low perfusion pressure, compromising patient prognosis. Therefore, it is important to monitor the fluid status of patients with thoracic trauma and ARDS.

Despite having been used for over 50 years, the usefulness of pulmonary artery catheters is disappointing [5]. The Pulse index Contour Continuous Cardiac Output (PiCCO) system from Pulsion Medical Systems (Feldkirchen, Germany) is based on transpulmonary thermodilution (TPTD) and continuous pulse contour analysis approaches. PiCCO is a minimally invasive technique and allows the monitoring of beat-by-beat cardiac output. In addition, volume status and pulmonary edema can be monitored, as well as the hemodynamic status

*Correspondence: shan928doctor@sina.com
Emergency Center, Shenzhen People's Hospital, Shenzhen 518020, China

[6]. The PiCCO system also allows for extravascular lung water (EVLW) monitoring [7]. Patients with acute severe thoracic trauma often have increased pulmonary EVLW. In addition, studies have demonstrated that ARDS is associated with elevated EVLW [8] and elevated EVLW is associated with an increased mortality rate [9, 10].

Optimizing the EVLW index (EVLWI) could be beneficial to patients with ARDS and severe thoracic trauma, but only one study investigated the outcomes of patients managed with PiCCO [11], while the other studies used intermediate parameters (fluid responsiveness, oxygenation, and pulmonary edema) only [12, 13]. Therefore, the present study aimed to examine the usefulness of a management algorithm based on the PiCCO system to improve the outcomes of patients with ARDS and severe thoracic trauma.

Methods

Study design

This study was performed prospectively and in consecutive 264 patients with severe thoracic trauma and acute respiratory distress syndrome (ARDS). All patients were admitted to the emergency intensive care unit (EICU) of Shenzhen People's Hospital, China, between March 2010 and April 2014. Thus, study was approved by the Ethics Committee of the Shenzhen People's Hospital. Written informed consent was obtained from the patients or their legal guardians/representatives.

Patients

Inclusion criteria were: (1) adult patients (≥18 years old); (2) thoracic trauma; and (3) met the clinical criteria of ARDS within 24 h after admission to the EICU. ARDS was defined according to the Berlin definition [14]: (1) onset within one week of a known clinical insult or new/worsening respiratory symptoms; (2) bilateral opacities on chest imaging that could not be fully explained; and (3) the respiratory failure event could not fully be explained by cardiac failure or fluid overload. Exclusion criteria were: (1) <18 years old or >60 years old; (2) traumatic brain or spinal injury, cardiac trauma, intrathoracic major arterial or venous injury, or abdominal visceral injury; (3) was moribund or informed consent could not be obtained; (4) any contraindications to catheter insertion; or (5) vascular conditions leading to inaccuracies of PiCCO measurements (e.g., intracardiac shunts, significant tricuspid regurgitation, or cooling/rewarming) [15–17].

Different treatments were administrated when the patients arrived at the EICU, according to the type of thoracic trauma. Patients with flail chest received chest external fixation. Patients with hemothorax or pneumothorax received closed drainage of the pleural cavity. For patients with massive hemothorax, thoracotomy hemostasis could be performed. During operation, topical or unilateral pneumonectomy was carried out if the lung tissue was completely destroyed by the trauma. Thereafter, patients began to receive their subsequent treatment in EICU or floor ward. Blood gas was routinely tested every 12 h, and chest X-ray or CT was checked every day until 5 days after injury to evaluate whether ARDS occurred. As soon as ARDS was diagnosed, the patient was enrolled in this study, sent to the EICU, and managed with mechanical ventilation.

All patients were randomized to the PiCCO or CVP group using a randomization sequence generated with Stata 12.0 (StataCorp, College Station, TX, USA). Randomization was stratified according to the presence of shock and using a 1:1 ratio.

All electrocardiogram (ECG) measurements in the study were taken using a single ECG monitor (Philips IntelliVue Patient Monitor with a PiCCO module). In the PiCCO group, cardiac output and lung water were measured every 8 h. Investigators who collected the baseline characteristics and follow-up results were blinded to grouping.

Interventions

In the PiCCO group, the PiCCO system was used within 2 h of enrollment. The aim of fluid management was to optimize the effective circulatory volume. If needed, hydroxyethyl starch 130/0.4 (Voluven®) and vasoactive agents were used to achieve a mean arterial blood pressure (MAP) of ≥60 mmHg. Diuretics were administrated to achieve a negative fluid balance, and PEEP would be increased when the volume status (ITBVI > 850 ml/m^2) was optimized but with an EVLWI of ≥10 ml/kg. If there were a suspicion that circulatory failure was the result of cardiac dysfunction (CI less than 2.5 l/m^2/min), dobutamine was started at 3.0 mg/kg/min. The use of the PiCCO system was discontinued after 48 h if the patient were clinically stable. Stability was determined by the attending physicians. Otherwise, the system was used for a maximum of 10 days.

For the patients in the CVP group, a central venous catheter was used, as per routine protocols. If the CVP was <8 mmHg, a 500-ml bolus of hydroxyethyl starch 130/0.4 (Voluven®) was infused over 20–30 min in order to achieve a CVP of 7–12 mmHg. The bolus was repeated if necessary. If the CVP exceeded 12 mmHg, the attending physician was allowed to use furosemide, at his discretion. If MAP was <60 mmHg, norepinephrine was infused at 0.05 μg/kg/min; the infusion could be increased by 0.05 μg/kg/min, at the discretion of the attending physician.

Therefore, the fluid management strategy was similar in the two groups. The main difference was the monitoring method. In the presence of a suspicion of catheter-related bloodstream infection (CRBSI), the central venous catheter was removed and analyzed to determine the causative agent, and a new catheter was indwelled.

The treatment algorithm was a circle that could be repeated if necessary, according to the condition of the patient. Without shock, volume expansion was not performed. The timing for the measurement of the hemodynamic parameters was at the discretion of the attending physician.

Outcome measures

The PaO_2/FiO_2 ratio was calculated according to blood gas analysis. Mechanical ventilation was terminated if: (1) the patient were cooperative; (2) the patient were hemodynamically stable; (3) the patient had adequate and strong cough reflex; (4) the patient had positive end-expiratory pressure <5 cmH_2O; (5) the patient had pressure support <10 cmH_2O; and (6) the patient had a successful spontaneous breathing trial.

The ICU length of stay was defined from the day of EICU admission to the day of ICU discharge. If there were no longer any need for vital organ support, the patient was considered ready for discharge.

EICU cost for monitoring and treatment was determined according to the expenses from EICU admission to leaving ICU. Operation cost for thoracic trauma was excluded.

The 28-day mortality was defined as death from any cause before day 28. Adverse events were monitored, including hematoma, pneumothorax, arterial emboli, catheter-related bloodstream infection, hemorrhage, pseudoaneurysm, and arrhythmia.

Statistical analysis

Normality of continuous variables was determined according to the graphical distribution of the values. Normally distributed continuous variables were analyzed using the one-sample *t* test for intergroup comparisons and using repeated measure ANOVA for intragroup analyses. Non-normally distributed continuous variables were analyzed using the Mann–Whitney *U* test. Categorical data were presented as frequencies and analyzed using the Pearson's Chi-square test. Multivariate logistic regression was used to adjust for confounding variables. Variables that were statistically different between the PiCCO and control groups in univariate analyses ($P < 0.05$) were entered into a multivariate model. The efficacy of treatment based on PiCCO monitoring was investigated in subgroups of ARDS and/or shock. Stata 12.0 (StataCorp, College Station, TX, USA) was used for statistical analysis. Two-sided P values <0.05 were considered statistically significant.

Results

Characteristics of the patients

Figure 1 presents the patient flowchart. The baseline characteristics of the patients are presented in Table 1. The ARDS severity parameters are presented in Additional file 1: Table S1. There were 126 patients in the PiCCO group and 138 in the CVP group. The patients were more critically ill in the PiCCO group than in the CVP group (median APACHE II score, 27 vs. 23, $P = 0.033$; and median ISS score, 14 vs. 13, $P = 0.038$). The PiCCO group showed lower PaO_2/FiO_2 ratio (185 ± 58 vs. 209 ± 90 mmHg, $P = 0.038$). There were no differences between the two groups for gender, age, cause of injury, time between injury and EICU admission, shock, and hemoglobin levels (all $P > 0.05$).

Outcomes

Fluid balance from day 1 to day 6 was similar between the two groups. On day 7, the amount of fluids received in the PiCCO group was significantly less than in the control group (median 188 vs. 644 ml, $P = 0.028$). Using repeated measures analysis, the test for a difference in PaO_2/FiO_2 ratio over time was statistically significant ($P < 0.001$) and the test for interaction between treatment and time was also significant ($P = 0.002$), indicating that the PaO_2/FiO_2 ratio increased over time in both groups, with a sharper increase in the PiCCO group (Fig. 2; Table 2), even though the PaO_2/FiO_2 ratio was lower in the CVP group on day 1.

As shown in Table 2, there was no difference in 28-day mortality between the two groups (3.2 vs. 3.6%, $P = 0.841$). However, days on mechanical ventilation (median 3 vs. 5 days, $P = 0.002$) and ICU length of stay (median 6 vs. 11 days, $P = 0.004$) were significantly lower in the PiCCO group than in the CVP group. EICU monitoring and treatment also showed significantly lower cost in the PiCCO group than in the CVP group.

Some complications associated with the placement of the femoral artery catheter for the PiCCO system were encountered and included 11 cases of venous puncture (4.2%), 4 of hematoma (1.5%), 2 of guide wire kinking (0.8%), and one of catheter malfunction (0.4%).

Multivariate analysis

The multivariate logistic regression model showed that the monitoring method (PiCCO vs. CVP) was independently associated with the length of ICU stay (odds ratio (OR) 3.16, 95% confidence interval (95% CI) 1.55–6.63, $P = 0.001$), as well as shock (OR 3.41, 95% CI 1.74–6.44, $P = 0.002$), shock and ARDS (OR 3.46, 95% CI 1.79–6.87, $P = 0.002$), and APACHE II score (OR 1.17, 95% CI 1.02–1.86, $P = 0.014$) (Table 3).

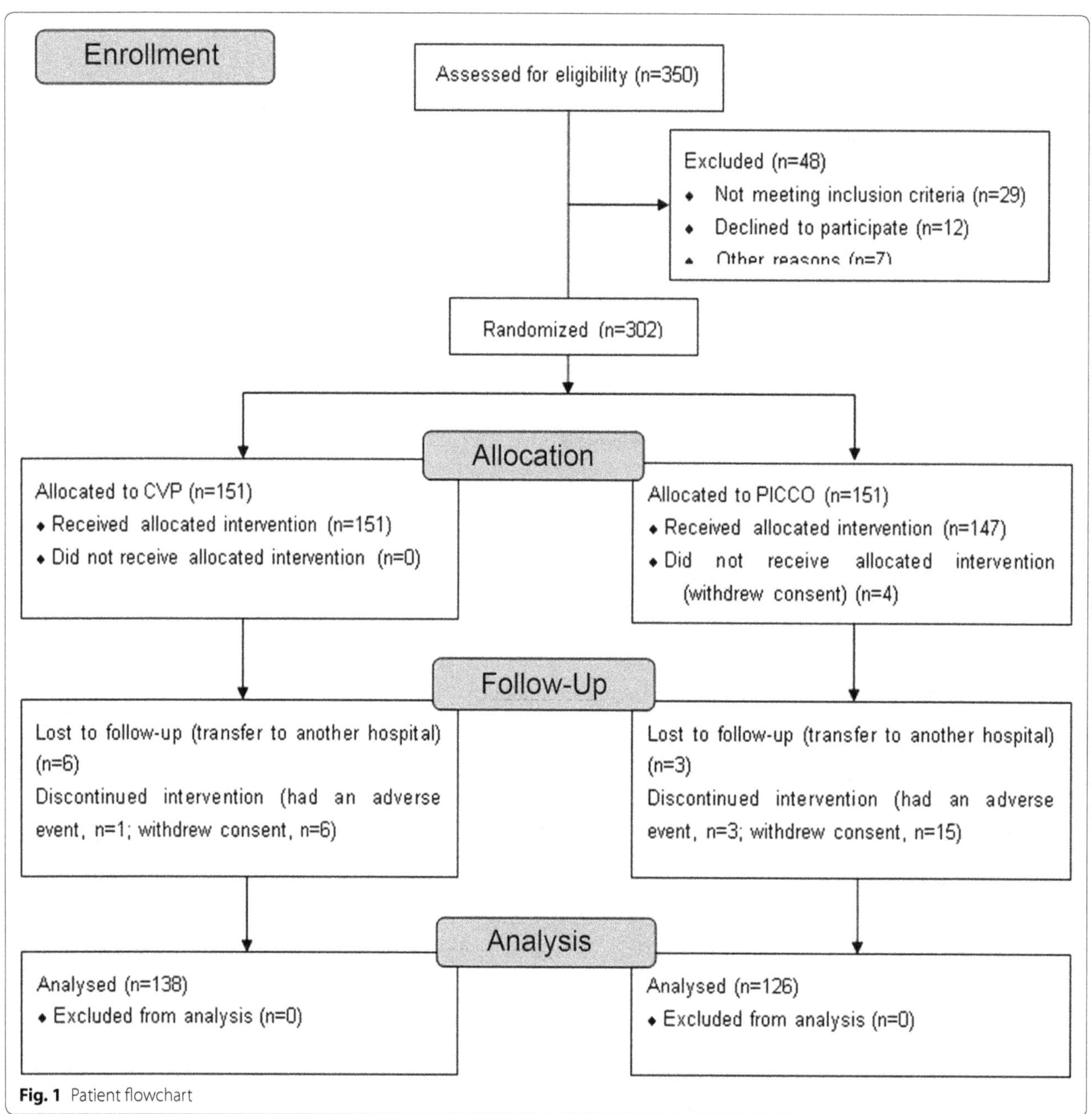

Fig. 1 Patient flowchart

Discussion

This study investigated the use of PiCCO-based or CVP-based fluid management for patients with severe thoracic trauma and ARDS. Results support the use of a PiCCO-based treatment algorithm. Indeed, the use of PiCCO significantly decreased the duration of mechanical ventilation and ICU length of stay without any major side effects. However, PiCCO-based fluid management did not improve mortality rate compared to CVP-based fluid management.

It is widely accepted and practiced in routine clinical practice that negative fluid balance benefits patients with ARDS [18]. Highly efficient diuretics have to be given if auscultation or chest X-ray suggests pulmonary edema and that ARDS is suspected. In the present study, the patients in the CVP group may actually experience similar levels of negative fluid balance despite unawareness of the exact amount of EVLW by the attending physician. Moreover, a substantial proportion of patients (>70%) had shock requiring massive blood or fluid transfusion on ICU admission for which the study protocol dictated positive fluid balance.

To the best of our knowledge, there are few studies exploring the effectiveness of treatment based on

Table 1 Characteristics of the patients at baseline

Characteristics	PiCCO group (*n* = 126)	CVP group (*n* = 138)	*P*
Male, *n* (%)	95 (75.4)	105 (76.1)	0.896
Age (years)	38.5 ± 7.6	37.9 ± 8.2	0.232
APACHE II, median (IQR)	27 (22–33)	23 (17–29)	0.033
ISS, median (IQR)	14 (12–16)	13 (12–15)	0.038
Type of injury cause, *n* (%)			0.578
Road traffic accident	66 (52.4)	71 (51.4)	
Falling injury	31 (24.6)	39 (28.3)	
Crush injury	20 (15.9)	19 (13.8)	
Explosive injury	9 (7.1)	9 (6.5)	
Time from acute onset to EICU admission, hours, median (IQR)	8 (2–31)	7 (2–24)	0.317
Shock, *n* (%)	90 (71.4)	94 (68.1)	0.559
ARDS severity[a] (by PaO_2/FiO_2, *n* (%))			0.025
Mild (200–300)	7 (5.6)	8 (5.8)	
Moderate (100–200)	86 (68.3)	112 (81.2)	
Severe (<100)	33 (26.2)	18 (13.0)	
Hemoglobin (g/L)	85 (62–109)	87 (65–107)	0.883

EICU emergency intensive care unit, *IQR* interquartile range, *APACHE II* Acute Physiology and Chronic Health Evaluation II; *ISS* injury severity score

[a] According to the Berlin definition

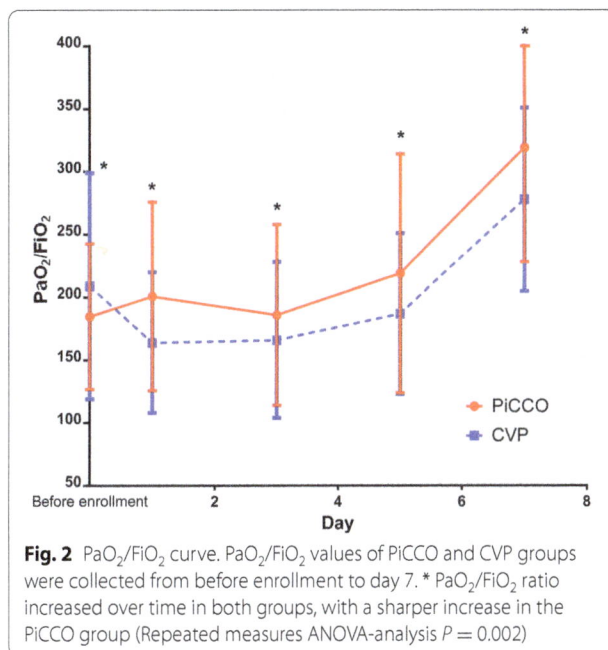

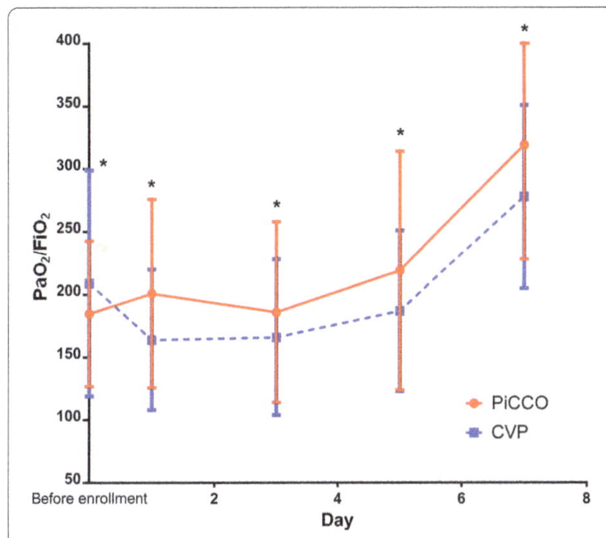

Fig. 2 PaO_2/FiO_2 curve. PaO_2/FiO_2 values of PiCCO and CVP groups were collected from before enrollment to day 7. * PaO_2/FiO_2 ratio increased over time in both groups, with a sharper increase in the PiCCO group (Repeated measures ANOVA-analysis $P = 0.002$)

PiCCO-derived physiological values on outcomes of patients with severe thoracic trauma and ARDS. Goepfert et al. [19] compared the effect of PiCCO-based treatment in cardiac surgery patients to historical controls and observed that fluid management based on PiCCO shortened the length of stay in ICU, supporting the present study. Lenkin et al. [20] compared the outcomes of goal-directed therapy guided using PAC or PiCCO and observed that PiCCO-based treatment increased the volume of fluid therapy, improved hemodynamics and oxygen delivery index, and reduced the duration of mechanical ventilation after complex valve surgery compared with PAC-guided management. Furthermore, several studies conducted among sepsis/shock patients also showed the potential usefulness of EVLW-directed fluid therapy according to improvements of the duration of mechanical ventilation, length of stay in ICU, and mortality [7, 21–23]. However, two recent studies carried out in critically ill patients with sepsis and/or shock reported that PiCCO-based fluid management failed to improve outcomes [3, 24]. Surgical patients (including cardiac surgery and thoracic trauma patients) usually have better pulmonary and circulatory functions compared with patients with septic shock and/or ARDS, which could partly explain these discrepancies. Indeed, trials with positive conclusions were conducted almost 8–10 years ago when the beneficial effect of a restrictive strategy had not yet been established. Currently, the beneficial effect of negative fluid balance is pretty well known and high doses of diuretics are given at a certain EVLWI threshold, even if no PiCCO system was used. In addition, studies with negative conclusions enrolled more severely and critically ill patients. As we know, for this type of patients, fatal outcomes are difficult to reverse even though a PiCCO-based treatment algorithm is administrated. In the present study, the mortality rate was low, which could

Table 2 Comparison of outcomes between the PiCCO and CVP groups

Outcome variables	PiCCO group ($n = 126$)	CVP group ($n = 138$)	*P*
PaO_2/FiO_2			
Before enrollment	185 ± 58	209 ± 90	0.038*
1 day after enrollment	201 ± 75	164 ± 56	0.022*
3 day after enrollment	186 ± 72	166 ± 62	0.047*
5 day after enrollment	219 ± 95	187 ± 64	0.037*
7 day after enrollment	319 ± 91	278 ± 73	0.042*
Days on MV, days, median (IQR)	3 (1–6)	5 (2–9)	0.002
Length of stay in EICU, days, median (IQR)	6 (4–8)	11 (6–16)	0.004
EICU cost for monitoring and treatment (RMB: yuan)	8.23 ± 3.25	12.87 ± 4.61	<0.001
28-day mortality, *n* (%)	4 (3.2)	5 (3.6)	0.841

* Post hoc *p* value in repeated measure of ANOVA

MV mechanical ventilation, *EICU* emergency intensive care unit, *IQR* interquartile range

Table 3 Multivariate logistic regression model for the length of ICU stay

Length of ICU stay (bivariate: >7 days or ≤7 days)	Odds ratio	Lower limit of 95% CI	Upper limit of 95% CI	*P*
Group (CVP vs. PiCCO)	3.16	1.55	6.63	0.001
Gender (male as the reference)	1.16	0.59	1.74	0.863
Age (with 1 year increase)	1.11	0.98	1.21	0.536
Time from acute onset to ICU admission	0.98	0.94	1.13	0.237
PaO_2/FiO_2	0.79	0.46	1.37	0.283
Type of patient (ARDS as reference)				
Shock	3.41	1.74	6.44	0.002
Both	3.46	1.79	6.87	0.002
APACHE II	1.17	1.02	1.86	0.014
ISS	1.15	0.89	1.24	0.176

APACHE II Acute Physiology and Chronic Health Evaluation II, *ISS* injury severity score, *ER* emergency room, *OR* operating room

be due to the patients being young and without severe trauma. This could also explain the lack of a statistically significant difference between the two groups.

In the present study, the multivariate analysis revealed that the monitoring method (PiCCO vs. CVP) was independently associated with the length of ICU stay, as well as shock, shock and ARDS, and APACHE II score. These results suggest that more critically ill patients will stay longer in the ICU compared with patients less critically ill and that the use of PiCCO could help shortening the ICU stay in all patients, independently of the illness severity. An ongoing clinical trial will help confirming these results [25].

Several limitations have to be acknowledged. First, there was a difference in the final number of patients between the two groups because more patients had to be excluded from the PiCCO group. In addition, there was an imbalance in the severity score between the two groups. Patients in the PiCCO group were more severely ill than in the CVP group, which would influence the outcomes. Despite this, positive conclusions could still be observed. Second, the treatment approach based on hemodynamic monitoring was largely relying on clinical experience and it will have to be confirmed by additional studies. Third, only patients with thoracic trauma were included and the impact of a PiCCO-based fluid approach on more severe trauma such as thoracic trauma accompanied by brain injury or abdominal visceral injury is largely unknown. Fourth, specific treatments were triggered by specific values of hemodynamic variables (e.g., ITBVI less than 850 was used to trigger fluid bolus) and it must be highlighted that the normal ranges of physiological values from the PiCCO system are not fixed but vary among subjects [26]; the algorithm had to be modified to accommodate the clinical condition of each patient. In real-world settings, we suggest that the clinical condition and clinicians' judgment should be considered rather than simply relying on PiCCO readings. Fifth, before admission, almost all patients had undergone operation and sedation. Therefore, it was often impossible to determine the real consciousness state of the patients. Therefore, we could only compute the APACHE II values according to what could be directly observed. Moreover, most patients (>90%) were directly sent to the operation room to receive emergency operation to control bleeding (damage control operation) and then were sent to the ICU. These patients who received emergency operation received 5 additional scores for APACHE II computation. Therefore, APACHE II scores could be overestimated. Lastly, the mortality rate was lower than expected, which may compromise the generalizability of the results. Additional studies are required to assess the usefulness of the PiCCO system in the management of fluids in trauma patients.

Conclusions

In conclusion, this study verified that the PiCCO system is able to improve outcomes for patient with ARDS and severe thoracic trauma. The results provide new evidence for fluid management in these patients.

Abbreviations

ARDS: acute respiratory distress syndrome; OR: odds ratio; TPTD: transpulmonary thermodilution technique; EVLW: extravascular lung water; EVLWI: EVLW index; ICU: intensive care unit; EICU: emergency intensive care unit; ECG: electrocardiogram; CRBSI: catheter-related bloodstream infection.

Authors' contributions

ZY and WJ contributed equally to the study and they coordinated, enrolled patients, and monitored the study, wrote the manuscript. SF contributed to the revision of the manuscript and acted as a statistical consultant. LL and LX collected data and were also responsible for monitoring safety. XS was responsible for the performance of PiCCO monitoring. SA designed the study and contributed to the study protocol. All authors read and approved the final manuscript

Acknowledgements

We are indebted to the nursing staff, especially Ludan Yang and Yueming Peng for coordinating the performance of PiCCO monitoring.

Competing interests

The authors declare that they have no competing interests.

Funding

The study was supported by the Science and Technology Planning Foundation of Shenzhen City (approval no. 201201011).

References

1. Zargar M, Khaji A, Karbakhsh Davari M. Thoracic injury: a review of 276 cases. Chin J Traumatol. 2007;10:259–62.
2. Simmons RS, Berdine GG, Seidenfeld JJ, Prihoda TJ, Harris GD, Smith JD, et al. Fluid balance and the adult respiratory distress syndrome. Am Rev Respir Dis. 1987;135:924–9.
3. Trof RJ, Beishuizen A, Cornet AD, de Wit RJ, Girbes AR, Groeneveld AB. Volume-limited versus pressure-limited hemodynamic management in septic and nonseptic shock. Crit Care Med. 2012;40:1177–85.
4. Boyd JH, Forbes J, Nakada TA, Walley KR, Russell JA. Fluid resuscitation in septic shock: a positive fluid balance and elevated central venous pressure are associated with increased mortality. Crit Care Med. 2011;39:259–65.
5. Rajaram SS, Desai NK, Kalra A, Gajera M, Cavanaugh SK, Brampton W, et al. Pulmonary artery catheters for adult patients in intensive care. Cochrane Database Syst Rev. 2013;2:CD003408.
6. Litton E, Morgan M. The PiCCO monitor: a review. Anaesth Intensive Care. 2012;40:393–409.
7. Tagami T, Tosa R, Omura M, Fukushima H, Kaneko T, Endo T, et al. Effect of a selective neutrophil elastase inhibitor on mortality and ventilator-free days in patients with increased extravascular lung water: a post hoc analysis of the PiCCO Pulmonary Edema Study. J Intensive Care. 2014;2:67.
8. Kushimoto S, Endo T, Yamanouchi S, Sakamoto T, Ishikura H, Kitazawa Y, et al. Relationship between extravascular lung water and severity categories of acute respiratory distress syndrome by the Berlin definition. Crit Care. 2013;17:R132.
9. Phillips CR, Chesnutt MS, Smith SM. Extravascular lung water in sepsis-associated acute respiratory distress syndrome: indexing with predicted body weight improves correlation with severity of illness and survival. Crit Care Med. 2008;36:69–73.
10. Zhang Z, Lu B, Ni H. Prognostic value of extravascular lung water index in critically ill patients: a systematic review of the literature. J Crit Care. 2012;27(420):e1–8.
11. Mutoh T, Kazumata K, Ishikawa T, Terasaka S. Performance of bed-side transpulmonary thermodilution monitoring for goal-directed hemodynamic management after subarachnoid hemorrhage. Stroke. 2009;40:2368–74.
12. Broch O, Renner J, Gruenewald M, Meybohm P, Hocker J, Schottler J, et al. Variation of left ventricular outflow tract velocity and global end-diastolic volume index reliably predict fluid responsiveness in cardiac surgery patients. J Crit Care. 2012;27(325):e7–13.
13. Zhang Z, Lu B, Sheng X, Jin N. Accuracy of stroke volume variation in predicting fluid responsiveness: a systematic review and meta-analysis. J Anesth. 2011;25:904–16.
14. Definition Task Force ARDS, Ranieri VM, Rubenfeld GD, Thompson BT, Ferguson ND, Caldwell E, et al. Acute respiratory distress syndrome: the Berlin Definition. JAMA. 2012;307:2526–33.
15. Heerdt PM, Pond CG, Blessios GA, Rosenbloom M. Inaccuracy of cardiac output by thermodilution during acute tricuspid regurgitation. Ann Thorac Surg. 1992;53:706–8.
16. Merrick SH, Hessel EA 2nd, Dillard DH. Determination of cardiac output by thermodilution during hypothermia. Am J Cardiol. 1980;46:419–22.
17. Giraud R, Siegenthaler N, Park C, Beutler S, Bendjelid K. Transpulmonary thermodilution curves for detection of shunt. Intensive Care Med. 2010;36:1083–6.
18. Roch A, Guervilly C, Papazian L. Fluid management in acute lung injury and ards. Ann Intensive Care. 2011;1:16.
19. Goepfert MS, Reuter DA, Akyol D, Lamm P, Kilger E, Goetz AE. Goal-directed fluid management reduces vasopressor and catecholamine use in cardiac surgery patients. Intensive Care Med. 2007;33:96–103.
20. Lenkin AI, Kirov MY, Kuzkov VV, Paromov KV, Smetkin AA, Lie M, et al. Comparison of goal-directed hemodynamic optimization using pulmonary artery catheter and transpulmonary thermodilution in combined valve repair: a randomized clinical trial. Crit Care Res Pract. 2012;2012:821218.
21. Bognar Z, Foldi V, Rezman B, Bogar L, Csontos C. Extravascular lung water index as a sign of developing sepsis in burns. Burns. 2010;36:1263–70.
22. Chung FT, Lin SM, Lin SY, Lin HC. Impact of extravascular lung water index on outcomes of severe sepsis patients in a medical intensive care unit. Respir Med. 2008;102:956–61.

23. Meyer NJ, Hall JB. Sizing up (or down) extravascular lung water as a predictor of outcome in acute lung injury/acute respiratory distress syndrome. Crit Care Med. 2008;36:337–8.
24. Zhang Z, Ni H, Qian Z. Effectiveness of treatment based on PiCCO parameters in critically ill patients with septic shock and/or acute respiratory distress syndrome: a randomized controlled trial. Intensive Care Med. 2015;41:444–51.
25. Zhang Z, Xu X, Yao M, Chen H, Ni H, Fan H. Use of the PiCCO system in critically ill patients with septic shock and acute respiratory distress syndrome: a study protocol for a randomized controlled trial. Trials. 2013;14:32.
26. Wolf S, Riess A, Landscheidt JF, Lumenta CB, Friederich P, Schurer L. Global end-diastolic volume acquired by transpulmonary thermodilution depends on age and gender in awake and spontaneously breathing patients. Crit Care. 2009;13:R202.

5

Prone positioning in acute respiratory distress syndrome after abdominal surgery

SAPRONADONF (Study of Ards and PRONe position After abDOmiNal surgery in France)

Stéphane Gaudry[1,2], Samuel Tuffet[1,3,4], Anne-Claire Lukaszewicz[3,4], Christian Laplace[5], Noémie Zucman[1], Marc Pocard[6,7], Bruno Costaglioli[8], Simon Msika[9,10], Jacques Duranteau[5], Didier Payen[3,4], Didier Dreyfuss[1,11,12], David Hajage[2,13] and Jean-Damien Ricard[1,11,12,14*]

Abstract

Background: The recent demonstration of prone position's strong benefit on patient survival has rendered proning a major therapeutic intervention in severe ARDS. Uncertainties remain as to whether or not ARDS patients in the postoperative period of abdominal surgery should be turned prone because of the risk of abdominal complications. Our aim was to investigate the prevalence of surgical complications between patients with and without prone position after abdominal surgery.

Methods: This study was a multicenter retrospective cohort of patients with ARDS in a context of recent abdominal surgery. Primary outcome was the number of patients who had at least one surgical complication that could be induced or worsened by prone position. Secondary outcomes included effects of prone position on oxygenation. Data from the prone group were compared with those from the supine group (not having undergone at least a prone position session).

Results: Among 98 patients included, 36 (37%) had at least one prone position session. The rate of surgical complications induced or worsened by prone position did not differ between prone and supine groups [respectively, 14 (39%) vs 27 (44%); $p = 0.65$]. After propensity score application, there was no significant difference between the two groups (OR 0.72 [0.26–2.02], $p = 0.54$). Revision surgery did not differ between the groups. The first prone session significantly increased PaO_2/FiO_2 ratio from 95 ± 47 to 189 ± 92 mmHg, $p < 0.0001$.

Conclusion: Prone position of ARDS patients after abdominal surgery was not associated with an increased rate of surgical complication. Intensivists should not refrain from proning these patients.

Keywords: Mechanical ventilation, ARDS, Prone position

Background

Prone positioning has been used for a long time to improve oxygenation in patients with acute respiratory distress syndrome (ARDS) [1]. The different mechanisms explaining its potential benefits include homogenization of ventilation–perfusion mismatch, redistribution of pleural pressure gradient, net alveolar recruitment and more harmonious alveolar inflation [2] and prevention and reduction of ventilator-induced lung injury (VILI) [3, 4]. Until recently, randomized controlled trials (RCT) on prone position failed to show a net benefit on survival [5–8] but had provided cues for a possible benefit among the most severe ARDS patients [9, 10]. Guerin et al. confirmed this hypothesis by demonstrating a strong survival benefit in a large RCT in patients with

*Correspondence: jean-damien.ricard@aphp.fr
[14] Service de Réanimation Médicale, 178 rue des Renouillers, 92701 Colombes Cedex, France
Full list of author information is available at the end of the article

PaO2/FiO2 ratio <150 mmHg [11]. This resounding demonstration, linked to the fact that prone positioning does not require any special equipment and is not associated with excess side effects (10), suggests all severe ARDS patients should be turned prone in case of refractory hypoxemia [12]. This is true irrespective of the origin (pulmonary or extra-pulmonary) of ARDS, with the exception of trauma patients with spinal instability or unmonitored increased intracranial pressure. Despite these evidences, a recent large international epidemiological study indicates that only 16% of severe ARDS patients are turned prone [13]. Among etiologies of extra-pulmonary origin, those consecutive to abdominal emergencies may constitute an obstacle to the use of prone position and lead to an even smaller percentage than above. In case of severe hypoxemia in the early postoperative period, intensivists could be reluctant to prone patients for fear of repercussions on scars, draining systems and stoma. Cases of midline abdominal wound dehiscence potentially related to prone positioning have been reported [14] but to what extent prone position may induce or worsen postsurgical complications remains unknown. Because prone position is now a major therapeutic intervention in the management of ARDS, it is crucial to determine whether prone position is associated or not with more complications in patients with ARDS after abdominal surgery.

Given that this population represents a minority of patients included the above-mentioned RCT and that there is no questioning of the efficacy of prone position in ARDS, yet another RCT is no desirable (nor feasible) to obtain such determination. We therefore conducted a retrospective, multicenter study to assess the prevalence of surgical complications that could be a priori induced or worsened by prone position among patients developing ARDS after abdominal or pelvic surgery.

Methods

Design and ethics

This was a retrospective study performed in three ICUs of Assistance Publique—Hôpitaux de Paris, University Hospitals (Louis Mourier, Lariboisière and Kremlin-Bicêtre) between March 2009 and March 2014 designed to compare the risk of surgical complications that could be a priori induced or worsened by prone position between patients who had at least one prone position session (prone group) and those who remained supine (supine group) after abdominal surgery. Admission of abdominal emergencies in these three ICUs is part of their routine activity. In case of ARDS, decision to prone patients was taken by the ICU physicians and the context of abdominal surgery was not considered as a contraindication.

The study was approved by the Ethics Committee of the French Intensive Care Society (project no. 14-31). We followed the Strengthening the Reporting of Observational Studies in Epidemiology (STROBE) statement guidelines for observational cohort studies [15].

Study population

Two independent searches on the ICU's electronic database were performed over the study period, one with the search label "ARDS" (ICD label J80) and the other with "acute respiratory failure" (ICD label J960). The two lists of patients were cross-checked to ensure exhaustibility and verify the final diagnosis of ARDS. Once extracted, medical records were reviewed. Patients were retained in the final analysis if they had an ARDS consistent with Berlin definition [16] (oxygenation criteria: PaO_2/FiO_2 <300 mmHg with PEEP or CPAP $\geq$5 cmH_2O) in a context of recent (less than 7 days) abdominal surgery. We did not include in the analysis patients who had just had a laparoscopy or who died in the next 48 h following surgery.

The day of inclusion (D0) in the analysis was defined as the day when ARDS occurred.

Main characteristics of protocol use for the prone positioning placement

During the study period, medical and paramedical teams followed protocol for prone positioning placement. A minimum of four persons were required for the procedure; one of them was placed at the patient's head to secure the endotracheal tube. Rotation to the left or to the right depended on the location of invasive arterial pressure and central venous lines. The upper limbs were placed alongside the body. Potential pressure points were protected using adhesive pads.

A circular pillow was used to ensure appropriate position of the head and the endotracheal tube. Pillows were placed under the thorax and pelvis in order to limit abdominal pressure.

Data collection

The data recorded from the files were the following:

Epidemiological data: age, sex, weight, body mass index (BMI), chronic obstructive pulmonary disease, ischemic heart disease, systemic hypertension and diabetes.

Characteristics of ICU severity: SAPS II [17], septic shock (at D0) defined by Bone's criteria [18] and catecholamine infusion (at D0).

Characteristics of ARDS and mechanical ventilation: lowest PaO_2/FiO_2 ratio at D0, highest plateau pressure (Pplat) at D0, lowest tidal volume at D0, highest PEEP at D0, use of adjunctive therapies (including neuromuscular blocking agents, inhaled nitric oxide, prone positioning) and duration of mechanical ventilation. For patients who had at least one prone position session (prone group), data collection included: time between surgery and first prone position session, number and duration of prone position session, PaO_2/FiO_2 before (measure on the last arterial blood gas before first prone session) and after (measure on the first arterial blood during the first prone position session) and hemodynamic changes after first prone session. To address this hemodynamic issue, we defined three categories depending on the changes in catecholamine dosage during the first 2 h of the first prone session: i/hemodynamic worsening (defined as increase in catecholamines), ii/hemodynamic improvement (decrease) and iii/hemodynamic stability (no change).

Characteristics of abdominal surgery: planned or emergent surgery, delay between surgery and ICU hospitalization, presence of peritonitis (defined according to the International Sepsis Forum Consensus Conference on Definitions of Infection in the Intensive Care Unit [19], type of surgical procedure, number and type of stoma. Not being a routine procedure, intra-abdominal pressure was not systematically measured.

Postoperative surgical complications: We defined a priori these complications: scar dehiscence, abdominal compartment syndrome (define as intra-abdominal hypertension >20 mmHg with new organ dysfunction or failure) [20], stoma leakage, stoma necrosis, scar necrosis, wound infection, displacement of a drainage system, removal of a gastro- or jejunostomy feeding tube and digestive fistula. The Clavien–Dindo classification for surgical complications was assessed. However, it was not discriminant since all the patients were *de facto* in the ICU and under invasive MV (≥IVa) [21].

Primary endpoint

The primary endpoint was the number of patients who had at least one surgical complication defined a priori (see above) that could be induced or worsened by prone position.

Secondary endpoints

Secondary endpoints were the number of revision operations due to complication induced or worsened by prone position. Other secondary endpoints were effect of prone position on oxygenation duration of mechanical ventilation, ICU mortality and ICU length of stay.

Statistical analysis

Statistical analysis was performed with GraphPad Prism 5 (GraphPad Software, San Diego, USA) and R version 3.1.2 (R Foundation for Statistical Computing, Vienna, Austria.). Categorical variables are described by their numbers and proportions and compared by the Fisher's exact test. The normality of continuous variables was tested by the Kolmogorov–Smirnov test. Continuous variables of normal distribution are described by mean and standard deviation and compared by Student's t test. Continuous variables of non-normal distribution are described by median and interquartile [25, 75%] range and compared by the Mann–Whitney test.

Primary endpoint was compared between the prone and supine groups using propensity score weighting to balance patient characteristics between the two groups. It was conducted in two stages. In the first stage, we performed a multivariate logistic regression to predict the probability of being in the prone group (i.e., the estimated propensity score (PS)), controlling for all the pre specified covariates (see above). In the second stage, we constructed logistic regression model to compare the risk of complication between prone and supine groups, using the inverse of the propensity score as a weight, targeting the average treatment effect in the whole population [22]. More precisely, a logistic model regressing the outcome with exposure (i.e., prone or supine group) as the only covariate was fitted, each subject being weighted according to its PS value, with a stabilized weight W equal to: $W = pT/PS$ if subject is in the prone group, and $(1 - pT)/(1 - PS)$ if subject is in the supine group, where pT is the is the overall probability of being in the prone group in the sample. Robust standard errors were used.

Variables considered for propensity score estimation were chosen based on empirical knowledge and included: age, weight, SAPS II, diabetes status, presence of a colonic stoma, of a small bowel stoma and of jejunostomy, use of catecholamines and delay from surgery to ICU hospitalization. No variable selection was performed. Balance on covariates between prone and supine groups was assessed and reported using absolute standardized differences (ASD) [23], and a sensitivity analysis with additional adjustment for covariates with ASD >10% after weighting was performed.

Results

Study population

Among the 10,039 patients admitted to the participating ICU during the study period, 1411 had ARDS consistent with the Berlin definition [16]. Of these, 98 patients had undergone an abdominal surgery in the last 7 days (Fig. 1). Thirty-six patients (37%) had at least one prone position session and 62 (63%) remained supine.

Table 1 shows that patients were severely ill as attested by high SAPS II scores and the requirement for catecholamine infusion at D0. Systemic hypertension and

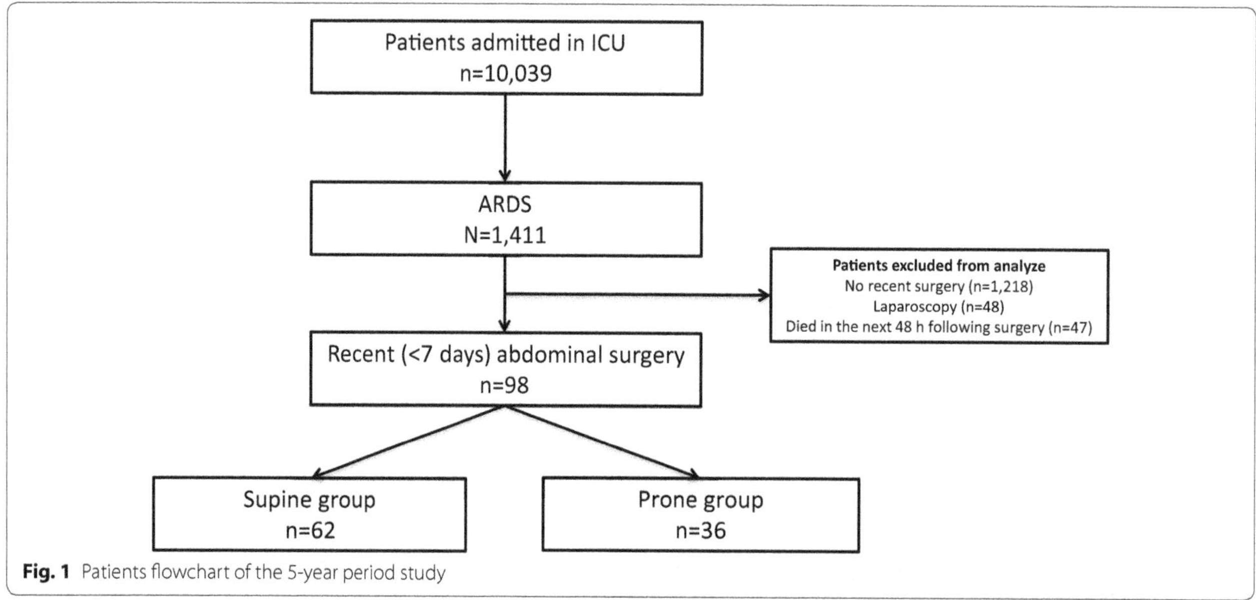

Fig. 1 Patients flowchart of the 5-year period study

diabetes were more frequent in the supine group, and those patients had a higher SAPS II.

Respiratory failure at D0 was more severe in the prone group with a lower PaO_2/FiO_2 (74 ± 24 mmHg vs 101 ± 43 mmHg, $p = 0.0005$), a higher PEEP level (13 ± 3 vs 10 ± 3 cm of water, $p = 0.0001$), a higher plateau pressure (26 ± 4 vs 23 ± 7 cm of water, $p = 0.02$) and a more frequent use of adjunctive therapies.

Characteristics of abdominal surgery were similar in the two groups except for colonic resection and colonic stoma (more frequent in supine group). The delay between surgery and ICU hospitalization was 0 [0–1] days.

Primary endpoint

Rate of surgical complications a priori induced or worsened by prone position did not differ between prone and supine groups [respectively: $n = 14$ (39%) vs $n = 27$ (44%); $p = 0.65$]. Details regarding these complications are summarized in Table 2.

After propensity score application, there was still no significant difference between the two groups (OR 0.72 [0.26–2.02], $p = 0.54$). Since an imbalance was detected after propensity score weighting for variable "colonic stoma" (Additional file 1: Figure 1E), an analysis adjusting for this covariate was also performed, with unchanged results (data not shown).

Secondary endpoint (Table 3)

Twenty-one (58%) patients were turned prone in the first 48 h following the surgery (median time between surgery and first prone session 2 [1–4] days). The median number of prone session was 1 [1–2] (1 session: 19 patients, 2 sessions: nine patients, 3 sessions: six patients, 4 sessions: one patient, 5 sessions: one patient). The duration of the first and second session were, respectively, 15.8 (±10.4) and 19.2 (±10.3) hours. PaO_2/FiO_2 ratio improves dramatically after the first prone session (Fig. 2).

During the first 2 h of the first prone session, 26 (72%) patients were hemodynamically stable, six (17%) experienced hemodynamic worsening and four (11%) experienced hemodynamic improvement.

Rate of revision surgery did not differ between the two groups. Duration of MV, ICU length of stay and ICU mortality were also not different (Table 3).

Discussion

This is the first retrospective multicentre study evaluating safety and efficacy of prone position for severe post-abdominal surgery ARDS patients. We found that early postoperative prone position was not associated with increased local or surgical complications and that oxygenation significantly improved after one session of proning. These results were found in a varied population of patients, in three distinct hospitals, which give credits to their generalizability. They may have an immediate and significant impact on patient outcome, given the recent demonstration of the strong survival benefit of prone position during ARDS [11].

Despite large RCT in this context [5–8, 11], data regarding post-abdominal surgery patients are missing. Indeed, although post-abdominal surgery is not stated as a contraindication to prone position, it is difficult to extract specific figures regarding this population from these studies. This is either due in part to the fact that

Table 1 Characteristics of patients

	Overall	Prone	Supine	p*
n	98	36	62	
Epidemiological data				
Age (years) (SD)	64 (18)	59 (19)	67 (17)	0.08
Male gender, *n* (%)	59 (60)	22 (61)	37 (60)	0.89
Weight (kg) (SD)	83 (24)	81 (26)	83 (24)	0.63
BMI (kg/m^2) (SD)	31 (9)	30 (10)	31 (10)	0.77
COPD, *n* (%)	15 (15)	6 (17)	9 (15)	0.77
Ischemic heart disease, *n* (%)	15 (15)	4 (11)	11 (18)	0.38
Systemic hypertension, *n* (%)	60 (61)	13 (36)	47 (76)	*0.001*
Diabetes, *n* (%)	29 (30)	5 (14)	24 (39)	*0.01*
Characteristics of ICU severity				
SAPS II (SD) [17]	53 (17)	47 (15)	56 (17)	*0.02*
Septic shock (at D0), *n* (%)	75 (77)	26 (72)	49 (79)	0.44
Catecholamine infusion (at D0)	87 (89)	33 (92)	54 (87)	0.74
PaO_2/FiO_2 and ventilator settings at D0				
PaO_2/FiO_2 (mmHg) (SD)	91 (39)	74 (24)	101 (43)	*0.0005*
Plateau pressure (cm of water) (SD)	24 (6)	26 (4)	23 (7)	*0.02*
Tidal volume (ml) [IQR]	446 [400–497]	444 [400–500]	448 [400–496]	0.57
PEEP (cm of water) (SD)	11 (4)	13 (4)	10 (3)	*0.0001*
Adjunctive therapies (during ICU stay)				
Inhaled nitric oxide, *n* (%)	24 (24)	13 (36)	11 (18)	*0.04*
NMBA, *n* (%)	59 (60)	32 (89)	27 (43)	*0.0001*
Characteristics of abdominal surgery				
Emergent surgery, *n* (%)	79 (81)	30 (83)	49 (79)	0.60
Peritonitis, *n* (%)	41 (42)	14 (39)	27 (43)	0.65
Colonic resection, *n* (%)	22 (22)	4 (11)	18 (29)	*0.04*
Small bowel resection, *n* (%)	27 (28)	9 (25)	18 (29)	0.67
Gastric resection, *n* (%)	8 (8)	4 (11)	4 (6)	0.46
Esophageal resection, *n* (%)	7 (7)	3 (8)	4 (6)	0.71
Cholecystectomy *n* (%)	11 (11)	5 (14)	6 (10)	0.53
Partial hepatectomy, *n* (%)	3 (3)	2 (6)	1 (2)	0.28
Splenectomy, *n* (%)	1 (1)	0 (0)	1 (2)	1.00
Partial pancreatectomy, *n* (%)	3 (3)	0 (0)	3 (5)	0.30
Hysterectomy, *n* (%)	1 (1)	0 (0)	1 (2)	1.00
Parietal resection, *n* (%)	8 (8)	5 (14)	3 (5)	0.14
Cesarean, *n* (%)	3 (3)	2 (6)	1 (2)	0.55
HIPEC, *n* (%)	1 (1)	0 (0)	1 (2)	1.00
$\geq$1 stoma, *n* (%)	34 (35)	10 (28)	24 (39)	0.27
Colonic stoma, *n* (%)	15 (15)	2 (6)	13 (21)	*0.04*
Small bowel stoma, *n* (%)	16 (16)	6 (17)	10 (16)	0.95
Jejunostomy, *n* (%)	5 (5)	2 (6)	3 (5)	1.00
Gastrostomy, *n* (%)	1 (1)	0 (0)	1 (2)	1.00
Open abdomen, *n* (%)	4 (4)	1 (3)	3 (5)	1.00

Italic values refer to a statistically significant p-value

BMI body mass index, *COPD* chronic obstructive pulmonary disease, SAPS II, *PEEP* positive end-expiratory pressure, *ICU* intensive care unit, *NMBA* neuromuscular blockade agent, *HIPEC* hyperthermic intraperitoneal chemotherapy, *SD* standard deviation, *IQR* interquartile [25, 75%]

* Prone versus supine

the precise number of patients with post-abdominal surgery is not provided [5, 7, 8] or because the definition of postoperative acute respiratory failure encompasses patients with very low risks of surgical complications

Table 2 Postoperative surgical complications

	Prone $n = 36$	Supine $n = 62$	p
Scar dehiscence, n (%)	3 (8)	15 (24)	0.06
Abdominal compartment syndrome, n (%)	1 (3)	6 (10)	0.26
Stoma leakage, n (%)	1 (3)	13 (2)	1.00
Stoma necrosis, n (%)	3 (8)	3 (5)	0.67
Scar necrosis, n (%)	1 (3)	1 (2)	1.00
Wound infection, n (%)	6 (17)	5 (8)	0.20
Displacement of a peritoneal drainage system	0 (0)	1 (2)	1.00
Displacement of a biliary drainage system	0 (0)	1 (2)	1.00
Removal of a gastrostomy feeding tube	0 (0)	0 (0)	1.00
Removal of a jejunostomy feeding tube	1 (3)	0 (0)	0.37
Digestive fistula	3 (8)	11 (18)	0.24

NB: one patient could have several complications. This explains that the total (19 for prone group and 56 for supine group) may be different than the number of primary endpoint (define as "at least one surgical complication")

Table 3 Primary and secondary endpoints

	Overall	Prone	Supine	p
Primary endpoint[a], n (%)	41 (42)	14 (39)	27 (44)	0.65
Revision surgery[b], n (%)	17 (17)	3 (8)	14 (23)	0.10
All revision surgery[c]	35 (36)	8 (22)	26 (42)	0.10
Duration of MV	10 [6–17]	9.5 [6–21]	11 [6–15]	0.72
ICU length of stay	13 [7–22]	13 [8–24]	13 [6–21]	0.77
ICU mortality[d], n (%)	43 (44)	15 (42)	28 (45)	0.43

MV mechanical ventilation, *ICU* intensive care unit

[a] At least one surgical complication that could be induced or worsened by prone position

[b] For primary endpoint

[c] Several patients had more than one revision surgery

[d] Five patients died in the first 48 h (two in the prone group and three in the supine group)

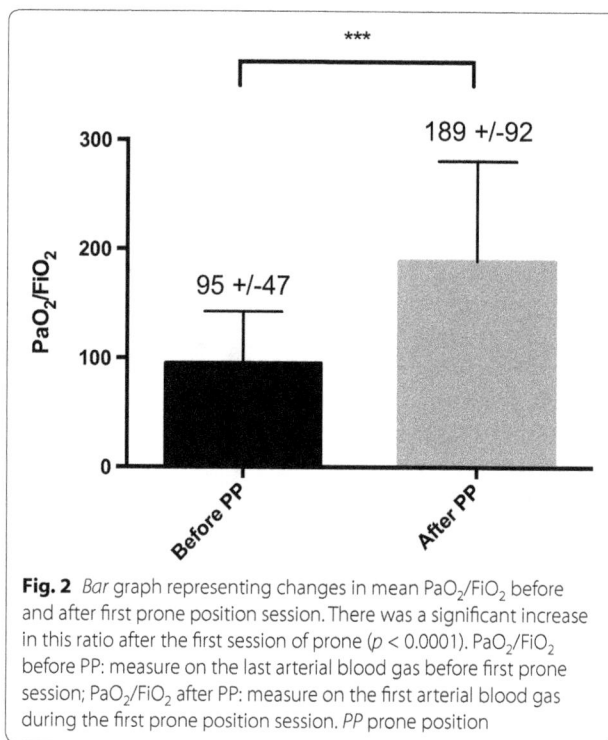

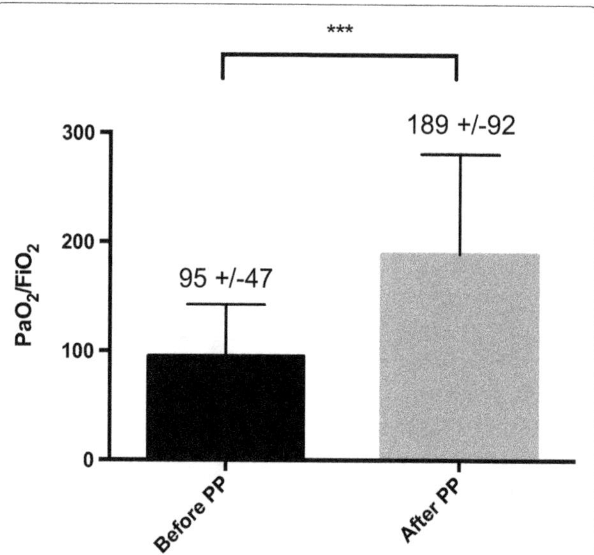

Fig. 2 *Bar* graph representing changes in mean PaO_2/FiO_2 before and after first prone position session. There was a significant increase in this ratio after the first session of prone ($p < 0.0001$). PaO_2/FiO_2 before PP: measure on the last arterial blood gas before first prone session; PaO_2/FiO_2 after PP: measure on the first arterial blood gas during the first prone position session. *PP* prone position

(endoscopic procedures and interventional radiological procedures) (6, 11). The lack of such available data led us to investigate the safety of prone position in abdominal postoperative ARDS patients. Our results could provide clinicians with answers to the following questions: is the prone position associated with a greater rate of surgical complications? Does it yet improve oxygenation?

We deliberately chose not to investigate other known adverse events related to prone position because these complications are not more frequent in patients turned prone [10].

Data on the rate of surgical complications are scarce. Offner et al. [14] described four patients with multisystem trauma placed prone after midline abdominal incisions for exploratory laparotomy. Among them, one experienced wound dehiscence. Authors suggested that careful consideration was required before turning prone this subset of patients. However, number of patients studied was very small and no comparison with patients kept supine was made, preventing any definite answer to the question. On the opposite, our results offer a clear answer: We found no increase in the number of complications even after using a propensity score. This result stemmed from an exhaustive analysis of the patients' charts and medical files, using an a priori a list of surgical complications possibly related to prone position, established in collaborations with surgeons at the participating centers and confronted to an analysis of the literature on the subject.

Regarding oxygenation, in this patient population, little is available in the literature. In a small retrospective study, Davis et al. [24] described trauma and surgical patients with acute lung injury and ARDS and questioned the benefit of prone position. Others found that oxygenation was improved by the prone position, which suggests the effectiveness of the technique in terms of oxygenation. However, numbers of patient were small and data regarding complications and more specifically surgical complications were not reported.

Our results confirm that in patients with postsurgical ARDS, prone positioning provides a clear benefit in terms of oxygenation. Compared to results from the large RCTs, we found a comparable if not greater improvement in PaO_2/FiO_2 ratio. Gattinoni et al. [5] and Guerin et al. [11] report a PaO2/FIO2 increase after the first prone session of approximately 60 and 50 mmHg, respectively.

Ours was almost 100 mmHg, which confirms and extends that patients with postsurgical ARDS are particularly responsive to prone position.

Strengths and weaknesses

Because Guerin et al. unambiguously demonstrated the clear benefit in terms of survival of prone position in a large population of very diverse etiologies of ARDS, there is obviously no case for another RCT in the specific setting of post-abdominal surgery (6). Indeed, we observed that 40% of patients had at least one surgical complication potentially related to position in the present study. To test the non-inferiority of prone position against supine position with a proper RCT, approximately 2400 subjects would be necessary to obtain a power of 80%, with a non-inferiority margin of 5%, and a type I error rate of 5%. It would take years to complete such a RCT. Given the small numbers of patients concerned by this condition, we felt that a retrospective study could help address our question. This choice has by design some limitations (including possible confounding effect, undisclosed bias in the decision of being or not turned prone). However, these were counterbalanced by the multicenter design of our study and the number of patients included which constitutes to date the largest study on the subset of postsurgical patients. Additionally, our database is part of a larger network used by many ICUs in Paris and its suburbs called CUB-Réa, and several publications have already been made with the data extracted from this database, so as to prove its efficacy and reliability [25, 26]. Although certain specifics of the prone sessions could not be traced in the records (e.g., staff required to turn the patient prone, number and location of pillows used), protocol used in the three ICUs was very similar and included placement of pillows under the thorax and pelvis in order to limit abdominal pressure [27]. We acknowledge the fact that the number of prone sessions was lower than in PROSEVA. The possibility that a greater number of prone sessions could be associated with an increased risk of surgical complication cannot be ruled out. However, intuitively, one can reason that the risk of complications specifically related to the surgery is greater in the early days after surgery. Because more than half the patients were turned prone within the first 48 h after surgery, we believe this limits the risks of having missed some complications because of insufficient number of prone sessions.

Baseline characteristics differed slightly between the two groups: Supine patients were older. This difference may impact related variables such as arterial hypertension, diabetes and SAPS II score. Nonetheless, the use of a propensity score analysis that takes into account these differences confirmed the initial findings.

Despite our conclusive results, the decision to turn a post-abdominal surgery patient prone should be taken on a case-by-case basis after discussion between the surgeons and the intensivists. Several issues could restrict use of prone position, such as multiple intra-hospital transport for CT scan, need for frequent revision surgery or presence of a Mikulicz drainage system. Nonetheless, we believe none of the above represents an absolute contraindication, and all are outweighed in case of life-threatening hypoxemia.

To conclude, our results confirm the effectiveness of prone positioning in terms of oxygenation in ARDS after abdominal surgery without significant increase in surgical complications and no effect on the need for surgical revisions. Hence, if necessary, our results suggest that clinicians should not refrain from proning patients with post-abdominal surgery ARDS.

Abbreviations

ARDS: acute respiratory distress syndrome; VILI: ventilator-induced lung injury; RCT: randomized controlled trials; STROBE: Strengthening the Reporting of Observational Studies in Epidemiology; ICU: intensive care units; BMI: body mass index.

Authors' contributions

SG, ST, DD and JDR wrote and reviewed the manuscript. DH performed the statistical analyses. ACL, CL, NZ, MP, BC, SM, JD and DP are investigators and were involved in critical review of the manuscript. All authors read and approved the final manuscript.

Author details

[1] Medico-Surgical Intensive Care Unit, Hôpital Louis Mourier, AP-HP, 178 rue des Renouillers, 92700 Colombes, France. [2] Sorbonne Paris Cité, ECEVE UMR 1123, Univ Paris Diderot, 75018 Paris, France. [3] Département d'Anesthésie Réanimation, Hôpital Lariboisière, AP-HP, 75010 Paris, France. [4] UMR U 1160, Université Paris-Diderot Paris 7, 75010 Paris, France. [5] Département d'Anesthésie Réanimation, Hôpital Bicêtre, AP-HP, 94270 Le Kremlin-Bicêtre, France. [6] Hôpital Lariboisière, Chirurgie digestive et cancérologique, AP-HP, 75010 Paris, France. [7] UMR U 965, Université Paris-Diderot Paris 7, 75010 Paris, France. [8] Hôpital Bicêtre, Chirurgie générale et digestive, AP-HP, 94270 Le Kremlin-Bicêtre, France. [9] Hôpital Louis Mourier, Chirurgie digestive, AP-HP, 178 rue des Renouillers, 92700 Colombes, France. [10] UMR 1149, Univ Paris Diderot, Sorbonne Paris Cité, 75018 Paris, France. [11] IAME,UMR 1137, INSERM, 75018 Paris, France. [12] IAME, UMR 1137, Univ Paris Diderot, Sorbonne Paris Cité, 75018 Paris, France. [13] Epidemiology and Clinical Research Department, Hôpital Louis Mourier, AP-HP, 178 rue des Renouillers, 92700 Colombes, France. [14] Service de Réanimation Médicale, 178 rue des Renouillers, 92701 Colombes Cedex, France.

Competing interests

The authors declare that they have no competing interests.

References

1. Piehl MA, Brown RS. Use of extreme position changes in acute respiratory failure. Crit Care Med. 1976;4:13–4.
2. Gattinoni L, Carlesso E, Taccone P, et al. Prone positioning improves survival in severe ARDS: a pathophysiologic review and individual patient meta-analysis. Minerva Anestesiol. 2010;76:448–54.
3. Valenza F, Guglielmi M, Maffioletti M, et al. Prone position delays the

progression of ventilator-induced lung injury in rats: does lung strain distribution play a role? Crit Care Med. 2005;33:361–7.
4. Broccard A, Shapiro RS, Schmitz LL, et al. Prone positioning attenuates and redistributes ventilator-induced lung injury in dogs. Crit Care Med. 2000;28:295–303.
5. Gattinoni L, Tognoni G, Pesenti A, et al. Prone-Supine Study Group: effect of prone positioning on the survival of patients with acute respiratory failure. N Engl J Med. 2001;345:568–73.
6. Guerin C, Gaillard S, Lemasson S, et al. Effects of systematic prone positioning in hypoxemic acute respiratory failure: a randomized controlled trial. JAMA. 2004;292:2379–87.
7. Mancebo J, Fernández R, Blanch L, et al. A multicenter trial of prolonged prone ventilation in severe acute respiratory distress syndrome. Am J Respir Crit Care Med. 2006;173:1233–9.
8. Taccone P, Pesenti A, Latini R, et al. Prone-Supine II Study Group: prone positioning in patients with moderate and severe acute respiratory distress syndrome: a randomized controlled trial. JAMA. 2009;302:1977–84.
9. Abroug F, Ouanes-Besbes L, Elatrous S, et al. The effect of prone positioning in acute respiratory distress syndrome or acute lung injury: a meta-analysis. Areas of uncertainty and recommendations for research. Intensive Care Med. 2008;34:1002–11.
10. Sud S, Taccone P, Polli F, et al. Prone ventilation reduces mortality in patients with acute respiratory failure and severe hypoxemia: systematic review and meta-analysis. Intensive Care Med. 2010;36:585–99.
11. Guerin C, Reignier J, Richard J-C, et al. Prone positioning in severe acute respiratory distress syndrome. N Engl J Med. 2013;368:2159–68.
12. Gattinoni L, Taccone P, Carlesso E, et al. Prone position in acute respiratory distress syndrome. Rationale, indications, and limits. Am J Respir Crit Care Med. 2013;188:1286–93.
13. Bellani G, Laffey JG, Pham T, et al. LUNG SAFE Investigators, ESICM Trials Group: epidemiology, patterns of care, and mortality for patients with acute respiratory distress syndrome in Intensive Care Units in 50 countries. JAMA. 2016;315:788–800.
14. Offner PJ, Haenel JB, Moore EE, et al. Complications of prone ventilation in patients with multisystem trauma with fulminant acute respiratory distress syndrome. J Trauma. 2000;48:224–8.
15. von Elm E, Altman DG, Egger M, et al. STROBE Initiative: the Strengthening the Reporting of Observational Studies in Epidemiology (STROBE) statement: guidelines for reporting observational studies. Ann Intern Med. 2007;147:573–7.
16. Definition Task Force ARDS, Ranieri VM, Rubenfeld GD, Thompson BT, et al. Acute respiratory distress syndrome: the Berlin definition. JAMA. 2012;307:2526–33.
17. Le Gall JR, Lemeshow S, Saulnier F. A new Simplified Acute Physiology Score (SAPS II) based on a European/North American multicenter study. JAMA. 1993;270:2957–63.
18. Bone RC, Balk RA, Cerra FB, et al. Definitions for sepsis and organ failure and guidelines for the use of innovative therapies in sepsis. The ACCP/SCCM Consensus Conference Committee. American College of Chest Physicians/Society of Critical Care Medicine. Chest. 1992;101:1644–55.
19. Calandra T, Cohen J. International sepsis forum definition of infection in the ICU consensus conference: the international sepsis forum consensus conference on definitions of infection in the intensive care unit. Crit Care Med. 2005;33:1538–48.
20. De Waele JJ, De Laet I, Kirkpatrick AW, et al. Intra-abdominal hypertension and abdominal compartment syndrome. Am J Kidney Dis Off J Natl Kidney Found. 2011;57:159–69.
21. Clavien PA, Barkun J, de Oliveira ML, et al. The Clavien-Dindo classification of surgical complications: five-year experience. Ann Surg. 2009;250:187–96.
22. Austin PC. A tutorial and case study in propensity score analysis: an application to estimating the effect of in-hospital smoking cessation counseling on mortality. Multivar Behav Res. 2011;46:119–51.
23. Ali MS, Groenwold RHH, Belitser SV, et al. Reporting of covariate selection and balance assessment in propensity score analysis is suboptimal: a systematic review. J Clin Epidemiol. 2015;68:112–21.
24. Davis JW, Lemaster DM, Moore EC, et al. Prone ventilation in trauma or surgical patients with acute lung injury and adult respiratory distress syndrome: is it beneficial? J Trauma. 2007;62:1201–6.
25. Zuber B, Tran T-C, Aegerter P, et al. CUB-Réa network: impact of case volume on survival of septic shock in patients with malignancies. Crit Care Med. 2012;40:55–62.
26. Annane D, Aegerter P, Jars-Guincestre MC, et al. CUB-Réa network: current epidemiology of septic shock: the CUB-Réa network. Am J Respir Crit Care Med. 2003;168:165–72.
27. Kirkpatrick AW, Pelosi P, De Waele JJ, et al. Clinical review: intra-abdominal hypertension: does it influence the physiology of prone ventilation? Crit Care. 2010;14:232.

6

Sound level intensity severely disrupts sleep in ventilated ICU patients throughout a 24-h period: a preliminary 24-h study of sleep stages and associated sound levels

Maxime Elbaz[1,2], Damien Léger[1,2*], Fabien Sauvet[2,3], Benoit Champigneulle[5], Stéphane Rio[1,2], Mélanie Strauss[1,4,6], Mounir Chennaoui[2,3], Christian Guilleminault[7] and Jean Paul Mira[5]

Abstract

Background: It is well recognized that sleep is severely disturbed in patients in intensive care units (ICU) and that this can compromise their rehabilitation potential. However, it is still difficult to objectively assess sleep quantity and quality and the determinants of sleep disturbance remain unclear. The aim of this study was therefore to evaluate carefully the impact of ICU sound intensity levels and their sources on ICU patients' sleep over a 24-h period.

Methods: Sleep and sound levels were recorded in 11 ICU intubated patients who met the criteria. Sleep was recorded using a miniaturized multi-channel ambulatory recording device. Sound intensity levels and their sources were recorded with the Nox-T3 monitor. A 30-s epoch-by-epoch analysis of sleep stages and sound data was carried out. Multinomial and binomial logistic regressions were used to associate sleep stages, wakefulness and sleep–wake transitions with sound levels and their sources.

Results: The subjects slept a median of 502.2 [283.2–718.9] min per 24 h; 356.9 [188.6–590.9] min at night (22.00–08.00) and 168.5 [142.5–243.3] during daytime (8 am–10 pm). Median sound intensity level reached 70.2 [65.1–80.3] dBC at night. Sound thresholds leading to disturbed sleep were 63 dBC during the day and 59 dBC during the night. With levels above 77 dBC, the incidence of arousals (OR 3.9, 95% CI 3.0–5.0) and sleep-to-wake transitions (OR 7.6, 95% CI 4.1–14) increased. The most disturbing noises sources were monitor alarms (OR 4.5, 95% CI 3.5–5.6) and ventilator alarms (OR 4.2, 95% CI 2.9–6.1).

Conclusions: We have shown, in a small group of 11 non-severe ICU patients, that sound level intensity, a major disturbance factor of sleep continuity, should be strictly controlled on a 24-h profile.

Keywords: Intensive care unit, Weaning, Sleep, Sound intensity, Monitoring

Background

Having a sufficient amount of sleep during a 24-h period is generally recommended as a major means of promoting health in adults [1, 2]. Sleep has a crucial role in many somatic, cognitive and psychological processes, and "sleeping well" appears to be a health imperative [3, 4]. Increasing evidence shows that sleeping too little impacts severely on health with an increasing risk of morbidity [5] and even mortality [6] across many groups. It may also affect memory and immunity, and can jeopardize safety [7, 8]. Chronic short sleep duration (<6 h) has been associated with an increased risk of obesity, diabetes, hypertension and other cardiovascular diseases [1, 9, 10]. Acute sleep deprivation (defined as sleeping 25–50% of a normal 8 h night's sleep) contributes to increased inflammation and disturbs the immunological response [11].

*Correspondence: damien.leger@aphp.fr; damien.leger@htd.aphp.fr
[2] EA 7330 VIFASOM Sommeil-Vigilance-Fatigue et Santé Publique, Hôtel Dieu de Paris, Université Paris Descartes, 1 place du Parvis Notre Dame, 75004 Paris, France
Full list of author information is available at the end of the article

Patients hospitalized in intensive care units (ICU) are likely to require support of two or more organ systems, including respiratory support. Such patients would clearly benefit from an optimal environment. However, patients often complain that their ICU stay was severely disturbed by noise, light and an inadequate environment to rest and sleep. Poor sleep is considered a major concern in ICU because of its potential interaction with other psychological and somatic diseases and its impact on rehabilitation [12–14]. However, previous studies have been limited at least by three major concerns:

- The quality of polysomnographic sleep recording (PSG) was traditionally considered poor due to interference from mechanical ventilators and alarms [12, 15–17] prior to the recent introduction of new technologies such as the ActiWave.
- There was an absence of precise analyses of how sound peaks may be linked to sleep arousals. Sound levels have been measured very accurately in ICU. However, few have made definitive assessments of potential associations between the overall level of sound (sound intensity) or sound peaks, and sleep arousals. This is principally because there are a large number of sound peaks in the environment and ICU patients experience many sleep arousals.

The goal of this study was therefore:

- To specifically characterize and classify the different sources of sounds peaks and significant sound intensity levels disturbing sleep.
- To analyze sleep quality on a 24-h basis.

Methods

Subjects

The eleven patients enrolled in this observational study were under mechanical ventilation and responded to the following inclusion criteria: resolution of disease for which the patient was intubated, cardiovascular stability with no need of vasopressors, no sedation for at least three days and adequate oxygenation defined as PaO_2/FiO_2 of at least 150 mmHg with positive end-expiratory pressure (PEEP) up to 8 cmH_2O. Exclusion criteria included a reported history of sleep disorders, including obstructive sleep apnea syndrome (OSAS) or insomnia, a diagnosed neurological disorder, renal insufficiency and any treatment with psychotropic drugs. The recruitment period was 16 months, and the data were collected over 7 months.

Patients were informed of the sleep protocol, received a written protocol and gave their informed consent to the study. Recording anonym data from the Cochin ICU patients has been approved by the National Ethical Data Protection Committee (CNIL) according to ethical committee procedures.

ICU

This study identifies that these particular ICU sound levels are above the limit recommended by the WHO and result in a higher incidence of disturbance of sleep patterns. Apart from the sound from alarms, other sounds coming from people around are implicated in the discussion of sleep continuity and quality.

The ICU department studied comprised 4 units of 6 beds with two nurses and one nursing auxiliary allocated to each. The nursing station was about 5 meters from the rooms. Patient were lying in bed the all day, but were mobilized by one medical intern and two physiotherapists (15 min each three times per day). Moreover, the ICU was open to visits regardless of time during the day and night with the median number of conversation noises per hour statistically higher during the day compared to the night. In emergencies, doctors and staff were called via a microphone system which may also disturb patients' sleep. This study did not identify a significant impact of conversation noise on sleep disturbances, but limiting voice loudness level and the frequency of conversations held by the bed side could certainly be recommended.

No specific instructions for patient sleep support (e.g., ear plugs, eye masks) were given to staff at the time of the study.

The rooms were lit by natural light from one window and artificial light at ceiling level. Lights were switched off manually by staff at night, with no specific schedule but depending on care intensity. The doors of the rooms were continually open day and night. The ICU unit had been refurnished recently to attenuate sound levels in ceilings and floors, with large specialist glass panels in order to improve supervision of patients.

Sleep recording and analysis

Sleep was recorded for 24 h, from 18.00 to 18.00 the following day, using a miniaturized multi-channel ambulatory recording device (ActiWave®, CamNtech Ltd England). This device collected three electroencephalogram (EEG) derivations (F1–M2, C3–M2 and O1–M2), two transversal electrooculogram (EOG) channels (E1–M2 and E2–M1) and one chin EMG channel. ActiWave is a miniaturized polysomnography device which is positioned directly onto the scalp using very short electrodes which eliminates interference in the signals. Three ActiWave devices were used, synchronized to within 1 ms and with the same time resolution criteria in order to get the final Polysomnographic file. This was validated against standard polysomnography of patients with a sleep disorder

[18]. Bio-electrical signals were digitized at a sampling frequency of 200 Hz with a 16-bit quantization between −500 and 500 μV, within a bandwidth of 0–48 Hz. All the data were stored in computer files using the standard EDF data format. EEG and EOG cup-electrodes (Ag–AgCl) were attached to the scalp and to the right and left cantus of the subjects using EC2 electrode cream (Grass Technologies, An Astro-Med, West Warwick, USA) according to the international 10–20 system for electrode placement. Sleep technicians tested each electrode at the start for signal quality in order to ensure clarity and easy interpretation over the 24-h period. Sleep analysis was performed in 30-s epochs according to the American Academy of Sleep Medicine's (AASM) [19] standardized rules for scoring sleep stages and classification of waking and sleep into five levels (awake, non-REM stage [N1, N2, N3] and REM sleep). Arousals were defined as "abrupt shifts in EEG frequency including alpha, theta and/or frequencies greater than 16 Hz (but not spindles) that lasted at least 3–15 s with at least 10 s of stable sleep preceding the change" [20]. Natural waking was also scored and included in the WASO (Wake After Sleep Onset) values.

Sound levels and assessment of their sources

Sound levels and their sources were positioned 40 cm from the subject's head and recorded simultaneously with PSG, using a microphone T3 device (NoxMedical®, Reykjavik, Iceland) with C-weighting (dBC) decibel calibrated sound. The Nox T3 signals were synchronized to the ActiWave montage signals by manual adjustment of the major sound pressure level events recorded by the Nox T3. The synchronized ActiWave signals were truncated to match Nox T3 recording times and fed through the Nox T3 software (Noxturnal 4.3) to output at 30-s intervals with sleep/wake and sound pressure levels.

Qualitative scoring of all sources of sound was done by two researchers listening continuously to each of the 24-h recordings obtained with the Noxturnal 3.2 software (NoxMedical®, Reykjavik, Iceland), and scoring was performed every 30 s. The most clearly identifiable sounds were classified into three main categories: monitor alarms, mechanical ventilator alarms and conversations. If none of these three categories was recognized, the sound was classified as "other." If many different types of sound were monitored during a given period, the most prevalent source was the one selected by the researchers.

One major aim of our study was to understand which sources of sound intensity, and at which decibel levels, were associated with arousals and/or change in sleep stages in order to calculate "cutoff values" above which sound level intensity disturbed sleep with a 95% confidence interval. Sleep, sound intensity levels and sound qualitative scoring were millisecond-synchronized and scored using the Noxturnal 3.2 software (NoxMedical®; Reykjavik, Iceland).

Statistics

Sleep and sound intensity sources were time-synchronized on the same software and analyzed epoch-by-epoch for each subject. For each 30-s period of sleep or waking, an average level of sound was calculated and the main source determined.

Statistical tests were performed using R studio (Version 0.99.175—© 2009–2014 RStudio, Inc.), and significance (α risk) was fixed at $p < 0.05$. Continuous variables were presented as mean ± standard deviation (m ± SD), and means were compared (day vs. night) using a paired 2-tailed t test. Dichotomous variables were presented as occurrence and percentage [n (%)]. A Chi-square was used to test the relationship between dichotomous variables. When significant, the odds ratio and its 95% confidence interval [OR (95% CI)] were calculated. Adjusted ORs (ORa) and 95% CI for subject, hour and age were also calculated. Dependence between quantitative variables was checked using a Pearson correlation test ($r \geq 0.6$, $p < 0.05$). Dependence between quantitative and qualitative variables was tested using an analysis of variance (ANOVA). A logistic regression was performed to estimate the probability for binary outcome (arousal, waking and sleep stage transitions) with noise level. A value of $p < 0.05$ for the Wald criterion was considered to denote regression coefficients significantly different from zero. The results are shown as ORs with 95% CIs. The fit of the models was judged using the Likelihood Ratio Test Statistic. Non-binary (more than 2 categories) dichotomous variables were analyzed using multinomial logistic regression models whereby noise level and hour were entered to predict awake and sleep stage.

Results

Eleven consecutive subjects were included in the study (patient's characteristics are shown in Table 1). Five patients had been hospitalized for septic shock, 4 for acute respiratory failure, 1 for hemorrhagic shock and 1 after major surgical procedure.

Sleep recordings (Table 2)

The quality of sleep recording was excellent for all 11 subjects, and no data were excluded based on reciprocal analysis of sleep signal quality with a final analysis of 95 040 PSG epochs of 30 s. Undetermined epochs due to artifacts or loss of signal represented <0.2% of the total scoring.

The median total sleep time (TST) over 24 h was 8.3 h (502 [283.2–718.9] min) with one-third of sleep (168.5 min [33%]) occurring during the daytime (i.e., 8 am–10 pm). REM sleep represented only 4% of TST during the 24 h and N3 sleep represented 9% of TST.

Table 1 Patient characteristics

Characteristics	Value
Age, yrs	64.2 ± 13.6
BMI, kg m^{-2}	29.2 ± 5.4
SAPSII score	74.3 ± 27.8
APACHE II score	30.1 ± 11.4
ICU LOS (days)	22.1 ± 18.5
MV duration (days)	15.2 ± 13.3

Key: yrs, years; BMI, body mass index; SAPSII, new simplified acute physiology score; APACHE II score, acute physiological score chronic health evaluation; ICU LOS, ICU length of stay; MV duration, mechanical ventilator duration

Percentages of N1, N2, N3 and REM sleep were not significantly different between night and day periods. But the median number of arousals per hour during the night was about tenfold those during the day (20 [6–32.6] vs. 2 [8–22.7]; $p = 0.03$).

Sound intensity level assessments (Table 3)

Sound characteristics, based on the analysis of 95 040 30-s epochs of recording per subject, are reported in Table 3 and Fig. 1.

The median level and interquartile range of noise in the rooms was 72.2 dBC [65.1–80.2] and was higher during the day than at night.

Qualitatively, the median number of alarm noises per hour (monitor or ventilator) was not significantly different between day and night. Conversely, the median number of conversation noises per hour was statistically higher during the day than during the night (28 [10–53], vs. 5 [4–12, 15, 16, 21], $p = 0.02$).

Impact of sound intensity on sleep

A significant increase (95% CI > 1) in waking time was observed with a cutoff sound greater than 63 dBC during the day and greater than 59 dBC at night (Fig. 2). Figure 2a, b shows the median percentage of each sleep stage for each median sound level for day and night periods. N3 and REM sleep occurred even when the sound intensity levels were greater than 80 dBC at night. During daytime, there was almost no REM sleep at sound levels greater than 80 dBC; however, N3 sleep persisted. Figure 2c, d shows the OR of triggers for awakening from sleep during the day and during the night. The curve profiles are very different for the day and the night, with a later and clear cutoff profile above 63 dBC during the day, and a lower and progressive OR increase above 59 dBC during the night.

The multinomial analysis of the effect of sound intensity levels on sleep stages is reported in Table 4. There was a globally significant effect of sound on N1, N2 and REM sleep whatever the period (night or day) but not on N3.

Table 2 Sleep characteristics (11 subjects)

Sleep values	24-h night and day sleep	Day (08h00–22h00)	Night (22h00–08h00)	Day vs. night *p*
TST, min	502.2 [283.2–718.9]	168.5 [142.5–243.3]	356.9 [188.6–590.9]	0.001
N1, min	112.1 [41.2–155.1]	32.1 [6.9–38.8]	98.2 [29.3–123.1]	0.002
N1, %TST	22.3 [14.6–30.7]	17.3 [4.6–21.7]	21.5 [7.5–28.5]	NS
N2, min	315.2 [242.1–480.3]	125.5 [52.3–144.7]	233.0 [143.3–364.0]	0.002
N2, %TST	62.7 [54.2–77.3]	68.7 [64.2–78.3]	62.1 [55.4–69.6]	NS
N3, min	55.2 [0–81.5]	23.5 [0–81.5]	39.7 [0–98.8]	NS
N3, %TST	9.0 [0–19.7]	3.5 [0–22.6]	6.5 [0–23.6]	NS
REM, min	20.1 [0–41.1]	5.3 [0–15.1]	19.8 [0–0.38]	0.04
REM, %TST	4.0 [0–9.7]	1.5 [0–3.9]	3.9 [0–10.1]	NS
Arousals, *n*/h	20 [6–32.6]	2 [0–16.6]	20 [8–22.7]	0.03

Data are median [interquartile range], TST = total sleep time, REM = rapid eye movement sleep, N1, N2, N3 = non-REM slow wave sleep stage N1, N2 and N3

Table 3 Sound characteristics (11 subjects)

Sound values	24-h night and day sleep	Day (08h00–22h00)	Night (22h00–08h00)	Day vs. night *p*
Sound level, dBC	72.2 [65.1–80.2]	74.2 [68.1–80.2]	70.2 [65.1–80.3]	0.01
Sound typology				
Alarm, *n*/h	38 [25–51]	22 [14–24]	18 [15–23]	NS
Mechanical respirators, *n*/h	101 [50–120]	55 [38–57]	49 [41–62]	NS
Talking; staff conversations, *n*/h	28 [10–53]	26 [9–43]	5 [4–15]	0.02
Other, *n*/h	15 [7–25]	10 [3–17]	7 [4–10]	NS

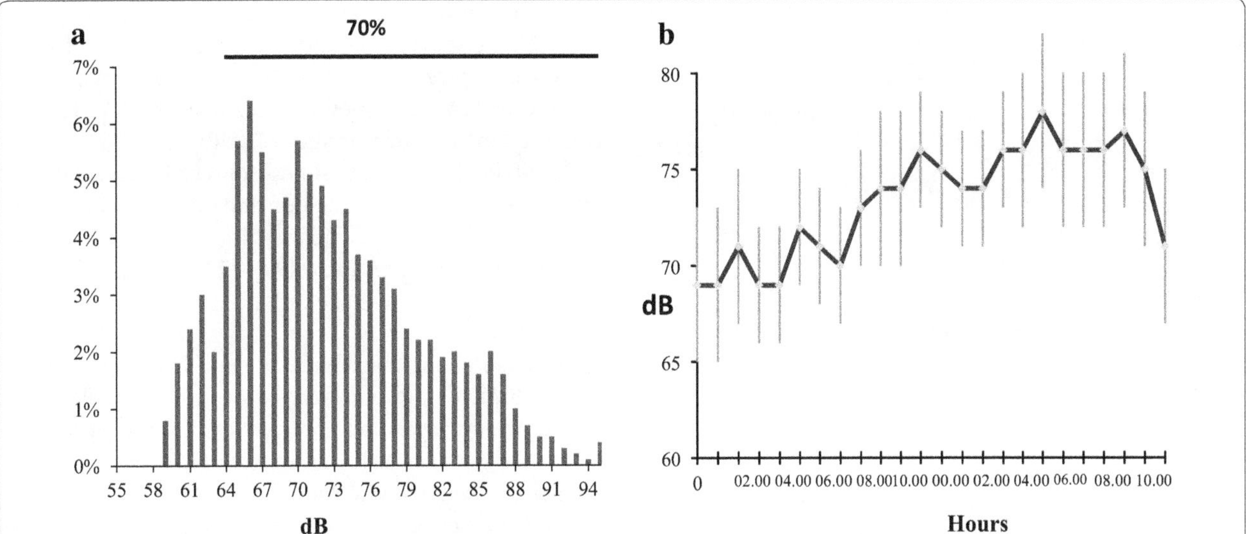

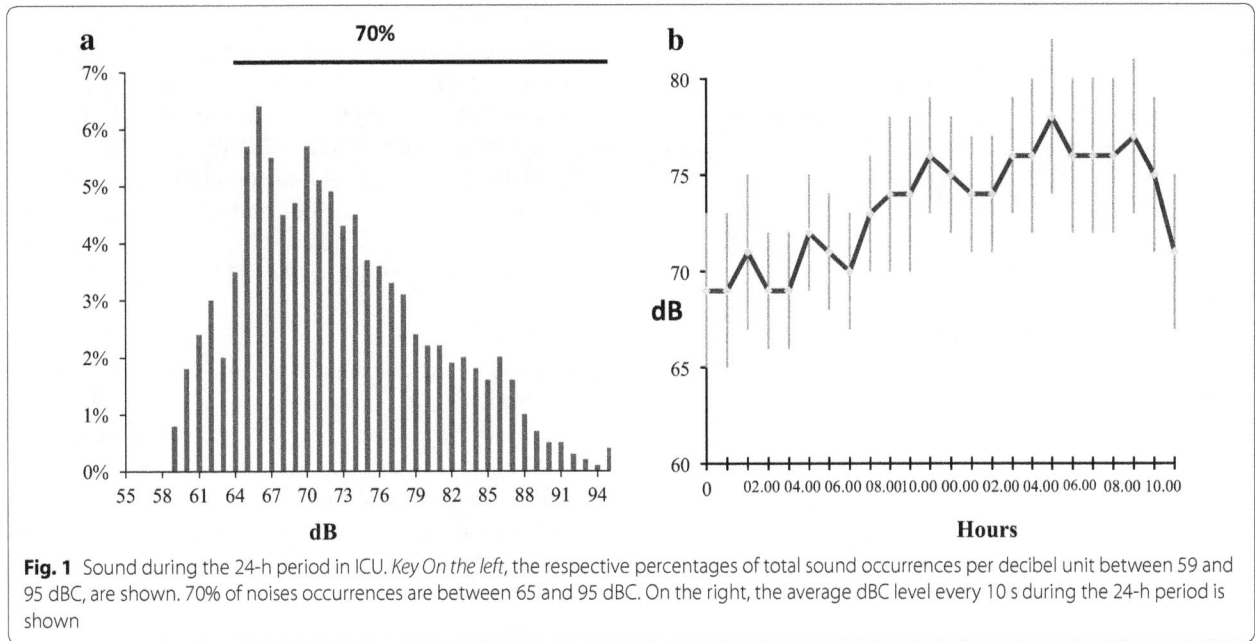

Fig. 1 Sound during the 24-h period in ICU. *Key On the left*, the respective percentages of total sound occurrences per decibel unit between 59 and 95 dBC, are shown. 70% of noises occurrences are between 65 and 95 dBC. On the right, the average dBC level every 10 s during the 24-h period is shown

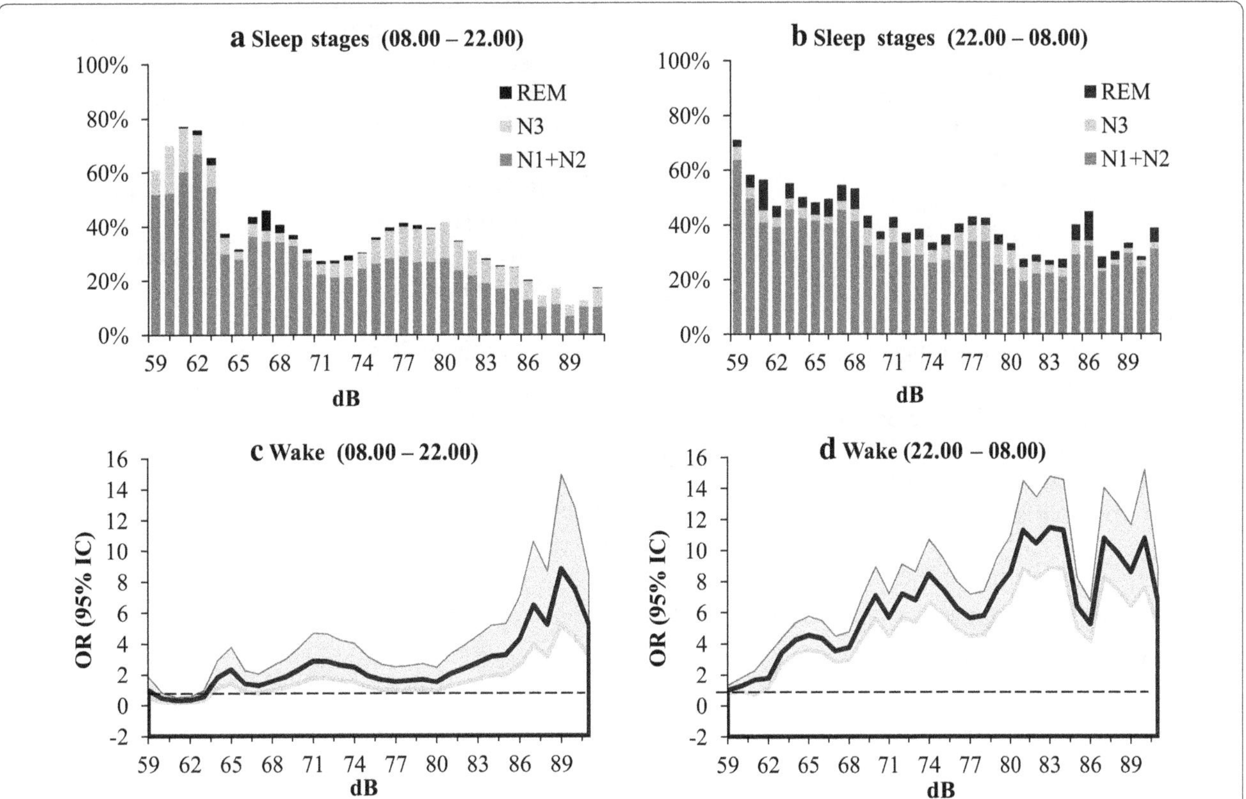

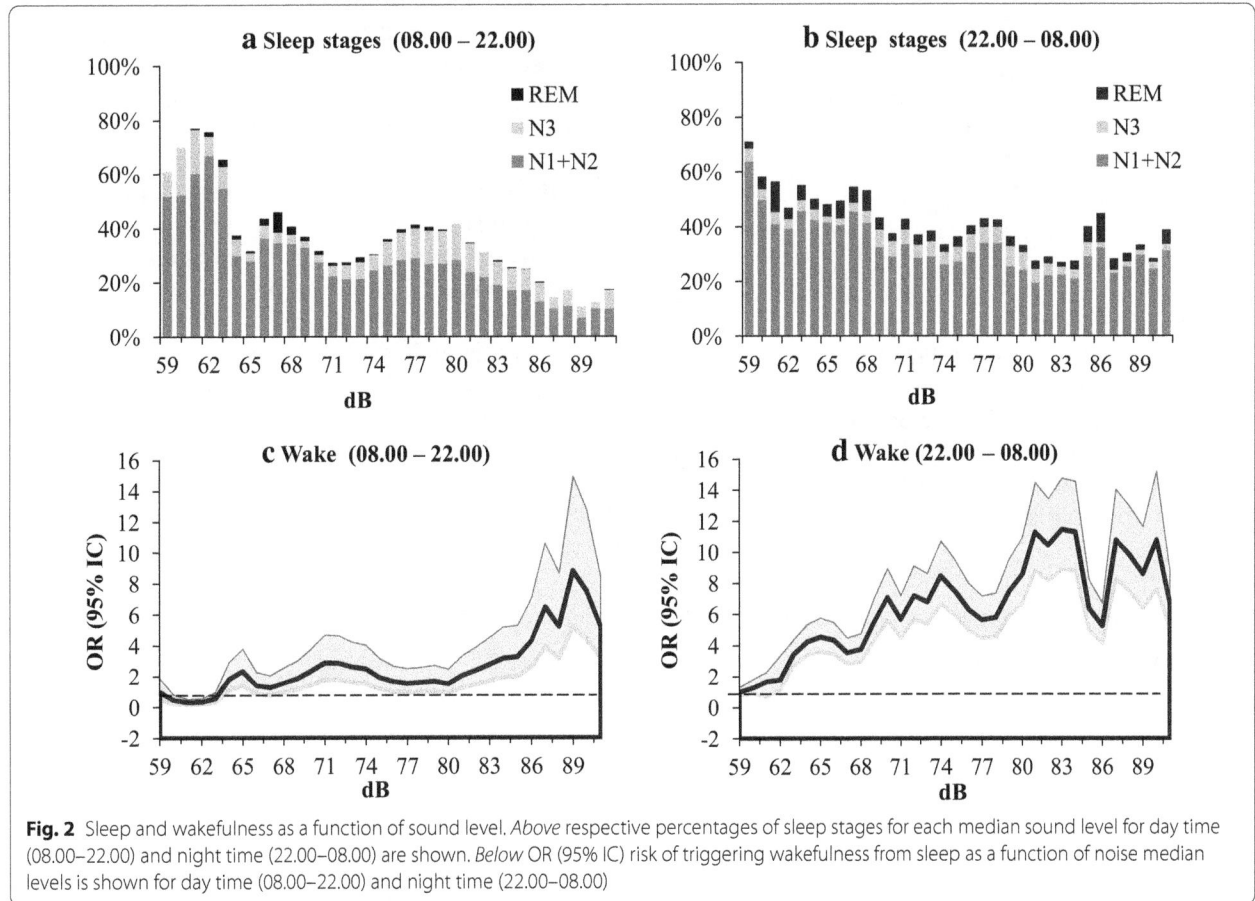

Fig. 2 Sleep and wakefulness as a function of sound level. *Above* respective percentages of sleep stages for each median sound level for day time (08.00–22.00) and night time (22.00–08.00) are shown. *Below* OR (95% IC) risk of triggering wakefulness from sleep as a function of noise median levels is shown for day time (08.00–22.00) and night time (22.00–08.00)

Table 4 Multinomial logistic regression between sleep stage and sound (dBC)

	Night (22h00–08h00) OR (95% CI)	Day (08h00–22h00) OR (95% CI)
Awakenings	1.0 (–)	1.0 (–)
N1	0.93 (0.93–0.94)***	0.97 (0.96–0.97)***
N2	0.95 (0.94–0.96)***	0.97 (0.96–0.97)***
N3	1.01 (1.00–1.02)	1.00 (0.99–1.01)
REM	0.91 (0.88–0.91)***	0.96 (0.95–0.97)***

OR (95% CI) odds ratio and 95% confidence interval

* $p < 0.05$; *** $p < 0.001$

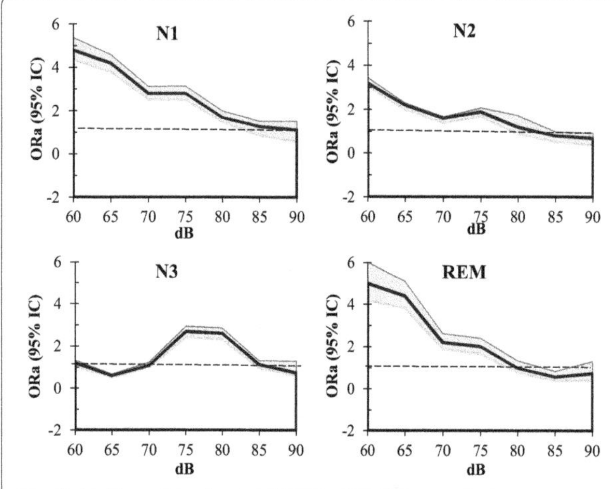

Fig. 3 Multinomial adjusted OR (ORa 95% CI) for each sleep stages as a function of sound levels. OR are adjusted for hours and subjects

Adjusted ORs (ORa) for each sleep stages as a function of sound levels are shown in Fig. 3. Sound intensity was significantly linked to waking (95% CI > from N1–N2 and REM sleep when the level was below 80 dBC and from N3 when the level was below 85 dBC). Logistic regression analyses showed that sound levels impacted significantly the occurrence of waking ($p < 0.001$), arousals ($p < 0.001$) and sleep-to-wake transitions for N2 to waking (see Table 5). No specific predictive awakening effect of sound level was observed for N1, N3 or REM sleep stages. The OR for arousals becomes significant (95% IC > 1) when sound intensity level was above 77 dBC.

Qualitatively, all of the sound sources had a significant impact on sleep stage transition and on arousal. However, ventilator alarms had the highest impact: 7.4 (6.1–8.7) on arousals in daytime and 10.9 (9.8–11.9) at night (Table 6).

Discussion

Knowledge about the impact of sound intensity in ICU is very limited, and our study aims to analyze sleep and sound objectively. A high prevalence of noise complaints from ICU patients has been reported in several previous studies [12–14, 22, 23]. Poor sleep is considered a major concern in the ICU because of its potential interaction with other psychological and somatic diseases and its impact on rehabilitation [14, 22, 23].

Sleep may be disturbed by multiple factors in ICU patients: pain [24, 25], high temperature [26], lighting [27], stress [24, 25], metabolic functions [28], the impact of mechanical ventilation [24, 29], adverse effects of some medications [30], and also by noise [31, 32]. However, it is unclear which sources of sound intensity are linked to the pathogenesis of sleep disturbance in ICU [33].

Using our miniaturized multi-channel ambulatory recording device, we succeeded in recording appropriately the different parameters necessary to score sleep in 30-s intervals in all our subjects. This miniaturized system is better tolerated than other standardized and larger PSG systems previously used in ICU and the shorter electrodes reduce interference.

Overall this study showed a fairly normal TST in subjects aged 64.2 ± 13.6 years—with a median of 502.2 [283.2–718.9] min and with a median nocturnal sleep of 356.9 min [188.6–590.9] and median daytime sleep of 168.5 [142.5–243.3] This TST is quite similar to the natural level (around 360 min per night) found in a

Table 5 Logistic regression between dependent variable and sound levels (dBC)

Dependant variable	Coefficient	SD	Wald statistics test	OR (95% CI)	Likelihood ratio test
Waking	0.049	0.009	1965***	1.05 (1.04–1.05)	206***
Arousal	0.018	0.004	15.4***	1.02 (1.01–1.03)	15.0***
Transitions	−0.028	0.004	58.8***	0.97 (0.96–0.98)	61.6***
N3 to W	0.052	0.031	1.7	1.05 (0.99–1.12)	2.7
N2 to W	0.048	0.009	27.6***	1.05 (1.03–1.07)	26.2***
N1 to W	−0.014	0.02	0.6	0.99 (0.95–1.02)	0.6
REM to W	0.066	0.05	1.8	1.07 (0.98–1.17)	1.6

OR (95% CI) odds ratio and 95% confidence interval

*** $p < 0.001$

Table 6 Influence of sound sources on sleep stages transitions and arousals. (Supplementary material)

	Day (08h00–22h00) ORa (95% IC)	Night (22h00–08h00) ORa (95% IC)
Alarm, *n*/h	1.9 (1.5–2.4)	1.9 (1.5–2.4)
Mechanical respirators, *n*/h	2.6 (2.3–2.9)	1.8 (2.3–2.9)
Talking; staff conversations, *n*/h	2.0 (1.6–2.4)	2.0 (1.6–2.4)
Other, *n*/h	1.9 (1.5–2.4)	1.8 (1.8–3.2)
Arousals		
Alarm, *n*/h	4.9 (3.4–6.7)	9.8 (8.6–11.3)
Mechanical respirators, *n*/h	7.4 (6.1–8.7)	10.9 (9.8–11.9)
Talking, staff conversations, *n*/h	3.0 (2.4–3.6)	5.2 (4.5–6.1)
Other, *n*/h	3.8 (2.3–6.3)	8.4 (6.9–10.1)

ORa OR adjusted for subject, hour and age

meta-analysis of 65 PSG studies including 3577 healthy subjects (ranging from 5 to 102 subjects, mean age 65 years old) [33]. Of note, this meta-analysis gave no reference to 24-h sleep, which has only been estimated subjectively by epidemiological surveys at around 440 min in the general adult population [33].

Twenty-four hour TST is arguably a better measurement to consider in ICU patients as they are on continuous bed rest (except when activated or mobilized by staff) and their sleep may not follow a mono-episodic profile. In our group as mentioned above, patients slept an average of 6 h at night, but also a median of 2.5 h during the day (168.5 min [142.5–243.3]). One previous study assessed day and night sleep over 24 h and found an altered circadian rhythm [23]. Assessing 24 h sleep is crucial to a better understanding of the impact of sleep on ICU prognosis as subjects clearly take daytime naps and promoting sleep in ICU patients may take advantage of this opportunity.

Sleep quality was disturbed more than sleep quantity in our patients. The median N3 percentage was 6.5% [0–23.6] compared to 26.1% [34], and median REM sleep 3.9% [0–10.1] vs. 20% [34]. This poor quality has been reported previously [10, 35, 36]. In our study, we observe a significant link between sleep changes and arousals and noise, suggesting a partial explanation for lack of N3 and REM sleep.

REM sleep represented only 4% of TST during the 24 h, which is lower than the usual rate in normal sleepers (15–20%) [3]. N3 sleep represented 9% of TST, also lower than the usual percentage in normal sleepers (15–20%) [2].

We used sleep analysis according to the American Academy Sleep of Medicine (AASM). Other studies have shown that AASM was often an insufficient monitor for sleep stages in critically ill patients. Therefore, a modified AASM has been proposed by Watson et al. which can be used in critically ill patients [37]. However, in our study, all the sleep stages in these ventilated patients could be pre-categorized as REM or non-REM, N1, N2, N3 and awake. No atypical patterns were observed, and absent signal was only 0.2%. One possible explanation for this finding could lie in the category of patients: the 11 patients included in the present study were highly selected. They were non-sedated, undergoing weaning and post-resolution of disease. In other words, they were long-term ventilated patients without a cute illness. They were ventilated and in the ICU, but not critically ill. The fact that these patients were not critically ill might be an explanation for the lack of atypical sleep patterns. Secondly, the ActiWave itself, with electrodes positioned close to the sleeping brain, may have delivered more accurate quality of sleep signals than previous studies.

Heightened sound intensity levels are considered to be a major sleep-disturbing factor, whatever the context. Sound levels in hospital should not exceed 35 dBA LAeq in areas where patients are being treated or observed, with a corresponding LAmax of 40 dBA [38].

Previous studies have already observed that sound is a significant sleep disturber in ICU [29, 33], but the authors [29, 33] reported that this was only responsible for <20, and 17% of awakenings. Our study shows that sound levels above 77 dBC are associated with awakenings 60% of the time during the night (Fig. 2b). The median noise level at night (70.2 dB [65.1–80.3]) is considerably greater than the WHO limit, and sound levels >59 dBC at night (10 pm–8 am) and >63 dBC during the day were significantly linked with awakenings in ICU patients. Interestingly, monitor alarms and mechanical ventilator alarms, integral to the ICU environment and used for patient safety, also significantly disturbed sleep. Currently, there are suggestions that "noise-alarms" be replaced with other emergency signals such as light at nursing stations. Our study only demonstrates the negative aspect of the "noise-alarm". This study identifies that these ICU and sound levels are above the limit recommended by the WHO and result in a higher incidence of disturbance of sleep patterns. Apart from alarms, other sounds coming from people around are implicated in the discussion of sleep continuity and quality.

We acknowledge that there are limitations to our study. For example, the evidence is based on a single 24-h PSG recording. It is known that the first PSG night is more disturbed than regular sleep, and two nights are required for pharmaceutical trials. Also we did not take into account the light environment of ICU rooms. Light at night is also known to alter the biological clock cycle and to disturb sleep. We recognize that concentrating on light and sleep in ICU is also a major issue in ICU [27, 29]. In our study, we did not assess the circadian factors that may influence the biological clock. Further research could record wrist actigraphy data from patients over a longer period.

Another potential limitation is that our study was limited to a group of 11 subjects who did not represent all patients hospitalized in the ICU. They had not received sedative medication recently and were not critically ill. However, in this preliminary study we deliberately concentrated on patients with an average of 22.1 ± 18.5 days stay in ICU, avoiding patients in the immediate post-diagnosis emergency period. We believe that our results reinforce and extend previous understanding of the fact that poor sleep is a persistent problem in ICU patients and that this is partly due to the negative effects of the immediate environment. Improving the physical and sensory aspects of the ICU environment represents an important and still under-researched potential for improving the sleep quality, and therefore the rehabilitation potential, of vulnerable patients.

Conclusions

In summary, our work shows, in a small sample of 11 non-severe ICU patients, that AW combined with T3 are good tools to record sleep and noise throughout a 24-h period in ICU patients. Sleep continuity is disturbed by alarms, particularly those of mechanical ventilators and monitors in ICU patients who are ventilated. Our study supports the need to evaluate alarms and emergency signaling in ICU. We found that 60% of awakenings are triggered by a noise higher than 77 dBC. However, further research is needed in order to be able to apply our conclusions to a wider population of ventilated critically ill patients.

Abbreviations

AASM: American Academy of Sleep Medicine; APACHE: acute physiology and chronic health evaluation scoring; BMI: body mass index; EEG: electroencephalogram; EOG: electrooculogram; EMG: electromyogram; ICU: intensive care unit; N1: non-REM sleep stage 1; N2: non-REM sleep stage 2; N3: non-REM sleep stage 3; OSAS: obstructive sleep apnea syndrome; PEEP: positive end-expiratory pressure; R: REM sleep; SAPSII: simplified acute physiology score; TST: total sleep time.

Authors' contributions

ME, DL, JPM were involved in conception and design; ME, SR, DL, JPM were involved in realization; ME, DL, JPM, FS, BC, MC, CG, MS, JPM analyzed and interpreted the data; ME, DL, CG, JPM drafted the manuscript for important intellectual content. All authors read and approved the final manuscript.

Author details

[1] Centre du Sommeil et de la Vigilance, Hôtel-Dieu de Paris, APHP, Université Paris Descartes, Paris, France. [2] EA 7330 VIFASOM Sommeil-Vigilance-Fatigue et Santé Publique, Hôtel Dieu de Paris, Université Paris Descartes, 1 place du Parvis Notre Dame, 75004 Paris, France. [3] Unité Fatigue et Vigilance, Institut de Recherche Biomédicale des Armées (IRBA), Brétigny-sur-Orge, France. [4] Cognitive Neuroimaging Unit, U992, INSERM, Gif/Yvette, France. [5] Service de Réanimation médicale, Hôpital Cochin, APHP, Université Paris Descartes, Paris, France. [6] NeuroSpin Center Institute of Bioimaging, Commissariat à l'Energie Atomique (CEA), Gif/Yvette, France. [7] Stanford University Sleep Disorders Clinic, Palo Alto, CA, USA.

Acknowledgements

Please acknowledge anyone who contributed to the article who does not meet the criteria for authorship including anyone who provided professional writing services or materials.

Competing interests

The authors declare that they have no competing interests.

Funding

This preliminary study received no funding.

References

1. Mukherjee S, Patel SR, Kales SN, Ayas NT, Strohl KP, Gozal D, et al. An official American thoracic society statement: the importance of healthy sleep. Recommendations and future priorities. Am J Respir Crit Care Med. 2015;191:1450–8.
2. Buysse DJ. Sleep health: can we define it? Does it matter? Sleep. 2014;37:9–17.
3. National Institute of Mental Health. Arousal and Regulatory Systems: Workshop Proceedings. 2013.
4. Strauss M, Sitt JD, King JR, Elbaz M, Azizi L, Buiatti M, et al. Disruption of hierarchical predictive coding during sleep. Proc Natl Acad Sci USA. 2015;112:E1353–62.
5. Kronholm E, Laatikainen T, Peltonen M, Sippola R, Partonen T. Self-reported sleep duration, all-cause mortality, cardiovascular mortality and morbidity in Finland. Sleep Med. 2011;12:215–21.
6. Ferrie JE, Shipley MJ, Cappuccio FP, Brunner E, Miller MA, Kumari M, et al. A prospective study of change in sleep duration: associations with mortality in the White-hall II cohort. Sleep. 2007;30:1659–66.
7. Spiegel K, Sheridan JF, Van Cauter E. Effect of sleep deprivation on response to immunizaton. JAMA. 2002;288:1471–2.
8. Faraut B, Nakib S, Drogou C, Elbaz M, Sauvet F, De Bandt JP, et al. Napping reverses the salivary interleukin-6 and urinary norepinephrine changes induced by sleep restriction. J Clin Endocrinol. 2015;100:E416–26.
9. Spiegel K, Tasali E, Leproult R, Van Cauter E. Effects of poor and short sleep on glucose metabolism and obesity risk. Nat Rev Endocrinol. 2009;5:253–61.
10. Faraut B, Touchette E, Gamble H, Royant-Parola S, Safar ME, Varsat B, et al. Short sleep duration and increased risk of hypertension: a primary care medicine investigation. J Hypertension. 2012;30:1354–63.
11. Faraut B, Boudjeltia KZ, Vanhamme L, Kerkhofs M. Immune, in-flammatory and cardiovascular consequences of sleep restriction and recovery. Sleep Med Rev. 2012;16:137–49.
12. Aurell J, Elmqvist D. Sleep in the surgical intensive care unit: continuous polygraphic recording of sleep in nine patients receiving postoperative care. BMJ. 1985;290:1029–32.
13. Valente M, Placidi F, Oliveira AJ, Bigagli A, Morghen I, Proietti R, et al. Sleep organization pattern as a prognostic marker at the subacute stage of post-traumatic coma. Clin Neurophysiol. 2002;113:1798–805.

14. Kamdar BB, Needham DM, Collop NA. Sleep deprivation in critical illness: its role in physical and psychological recovery. J Intensive Care Med. 2012;27:97–111.
15. Gottschlich MM, Jenkins ME, Mayes T, Khoury J, Kramer M, Warden GD, et al. The 1994 clinical research award. A prospective clinical study of the polysomnographic stages of sleep after burn injury. J Burn Care Rehabil. 1994;15:486–92.
16. Cooper AB, Thornley KS, Young GB, Slutsky AS, Stewart TE, Hanly PJ. Sleep in critically ill patients requiring mechanical ventilation. Chest. 2000;117:1809–18.
17. Orwelius L, Nordlund A, Nordlund P, Edéll-Gustafsson U, Sjöberg F. Prevalence of sleep disturbances and long-term reduced health-related quality of life after critical care: a prospective multicenter cohort study. Crit Care. 2008;12:R97.
18. Elbaz M, Léger D, Purday M, Rouffret G, Raffray T. Validation of the ActiWave mini polysomnogram (associated with Embletta Gold) versus complete polysomnography. Eur Sleep Res Soc JSR. 2010;19(Suppl. 2):1–378.
19. Iber C, Ancoli-Israel S, Chesson A, Quan SF. The AASM the manual for scoring of sleep and associated events: rules, terminology and technical specification. 1st ed. Westchester: American Academy of Sleep Medicine; 2007.
20. Tembo AC, Parker V, Higgins I. The experience of sleep deprivation in intensive care patients: findings from a larger hermeneutic phenomenological study. Intensive Crit Care Nurs. 2013;29:310–6.
21. Vgontzas AN, Liao D, Pejovic S, Calhoun S, Karataraki M, Bixler EO. Insomnia with objective short sleep duration is associated with type 2 diabetes: a population-based study. Diabetes Care. 2009;32:1980–5.
22. Knauert MP, Yaggi HK, Redeker NS, Murphy TE, Araujo KL, Pisani MA. Feasibility study of unattended polysomnography in medical intensive care unit patients. Heart Lung. 2014;43:445–52.
23. Elliott R, McKinley S, Cistulli P, Fien M. Characterisation of sleep in intensive care using 24-hour polysomnography: an observational study. Crit Care. 2013;17:R46.
24. Bihari S, Doug McEvoy R, Matheson E, Kim S, Woodman RJ, Bersten AD. Factors affecting sleep quality of patients in intensive care unit. J Clin Sleep Med. 2012;8:301–7.
25. Gazendam JA, Van Dongen HP, Grant DA, Freedman NS, Zwavelling JH, Schwab RJ. Altered circadian rhythmicity in patients in the ICU. Chest. 2013;144:483–9.
26. Gabor JY, Cooper AB, Crombach SA, et al. Contribution of the intensive care unit environment to sleep disruption in mechanically ventilated patients and healthy subjects. Am J Respir Crit Care Med. 2003;167:708–15.
27. Drouot X, Cabello B, d'Ortho MP, Brochard L. Sleep in the intensive care unit. Sleep Med Rev. 2008;12:391–403.
28. Kress JP, Pohlman AS, Hall JB. Sedation and analgesia in the intensive care unit. Am J Respir Crit Care Med. 2002;166:1024–8.
29. Bano M, Chiaromanni F, Corrias M, et al. The influence of environmental factors on sleep quality in hospitalized medical patients. Front Neurol. 2014;5:267.
30. Freedman NS, Gazendam JA, Levan L, Richard AP, Schawb J. Abnormal sleep/wake cycles and the effect of environmental noise on sleep disruption in the intensive care unit. Am J Respir Crit Care Med. 2001;163:451–7.
31. Wang J, Greenberg H. Sleep and the ICU. Open Crit Care Med J. 2013;6:80–7.
32. Delaney LJ, Van Haren F, Lopez V. Sleeping on a problem: the impact of sleep disturbance on intensive care patients—a clinical review. Ann Intensive Care. 2015;5:3.
33. Ohayon MM, Carskadon MA, Guilleminault C, Vitiello MV. Meta-analysis of quantitative sleep parameters from childhood to old age in healthy individuals: developing normative sleep values across the human lifespan. Sleep. 2004;27:1255–73.
34. Vernet C, Arnulf I. Idiopathic hypersomnia with and without long sleep time: a controlled series of 75 patients. Sleep. 2009;32:753–9.
35. Parthasarathy S, Tobin MJ. Effect of ventilator mode on sleep quality in critically ill patients. Am J Respir Crit Care Med. 2002;166:1423–9.
36. Bosma K, Ferreyra G, Ambrogio C, Pasero D, Mirabella L, Braghiroli A, et al. Patient-ventilator interaction and sleep in mechanically ventilated patients: pressure support versus proportional assist ventilation. Crit Care Med. 2007;35:1048–54.
37. Watson PL, Pandharipande P, Gehlbach BK, Thompson JL, Shintani AK, Dittus BS, et al. Atypical sleep in ventilated patients: empirical electroencephalography findings and the path toward revised ICU sleep scoring criteria. Crit Care Med. 2013;41:1958–67.
38. Berglund B, Lindvall T, Schwela DH. Guidelines for community noise. Geneva: World Health Organization; 1999.

7

High-flow nasal cannula to prevent postextubation respiratory failure in high-risk non-hypercapnic patients

Rafael Fernandez[1*], Carles Subira[1], Fernando Frutos-Vivar[2], Gemma Rialp[3], Cesar Laborda[4], Joan Ramon Masclans[5], Amanda Lesmes[2], Luna Panadero[2] and Gonzalo Hernandez[6]

Abstract

Background: Extubation failure is associated with increased morbidity and mortality, but cannot be safely predicted or avoided. High-flow nasal cannula (HFNC) prevents postextubation respiratory failure in low-risk patients.

Objective: To demonstrate that HFNC reduces postextubation respiratory failure in high-risk non-hypercapnic patients compared with conventional oxygen.

Methods: Randomized, controlled multicenter trial in patients who passed a spontaneous breathing trial. We enrolled patients meeting criteria for high-risk of failure to randomly receive HFNC or conventional oxygen for 24 h after extubation. Primary outcome was respiratory failure within 72-h postextubation. Secondary outcomes were reintubation, intensive care unit (ICU) and hospital lengths of stay, and mortality. Statistical analysis included multiple logistic regression models.

Results: The study was stopped due to low recruitment after 155 patients were enrolled (78 received high-flow and 77 received conventional oxygen). Groups were similar at enrollment, and all patients tolerated 24-h HFNC. Postextubation respiratory failure developed in 16 (20%) HFNC patients and in 21 (27%) conventional patients [OR 0.69 (0.31–1.54), $p = 0.2$]. Reintubation was needed in 9 (11%) HFNC patients and in 12 (16%) conventional patients [OR 0.71 (0.25–1.95), $p = 0.5$]. No difference was found in ICU or hospital length of stay, or mortality. Logistic regression models suggested HFNC [OR 0.43 (0.18–0.99), $p = 0.04$] and cancer [OR 2.87 (1.04–7.91), $p = 0.04$] may be independently associated with postextubation respiratory failure.

Conclusion: Our study is inconclusive as to a potential benefit of HFNC over conventional oxygen to prevent occurrence of respiratory failure in non-hypercapnic patients at high risk for extubation failure.

Keywords: Mechanical ventilation, Weaning, Reintubation, High-flow oxygen

Background

The need for mechanical ventilation (MV) is one of the main reasons for admission to intensive care units (ICU). Once patients recover from critical illness, they need to be extubated and resume spontaneous breathing. It is difficult to predict whether a patient is ready to be extubated [1, 2], and physicians must balance the benefits of prolonging MV allowing for better recovery, against the associated risks, mainly pulmonary infections, delirium, and muscle atrophy. Between 10 and 20% of attempts to extubate fail [3], and extubation failure is associated with

*Correspondence: rfernandezf@althaia.cat
[1] Critical Care Department, Hospital Sant Joan de Deu- Fundacio Althaia, CIBERES, Universitat Internacional de Catalunya, Dr Joan Soler 1, 08243 Manresa, Spain
Full list of author information is available at the end of the article

increased morbidity and mortality [4]. Thus, there is a need for strategies that can reduce the rate of extubation failure [5].

After extubation, patients routinely receive oxygen-enriched air through nasal prongs or masks; the concentration of oxygen is controlled and progressively tapered off within hours or days based on patients' tolerance.

Recently, a new method to deliver oxygen, high-flow nasal cannula (HFNC), reached the clinical arena [6, 7]. HFNC devices supply between 30 and 60 L/min of a controlled mixture of actively warmed (32–37 °C) and humidified (up to 100% relative humidity) oxygen and air through modified nasal prongs, producing a moderate positive end-expiratory pressure (PEEP) [8]. HFNC might help prevent extubation failure through different mechanisms. First, the controlled oxygen concentration may reduce transient hypoxemic episodes [9]. Second, the high flow washes the nasopharyngeal dead space, thus reducing CO_2 re-breathing; this effect reduces respiratory rate and minute ventilation [10]. Third, the small amount of PEEP may reduce lung collapse [11], enabling better gas exchange and reduced work of breathing; moreover, in patients with chronic obstructive pulmonary disease (COPD), this level of PEEP may counterbalance autoPEEP, further reducing the work of breathing [12–14]. Finally, humidification may improve mucus drainage and reduce mucus retention, alleviating the associated atelectasis [15, 16].

HFNC after extubation has shown benefits in patients at low risk for extubation failure [17], in mixed populations of critically ill patients [9, 18], and in patients after cardiothoracic surgery [19], but not in post-cardiac obese patients [20]. We hypothesized that HFNC as compared to standard oxygen may reduce postextubation respiratory failure in non-hypercapnic patients at high risk for extubation failure. We focused the current study on patients with high risk for extubation failure excluding hypercapnic patients in whom the use of noninvasive ventilation (NIV) may be beneficial [21, 22].

Methods

This randomized trial (Clinicaltrials.gov NCT01820507) was conducted in four general ICUs in Spain in 2013–2014. Approval for involvement of human subjects was obtained from institutional review boards (IRBs) at each study sites [FA IRB No. CEIC 12/85, HG IRB No. A06-13, HSLl IRB No. 2105/13, HVH IRB No. PR(AG)116/2013]. Written informed consent was obtained from patients' relatives.

We screened adult patients receiving MV >12 h deemed ready for scheduled extubation after a spontaneous breathing trial (SBT). We included patients fulfilling at least one of the following high-risk criteria for extubation failure [20–24]: older than 65 years, heart failure as cause of intubation, non-hypercapnic moderate-to-severe COPD, APACHE II score >12 points at extubation, body mass index >30 kg/m^2, weak cough and copious secretions, more than one SBT failure, or MV >7 days. We excluded patients with tracheotomy, inability to follow commands, or do-not-reintubate orders, as well as those who developed hypercapnia during the SBT because they required NIV immediately after extubation.

Weaning protocol

Patients fulfilling the criteria for tolerance of spontaneous ventilation underwent an SBT following the local protocols. The SBT ranged from 30 to 120 min and was performed with 5-cmH_2O continuous positive airway pressure, 7-cmH_2O pressure support, or T-tube.

Criteria for SBT failure were agitation, anxiety, depressed mental status, diaphoresis, cyanosis, evidence of increasing respiratory effort, increased accessory muscle activity, facial signs of distress, dyspnea, $PaO_2 \leq 60$ mmHg or SpO_2 <90% on $FiO_2 \geq 0.5$, $PaCO_2$ >50 mmHg or >8 mmHg increase, arterial pH <7.32 or ≥0.07 decrease, respiratory rate >35 breaths min^{-1} or ≥50% increase, heart rate >140 beats min^{-1} or ≥20% increase, systolic arterial pressure >180 mmHg or ≥20% increase, systolic arterial pressure <90 mmHg, or cardiac arrhythmia.

Patients who failed the SBT were reconnected to the ventilator for an additional 24-h rest period before a new SBT. Patients who tolerated the SBT were directly extubated and randomized to receive either high-flow or conventional oxygen therapy for a fixed 24-h period. Randomization was performed via a computerized random-number table in blocks of four for each hospital; allocation was concealed through numbered opaque envelopes.

Interventions

Conventional group

Oxygen after extubation was supplied either by nasal prongs or facial mask with oxygen concentration regulated by Venturi effect.

HFNC group

Oxygen after extubation was supplied by Optiflow® (Fisher&Paykel, New Zealand). Flow was started at 40 L/min and was adjusted according to patients' subjective tolerance. The humidifier was set in the invasive mode (37 °C), but was switched to noninvasive mode (34 °C) if the patient felt excessive warmth.

In both groups, oxygen supply was continuously adjusted to achieve SpO2 between 92 and 95%. At the end of the 24-h study period, all patients received conventional oxygen therapy when needed and were followed up to hospital discharge.

The primary outcome variable was respiratory failure within 72 h postextubation, defined as the presence and persistence of any of the following: respiratory acidosis (pH <7.35 with $PaCO_2$ >45 mmHg), hypoxemia (SpO_2 <90% or PaO_2 <60 mmHg with $FiO_2 \geq 0.5$), tachypnea >35 breaths/min and/or signs of respiratory muscle fatigue, and/or low level of consciousness or agitation.

Patients were continuously monitored by electrocardiography and pulse oximetry. For the purpose of this trial, NIV as rescue treatment for extubation failure was discouraged, but remained available at the discretion of the attending team.

Secondary outcome variables were reintubation, ICU and hospital lengths of stay, and survival. Criteria for immediate reintubation were cardiac or respiratory arrest, respiratory pauses with neurological deterioration, massive aspiration, uncontrollable agitation, sputum retention, and hemodynamic deterioration unresponsive to vasoactive drugs. Patients were also reintubated when they needed it for non-respiratory reasons, such as emergency surgery or when postextubation respiratory failure did not improve after 12 h.

Statistical analysis

With an expected extubation failure rate of 28% in the control group and an absolute expected improvement with HFNC of 7% (25% relative reduction) [25], the planned sample was 592 patients in each arm, for an alpha error of 5% and a power of 80%.

Because it was impossible to mask patients and staff to treatment and outcome, we used the following measures to minimize bias in assessing results: The database was monitored by third parties with no direct involvement in the study procedures and no interest in outcome, and the data were analyzed exactly according to the statistical analysis plan decided on before the study started.

Data were analyzed with an intention-to-treat approach. Categorical variables were compared by Chi-square or Fisher's exact test, as appropriate. Continuous variables were compared by Student's t test. Kaplan–Meier survival analyses were done for extubation failure, reintubation, and mortality, and the log-rank test was used for comparisons.

To determine factors independently associated with postextubation respiratory failure, we elaborated a multivariable logistic regression model using a backward procedure, including HFNC and all non-redundant variables associated with postextubation respiratory failure (p < 0.1). Statistics were analyzed with STATA 10.0® (StataCorp, TX) and EpiInfo-7® (CDC, GA).

Results

When after 18 months only 155 patients had been recruited (78 randomized to receive high-flow oxygen and 77 conventional oxygen), the investigators stopped the trial due to low recruitment (Fig. 1).

The two groups were not different at inclusion (Table 1). The most common criteria for high-risk for postextubation respiratory failure were age >65 years and abundant secretions. All patients tolerated 24-h HFNC, but 14 (18%) reported some kind of discomfort, mainly noise, and 2 (2.6%) developed small nostril skin lesions. Pneumonia after extubation was the only reported adverse event, affecting only 2 (2.6%) patients, both in the conventional group.

Postextubation respiratory failure developed in 16 (20%) HFNC patients and in 21 (27%) conventional patients [OR 0.69 (95% CI 0.31–1.54), $p = 0.2$] (Table 2; Fig. 2). Time-to-failure was not different in the two groups [17 (7, 44) h vs. 21 (6, 44) h, $p = 0.7$]. The criteria identifying respiratory failure were not different between groups. NIV was used as rescue therapy for respiratory failure in 10 (62%) HFNC patients and 12 (57%) conventional patients ($p = 0.9$).

Reintubation was needed in 9 (11%) HFNC patients and in 12 (16%) conventional patients [OR 0.71 (95% CI 0.25–1.95), $p = 0.5$]. Reintubation was needed in 3 (30%) HFNC patients treated with NIV and in 7 (58%) conventional patients treated with NIV ($p = 0.18$).

Length of ICU and hospital stays and mortality were not different between the two groups. Mortality in patients exhibiting postextubation respiratory failure did not differ between those treated with NIV and those without (10/22, 45% and 3/15, 20%; $p > 0.1$, respectively).

The multivariable logistic regression model identified HFNC [OR 0.43 (0.18–0.99), $p = 0.04$) and cancer [OR

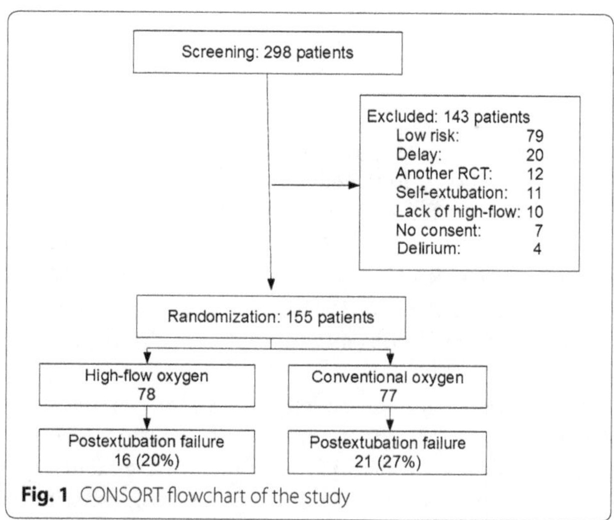

Fig. 1 CONSORT flowchart of the study

Table 1 Characteristics at randomization of patients in the HFNC group versus those in the conventional oxygen therapy group

Baseline variables	HFNC $n = 78$	Conventional $n = 77$	p
Age (years)	67.3 ± 12.1	69.7 ± 13.0	0.2
Female sex	32 (41%)	22 (29%)	0.1
Height (cm)	168 ± 9	168 ± 21	0.2
APACHE II on admission, points	21 ± 8.8	21 ± 8.2	0.9
APACHE II at extubation, points	11 ± 5.5	10 ± 6.7	0.2
Length of mechanical ventilation before extubation (days)	8.2 ± 5.9	7.4 ± 3.6	0.3
High-risk criteria[a]			
Age >65 years	49 (67%)	55 (75%)	0.4
Abundant secretions	33 (47%)	35 (51%)	0.7
>2 comorbidities	31 (43%)	34 (49%)	0.5
APACHE II >12 points	24 (34%)	31 (45%)	0.2
Body mass index >30 kg/m^2	14 (20%)	18 (25%)	0.5
Chronic obstructive pulmonary disease	12 (18%)	10 (15%)	0.8
Weak cough	10 (15%)	14 (21%)	0.4
Congestive heart failure	9 (14%)	9 (14%)	1
Failed spontaneous breathing trial	6 (9%)	5 (7%)	1
Pre-SBT respiratory rate (min^{-1})	21.7 ± 6.0	21.8 ± 5.8	0.8
Pre-SBT FiO_2	0.30 ± 0.08	0.30 ± 0.08	0.9
Pre-SBT SpO_2 (%)	96.5 ± 1.9	96.0 ± 2.3	0.8

HFNC high-flow nasal cannula, *APACHE II* Acute Physiology and Chronic Health Evaluation, *SBT* spontaneous breathing trial

[a] More than one criteria can be present

Table 2 Outcome variables in the two groups

Outcome variables	HFNC $n = 78$	Conventional $n = 77$	p
Postextubation respiratory failure	16 (20%)	21 (27%)	0.2
Causes of respiratory failure			
Hypoxemia	11 (65%)	14 (67%)	0.6
Respiratory rate >35	9 (54%)	14 (67%)	0.3
Respiratory muscle fatigue	7 (47%)	8 (53%)	0.5
Respiratory acidosis	2 (12%)	8 (36%)	0.08
Low level of consciousness	3 (18%)	1 (5%)	0.2
Time-to-failure (h)	17 [7, 44]	21 [6, 44]	0.7
Reintubation within 72 h	9 (11%)	12 (16%)	0.5
Intensive care unit length of stay (days)	12 [7, 25]	14 [9, 17]	0.8
Intensive care unit mortality	6 (7.7%)	7 (9.0%)	0.9
Hospital length of stay (days)	27 [18, 54]	27 [18, 47]	1
Hospital mortality	12 (15.4%)	12 (15.6%)	1

2.87 (1.04–7.91), $p = 0.04$] as independently associated with postextubation respiratory failure (see Additional file 1). Due to the limited sample size, the multivariable logistic regression must be considered as exploratory. In order to explore the likelihood of a clinically sound effect of HFNC, a sensitivity analysis with four different regression models is shown in the Additional file 1.

Discussion

Given our small sample, postextubation respiratory failure with HFNC was not significantly different than with conventional oxygen. Nevertheless, after adjustment for confounding variables in four multivariable regression models, HFNC might be independently associated with lower postextubation failure.

Extubation failure remains one of the most pressing issues in MV. Despite advances in protective ventilation, sedation practices, and early mobilization, 10–20% of patients experience extubation failure [3]. Moreover, extubation failure is clearly associated with increased morbidity and mortality. Mortality rate may indeed reach 50% in patients that require reintubation [24]. The incidence of postextubation respiratory failure is clearly dependent on ICU case-mix, being lower in patients intubated for scheduled surgery and higher in medical and debilitated patients. Therefore, it is essential to classify patients according to risk when testing any preventive treatment. There is no general consensus about the risk factors that predict extubation failure [1, 2, 23], and different investigators have defined their own criteria.

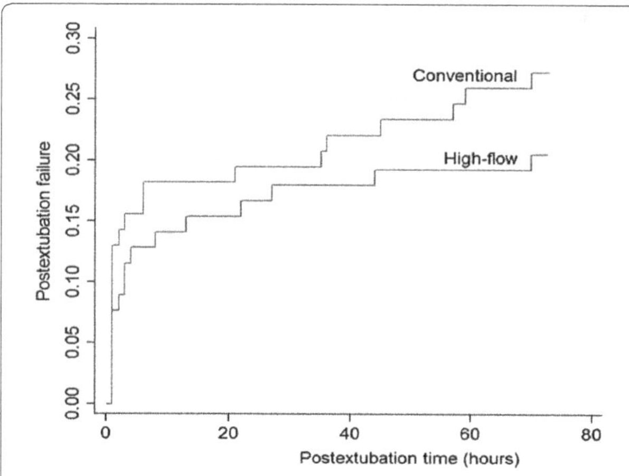

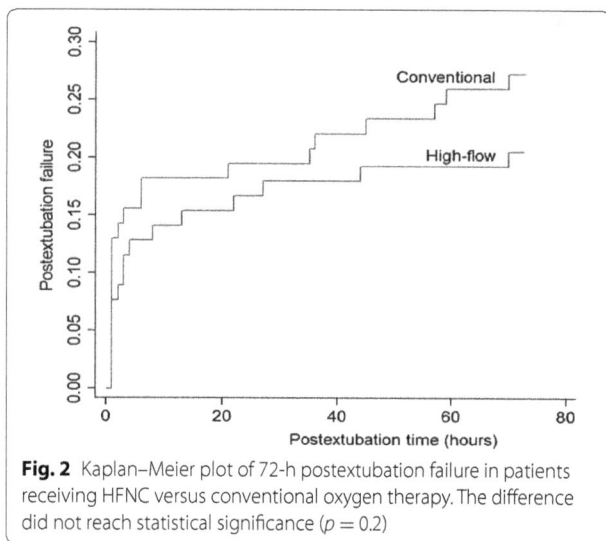

Fig. 2 Kaplan–Meier plot of 72-h postextubation failure in patients receiving HFNC versus conventional oxygen therapy. The difference did not reach statistical significance ($p = 0.2$)

Recently, Thille et al. [24] demonstrated that caregivers' experience is of limited value in predicting extubation failure; only one-third of the patients who required reintubation were considered at high risk for extubation failure in a very experienced ICU. In our study, we used nine criteria to select patients with higher likelihood of failure. Our 27% postextubation respiratory failure rate in the conventional group is very close to our anticipated rate and suggests that less sick patients were excluded.

Although supportive treatments may help prevent respiratory failure, they may also delay intubation in patients who develop respiratory failure. Esteban et al. [26] found increased mortality rate in patients receiving NIV to treat postextubation respiratory failure and attributed this finding mainly to a delay in reintubation. In a different scenario, Kang et al. [27] reported that patients intubated after 120 h of HFNC had a higher mortality than those intubated before 48 h, thereby suggesting that prolonging HFNC unduly is clearly detrimental to the patients [28]. However, these studies focused on supportive treatment used to treat respiratory failure rather than to prevent it. Although supportive treatment might mask signs and symptoms of respiratory failure that might delay intubation, our data showed no delays in reintubation in high-flow patients.

Our study might also shed light on the role of NIV as rescue treatment for postextubation respiratory failure. The literature supports NIV in hypercapnic patients [22], and this was the rationale for excluding them in our trial. By contrast, studies on the use of NIV as rescue treatment for patients without hypercapnia have found discrepant results; thus, we discouraged its use, but allowed it at the discretion of the attending team. Nevertheless, nearly half the patients who developed postextubation respiratory failure received NIV. There was a trend toward a lower reintubation rate in patients rescued with NIV, but there was also a trend toward higher mortality. One can speculate that physicians commonly offered NIV to the sickest patients, precluding any conclusion about the beneficial or harmful effect of NIV in this setting.

Limitations of the study

The small sample size is the major limitation of our study. Enrollment was much lower than expected for various reasons. First, after their initial commitment to participate, some centers decided to opt out due to workforce reductions. Second, number of devices were insufficient at some centers. Third, budget constraints at some centers resulted in a shortage of circuits and disposables. Nevertheless, there is growing evidence that robust statistical analyses with covariate adjustment in multiple regression models can help reduce sample size requirements [29]. All our exploratory regression models are prone to "overfitting" due to sample size, but they may offer some insights about the likelihood of a real effect of high flow. Additionally, very recently Hernandez et al. [17] demonstrated similar results in low-risk patients in a study with an adequate sample size.

The optimal length of HFNC treatment after extubation is not yet known. We decided upon a 24-h interval for practical reasons. Others have used HFNC for 48-h [9]. Further studies are required to determine the adequate length of HFNC duration after extubation. Availability of the device in the ICUs may be a limiting factor for a prolonged used of HFNC in this indication.

Our use of conventional oxygen in the control arm also deserves comment. Some studies suggest that high-risk patients have better outcome after extubation if routinely treated with NIV [10, 30], but others suggest otherwise [26, 31]. This issue remains controversial, and NIV has a definite indication only in hypercapnic patients [22, 32]. Thus, we excluded hypercapnic patients from our study. Some ongoing trials comparing HFNC with NIV in postextubation failure may help define the best comparison arm.

Our lack of sequential recordings of arterial blood gases and respiratory variables precludes any speculation about the physiological features involved in the improvement in respiratory failure, but published studies show HFNC improves oxygenation and thoracoabdominal synchrony and decreases respiratory rate and dyspnea [8–11, 33, 34].

Conclusion

Although exploratory multivariable logistic regression analysis found a protective effect of HFNC against postextubation respiratory failure, our study is inconclusive as to a potential benefit of HFNC over conventional oxygen to prevent occurrence of respiratory failure in non-hypercapnic patients at high risk for extubation failure.

Abbreviations

COPD: chronic obstructive pulmonary disease; HFNC: high-flow nasal cannula; ICU: intensive care unit; MV: mechanical ventilation; NIV: noninvasive ventilation; PEEP: positive end-expiratory pressure; SBT: spontaneous breathing trial.

Authors' contributions

RF and GH conceived of the study, and participated in its design and coordination and helped to draft the manuscript. RF, CS, FF, GR analyzed and interpreted the results; JRM, CL, AL, LP participated in drafting the manuscript for important intellectual content. All authors read and approved the final manuscript.

Author details

[1] Critical Care Department, Hospital Sant Joan de Deu- Fundacio Althaia, CIBERES, Universitat Internacional de Catalunya, Dr Joan Soler 1, 08243 Manresa, Spain. [2] CIBERES, Hospital de Getafe, Madrid, Spain. [3] Hospital Son Llatzer, Majorca, Spain. [4] Hospital Valle Hebron, Barcelona, Spain. [5] Hospital del Mar, CIBERES, IMIM, Pompeu Fabra University, Barcelona, Spain. [6] Hospital Virgen de la Salud, Toledo, Spain.

Competing interests

RF has received fees for conferences by Fisher & Paykel Healthcare. JRM has received a postdoctoral Grant from Fisher & Paykel Healthcare.

References

1. McConville JF, Kress JP. Weaning patients from the ventilator. N Engl J Med. 2012;367:2233–9.
2. Saugel B, Rakette P, Hapfelmeier A, Schultheiss C, Phillip V, Thies P, Treiber M, Einwächter H, von Werder A, Pfab R, Eyer F, Schmid RM, Huber W. Prediction of extubation failure in medical intensive care unit patients. J Crit Care. 2012;27:571–7.
3. Esteban A, Frutos-Vivar F, Muriel A, Ferguson ND, Peñuelas O, Abraira V, Raymondos K, Rios F, Nin N, Apezteguía C, Violi DA, Thille AW, Brochard L, González M, Villagomez AJ, Hurtado J, Davies AR, Du B, Maggiore SM, Pelosi P, Soto L, Tomicic V, D'Empaire G, Matamis D, Abroug F, Moreno RP, Soares MA, Arabi Y, Sandi F, Jibaja M, Amin P, Koh Y, Kuiper MA, Bülow HH, Zeggwagh AA, Anzueto A. Evolution of mortality over time in patients receiving mechanical ventilation. Am J Respir Crit Care Med. 2013;188:220–30.
4. Thille AW, Harrois A, Schortgen F, Brun-Buisson C, Brochard L. Outcomes of extubation failure in medical intensive care unit patients. Crit Care Med. 2011;39:2612–8.
5. Thille AW, Richard JCh, Brochard L. The decision to extubate in the intensive care unit. Am J Respir Crit Care Med. 2013;187:1294–302.
6. Ricard JD. High flow nasal oxygen in acute respiratory failure. Minerva Anestesiol. 2012;78:836–41.
7. Papazian L, Corley A, Hess D, Fraser JF, Frat JP, Guitton C, Jaber S, Maggiore SM, Nava S, Rello J, Ricard JD, Stephan F, Trisolini R, Azoulay E. Use of high-flow nasal cannula oxygenation in ICU adults: a narrative review. Intensive Care Med. 2016;42:1336–49.
8. Roca O, Riera J, Torres F, Masclans JR. High-flow oxygen therapy in acute respiratory failure. Respir Care. 2010;55:408–13.
9. Maggiore SM, Idone FA, Vaschetto R, Festa R, Cataldo A, Antonicelli F, Montini L, De Gaetano A, Navalesi P, Antonelli M. Nasal high-flow versus venture mask oxygen therapy after extubation. Effects on oxygenation, comfort, and clinical outcome. Am J Respir Crit Care Med. 2014;190:282–8.
10. Rittayamai N, Tscheikuna J, Rujiwit P. High-flow nasal cannula versus conventional oxygen therapy after endotracheal extubation: a randomized crossover physiologic study. Respir Care. 2014;59:485–90.
11. Riera J, Perez P, Cortes J, Roca O, Masclans JR, Rello J. Effect of high flow nasal cannula and body position on end-expiratory lung volume: a cohort study using electrical impedance tomography. Respir Care. 2013;58:589–96.
12. Parke RL, McGuinness SP. Pressures delivered by nasal high flow therapy during all phases of the respiratory cycle. Respir Care. 2013;58:1621–4.
13. Lee JH, Rehder KJ, Williford L, Cheifetz IM, Turner DA. Use of high flow nasal cannula in critically ill infants, children and adults: a critical review of the literature. Intensive Care Med. 2013;39:247–57.
14. Vargas F, Saint-Leger M, Boyer A, Bui NH, Hilbert G. Physiologic effects of high-flow nasal cannula oxygen in critical care subjects. Respir Care. 2015;60:1369–76.
15. Girault C, Breton L, Richard JC, Tamion F, Vandelet P, Aboab J, Leroy J, Bonmarchand G, Vandelet P, Aboba J. Mechanical effects of airway humidification devices in difficult-to-wean patients. Crit Care Med. 2003;31:1306–11.
16. Chanques G, Constantin JM, Sauter M, Jung B, Sebbane M, Verzilli D, Lefrant JY, Jaber S. Discomfort associated with underhumidified high-flow oxygen therapy in critically ill patients. Intensive Care Med. 2009;35:996–1003.
17. Hernandez G, Vaquero C, González P, Subira C, Frutos-Vivar F, Rialp G, Laborda C, Colinas L, Cuena R, Fernandez R. Effect of postextubation high-flow nasal cannula vs conventional oxygen therapy on reintubation in low-risk patients. A randomized clinical trial. JAMA. 2016;315:1354–61.
18. Brotfain E, Zlotnik A, Schwartz A, Frenkel A, Koyfman L, Gruenbaum SE, Klein M. Comparison of the effectiveness of high flow nasal oxygen cannula vs. standard non-rebreather oxygen face mask in post-extubation intensive care unit patients. Isr Med Assoc J. 2014;16:718–22.
19. Stéphan F, Barrucand B, Petit P, Rézaiguia-Delclaux S, Médard A, Delannoy B, Cosserant B, Flicoteaux G, Imbert A, Pilorge C, Bérard L, BiPOP Study Group. High-flow nasal oxygen vs noninvasive positive airway pressure in hypoxemic patients after cardiothoracic surgery: a randomized clinical trial. JAMA. 2015;313:2331–9.
20. Corley A, Bull T, Spooner AJ, Barnett AG, Fraser JF. Direct extubation onto high-flow nasal cannulae post-cardiac surgery versus standard treatment in patients with a BMI ≥30: a randomised controlled trial. Intensive Care Med. 2015;41:887–94.
21. Nava S, Gregoretti C, Fanfulla F, Squadrone E, Grassi M, Carlucci A, Beltrame F, Navalesi P. Noninvasive ventilation to prevent respiratory failure after extubation in high-risk patients. Crit Care Med. 2005;33:2465–70.
22. Ferrer M, Sellares J, Valencia M, Carrillo A, Gonzalez G, Badia JR, Nicolas JM, Torres A. Non-invasive ventilation after extubation in hypercapnic patients with chronic respiratory disorders: randomised controlled trial. Lancet. 2009;374:1082–8.
23. Brown CV, Daigle JB, Foulkrod KH, Brouillette B, Clark A, Czysz C, Martinez M, Cooper H. Risk factors associated with early reintubation in trauma patients: a prospective observational study. J Trauma. 2011;71:37–41.
24. Thille AW, Boissier F, Ghezala HB, Razazi K, Mekontso-Dessap A, Brun-Buisson C. Risk factors for and prediction by caregivers of extubation failure in ICU patients: a prospective study. Crit Care Med. 2015;43:613–20.
25. Hernandez G, Vaquero C, Garcia S, Villasclaras A, Pardo C, de la Fuente E, Cuena R, Gonzalez P, Fernandez R. High flow conditioned oxygen therapy for prevention of reintubation in critically ill patients: a preliminary cohort study. Int J Crit Care Emerg Med. 2015;1(2):1–6.
26. Esteban A, Frutos-Vivar F, Ferguson ND, Arabi Y, Apezteguía C, González M, Epstein SK, Hill NS, Nava S, Soares MA, D'Empaire G, Alía I, Anzueto A. Noninvasive positive-pressure ventilation for respiratory failure after extubation. N Engl J Med. 2004;350:2452–60.
27. Kang BJ, Koh Y, Lim CM, Huh JW, Baek S, Han M, Seo HS, Suh HJ, Seo GJ, Kim EY, Hong SB, Han M. Failure of high-flow nasal cannula therapy may delay intubation and increase mortality. Intensive Care Med. 2015;41:623–32.
28. Ricard JD, Messika J, Sztrymf B, Gaudry S. Impact on outcome of delayed intubation with high-flow nasal cannula oxygen: is the device solely responsible? Intensive Care Med. 2015;41:1157–8.
29. Turner EL, Perel P, Clayton T, Edwards P, Hernández AV, Roberts I, Shakur H, Steyerberg EW, CRASH trial collaborators. Covariate adjustment increased power in randomized controlled trials: an example in traumatic brain injury. J Clin Epidemiol. 2012;65:474–81.

30. Glossop AJ, Shepherd N, Bryden DC, Mills GH. Non-invasive ventilation for weaning, avoiding reintubation after extubation and in the postoperative period: a meta-analysis. Br J Anaesthesia. 2012;109:305–14.
31. Burns KE, Meade MO, Premji A, Adhikari NK. Noninvasive ventilation as a weaning strategy for mechanical ventilation in adults with respiratory failure: a Cochrane systematic review. CMAJ. 2014;186:E112–22.
32. Hilbert G, Gruson D, Portel L, Gbikpi-Benissan G, Cardinaud JP. Noninvasive pressure support ventilation in COPD patients with postextubation hypercapnic respiratory insufficiency. Eur Respir J. 1998;11:1349–53.
33. Itagaki T, Okuda N, Tsunano Y, Kohata H, Nakataki E, Onodera M, Imanaka H, Nishimura M. Effect of high-flow nasal cannula on thoraco-abdominal synchrony in adult critically ill patients. Respir Care. 2014;59:70–4.
34. Sztrymf B, Messika J, Bertrand F, Hurel D, Leon R, Dreyfuss D, Ricard JD. Beneficial effects of humidified high flow nasal oxygen in critical care patients: a prospective pilot study. Intensive Care Med. 2011;37:1780–6.

8

Nasal high flow in management of children with status asthmaticus

Florent Baudin[1,2*], Alexandra Buisson[1], Blandine Vanel[1], Bruno Massenavette[1], Robin Pouyau[1] and Etienne Javouhey[1,2]

Abstract

Background: Asthma is the most common obstructive airway disease in children and adults. Nasal high flow (NHF) is a recent device that is now used as a primary support for respiratory distress. Several studies have reported use of NHF as a respiratory support in status asthmaticus; however, there are no data to recommend such practice. We therefore conducted this preliminary study to evaluate NHF therapy for children with status asthmaticus admitted to our PICU in order to prepare a multicentre randomized controlled study.

Results: Between November 2009 and January 2014, 73 patients with status asthmaticus were admitted to the PICU, of whom 39 (53%) were treated with NHF and among these 10 (26%) presented severe acidosis at admission (pH < 7.30). Thirty-four less severe children (41%) were treated with standard oxygen. For one child (2.6%) NHF failed and was then switched to non-invasive ventilation. NHF was discontinued in another patient because of the occurrence of pneumothorax after 31 h with NHF; the patient was then switched to standard oxygen therapy. Mean ± SD heart rate (165 ± 21 vs. 141 ± 25/min, $p < 0.01$) and respiratory rate (40 ± 13 vs. 31 ± 8/min, $p < 0.01$) decreased significantly, and blood gas improved in the first 24 h. In the subgroup of patients with acidosis, median [IQR] pH increased significantly between hour 0 and 2 (7.25 [7.21–7.26] vs. 7.30 [7.27–7.33], $p = 0.009$) and median [IQR] pCO_2 decreased significantly (7.27 kPa [6.84–7.91 vs. 5.85 kPa [5.56–6.11], $p = 0.007$). No patient was intubated.

Conclusion: This retrospective study showed the feasibility and safety of NHF in children with severe asthma. Blood gas and clinical parameters were significantly improved during the first 24 h. NHF failed in only two patients, and none required invasive ventilation.

Keywords: Asthma, Children, High-flow nasal cannula, Non-invasive ventilation, Paediatric intensive care unit

Background

Asthma is the most common obstructive airway disease in children and adults. Approximately 334 million people around the world and 2.5 million people in France suffer from asthma [1], a third of whom are children [1, 2], and the prevalence of asthma in this subpopulation has increased in recent decades [2]. Supplemental oxygen is commonly administered to children with an asthma exacerbation in the emergency department or intensive care unit in association with beta 2 agonist nebulization [3–5]. Non-invasive ventilation (NIV) may be used as respiratory support in children with status asthmaticus in case of standard treatment failure [6–9]. However, the level of evidence of its efficacy remains low according to the grade system of evidence quality [10].

Nasal high flow (NHF) is a recent device, now used as a primary support for respiratory distress in paediatric and adult intensive care units and in emergency departments [11–16]. It is increasingly used because it is well tolerated [11, 12, 17, 18] especially in infants with bronchiolitis [11, 17, 18]. NHF delivers humidified and heated gas at a rate greater than inspiratory flow [14, 19]. It reduces

*Correspondence: florent.baudin@chu-lyon.fr
[1] Réanimation pédiatrique, Hôpital Femme Mère Enfant, Hospices Civils de Lyon, 69500 Bron, France
Full list of author information is available at the end of the article

anatomical dead space by flushing the nasopharyngeal cavity and may improve CO_2 clearance. It also provides a certain level of positive end-expiratory pressure (PEEP), between 2 and 7 cm H_2O, depending on the flow rate used [14, 19–22] that may reduce resistance. In children with status asthmaticus, external PEEP may decrease work of breathing [23] based on the "waterfalls" principle published by Tobin and Lodato [24]. HFNC may also reduce the metabolic cost of breathing by supplying adequately warmed and humidified gas. Similarly, in infants with severe bronchiolitis, Milesi et al. demonstrated that HFNC significantly reduced work of breathing, respiratory rate, and Ti/Ttot ratio [25]. By increasing the expiratory time, HFNC may decrease dynamic hyperinflation in patients with obstructive lung disease and break the vicious circle.

There are, however, very few data reported NHF as a primary respiratory support for status asthmaticus, even though some studies have reported its use in the emergency department or intensive care unit in children [11, 12, 15, 16, 26, 27] as in adult patients [28, 29]. Over the previous five years NHF has been commonly used for children admitted to our PICU for acute respiratory failure (ARF) including patients with lower airway obstruction (bronchiolitis or asthma). We therefore conducted this preliminary study to evaluate NHF therapy for children admitted to our PICU with status asthmaticus in order to prepare a multicentre randomized controlled study.

Methods

Study design

We conducted a retrospective observational study in a 23-bed PICU of a tertiary university hospital (Hôpital Femme Mère Enfant, Lyon University Hospital, France). Children aged between 1 and 18 years, without severe comorbidities, admitted between November 2009 and January 2014 to the PICU, and with a diagnosis of status asthmaticus were included. The study was approved by our institutional review board and a waiver of consent given (CPP Sud-Est II N°00009118—2016-08).

Population

Patients were identified in the French hospital information system (PMSI) and the PICU database by using the primary diagnosis of status asthmaticus (International Classification of Diseases—ICD 10 code J46) or ARF associated with asthma (ICD 10 J96.0/J45). Based on the local protocol and French recommendations [5], children were admitted to the PICU after at least 1 h in the emergency department during which they did not response to standard therapy, based on at least three successive beta agonist nebulizations, supplemental oxygen, and oral or intravenous corticosteroids at 2 mg/kg.

In PICU, respiratory support (oxygen, HFNC, NIV, or invasive ventilation—IV) and additional therapy (intravenous salbutamol, magnesium sulphate) were left to the physician's judgment. Patients with severe comorbidities were excluded: cardiopulmonary disease, neuromuscular or metabolic disease, restrictive or chronic respiratory disease (pulmonary fibrosis, cystic fibrosis, bronchodysplasia), ENT disease (laryngo- or tracheo- or broncho-malacia) or children with tracheotomy. For NHF, Optiflow RT330 (Fisher & Paykel Healthcare, Auckland, New Zealand) circuit and nasal prong adapted to the age and the size of the nose were used. The nebulizer system (Aerogen, Inc., Mountain View, CA, USA) was inserted upstream from the electrically heated humidifier [30–32].

Data and outcome

Data were retrospectively collected using the electronic medical record IntelliSpace Critical Care and Anesthesia (Philips Healthcare, Suresnes, France). A patient was attributed to only one group (NHF or standard oxygen), and in case of multiple stays during the period, only the first one was analysed. The primary outcome was defined as failure of the NHF therapy and described as a proportion of all children with asthma having received NHF therapy. The secondary outcome was the change of clinical parameters (respiratory rate, heart rate, SpO_2/FiO_2 ratio) from NHF initiation to 6, 12, 24, and 48 h later, as well as blood gas parameters in children treated with NHF.

Baseline characteristics of the population (age, weight, comorbidity, history of asthma) were collected at admission and compared to those of the standard oxygen group. Data on the medication used before and during PICU stay, and the duration of NHF use and of supplemental oxygen therapy, and length of PICU stay were also collected. Safety of HFNC treatment was assessed by the number of patients with air-leak complications and by the tolerance of the system according to nurse reports. A subgroup analysis of children with severe acidosis treated with NHF was also performed.

Statistical analysis

Qualitative variables are reported as numbers and percentages, and quantitative variables are reported as mean ± standard deviation (SD) or confidence intervals, or as median with interquartile range [IQR], when appropriate. Chi-square test or Fisher's exact test for qualitative variables and Mann–Whitney *U* test for nonparametric independent sample were used to compare the data between NHF and standard oxygen groups, when appropriate. Repeated-measures analysis of variance (ANOVA) was used to compare clinical variables over time. The assumption of sphericity was tested using Mauchly's test of sphericity; if sphericity was violated epsilon (ε) was calculated according to Greenhouse and Geisser and used to correct the one-way repeated-measures ANOVA [33]. Post hoc analysis was performed with a Bonferroni adjustment. Wilcoxon signed-rank test was used for non-parametric paired samples. Differences were considered statistically significant at $p < 0.05$. Statistical analysis was performed using SPSS Statistics (V22, IBM, Armonk, NY, US).

Results

Between November 2009 and January 2014, 91 children with diagnosis of status asthmaticus were admitted in our PICU. Sixteen children were excluded because of the presence of severe comorbidities and one because the primary diagnosis was hypoxemic pneumonia. Among the 73 children admitted for status asthmaticus, 39 (53%) were treated with NHF and 30 (41%) received only standard supplemental oxygen therapy (16 with non-rebreathing mask and 14 with standard nasal cannula, Fig. 1). The proportion of children treated by standard oxygen and NHF in each year of the study period was similar ($p = 0.66$) (Fig. 2). A further two children were intubated before admission to PICU (for transport): one was treated with NIV, and one was admitted in the PICU more than 24 h after starting NHF in an intermediate care unit outside of the university hospital (Fig. 1). The median [IQR] age of children treated with NHF was 3.6 years [1.6–5.6], which was similar to that of children treated with standard oxygen (3.6 [2.2–6.7]; $p = 0.72$). All

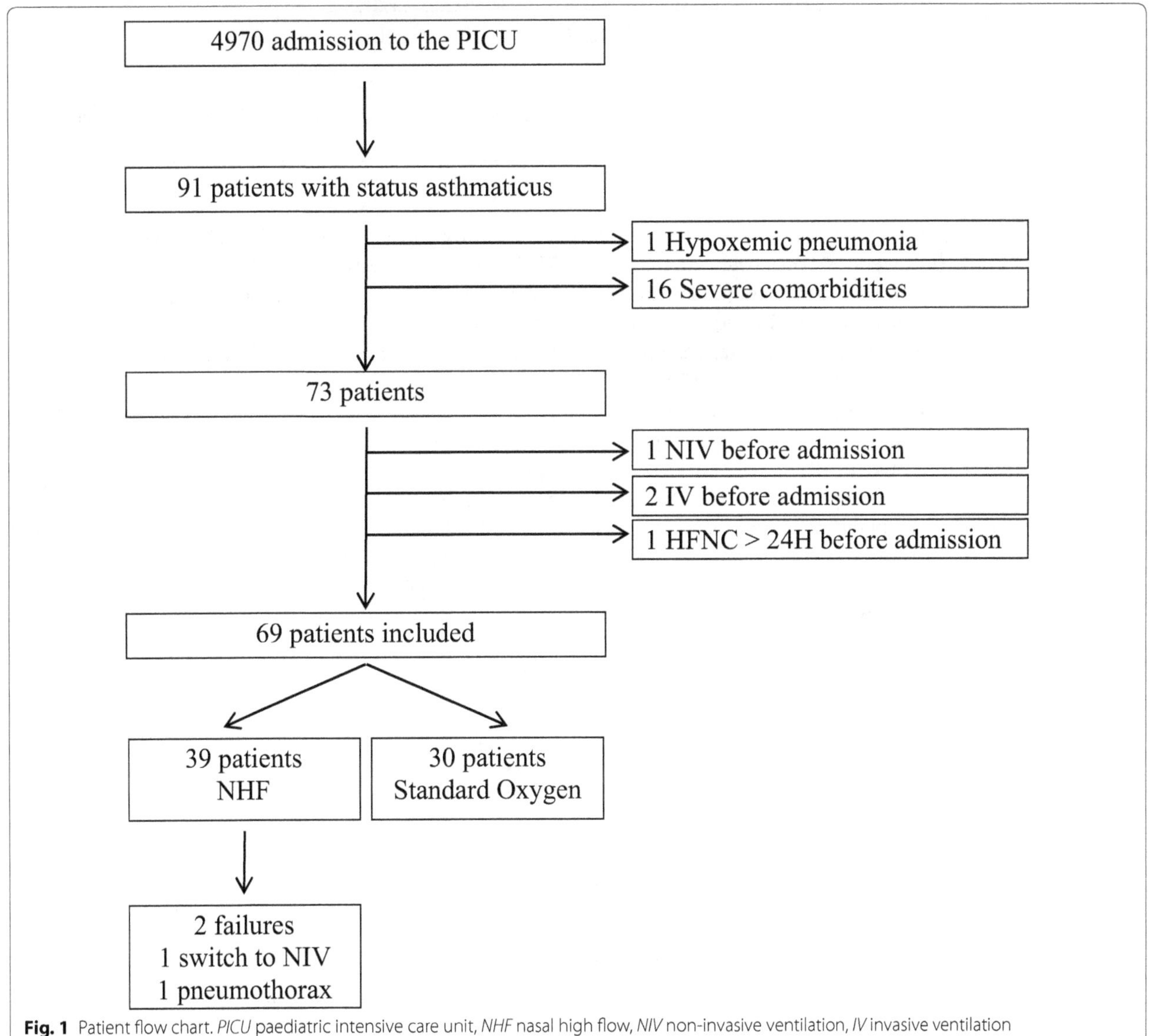

Fig. 1 Patient flow chart. *PICU* paediatric intensive care unit, *NHF* nasal high flow, *NIV* non-invasive ventilation, *IV* invasive ventilation

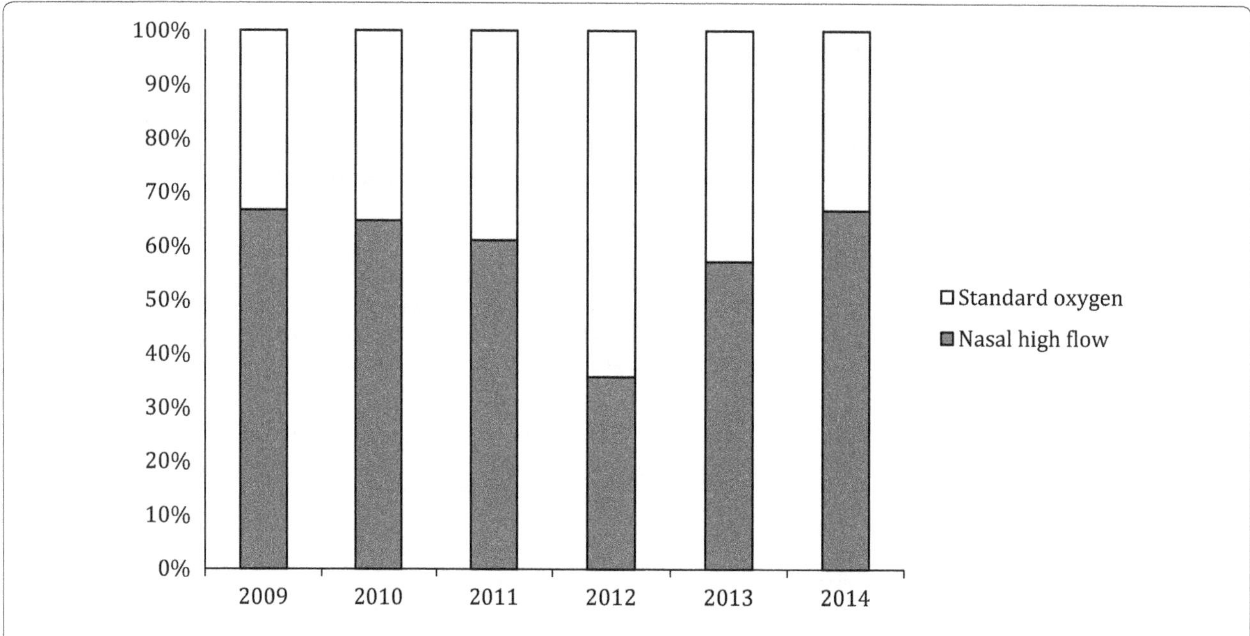

Fig. 2 Proportion of children treated by nasal high flow and standard oxygen from 2009 to 2014 ($p = 0.66$ with Fisher's exact test). *NHF* nasal high flow

children in the two groups received nebulized salbutamol and corticosteroids (intravenous corticosteroid for 79% in NHF and 63% in standard oxygen group). Continuous intravenous salbutamol was used in 13 children (33%) in the NHF group and in 5 (17%); $p = 0.12$. Magnesium sulphate was more often used in the NHF group (59%) than in standard oxygen group (27%, $p = 0.007$; Table 1).

The median [IQR] flow of NHF was initially set at 0.9 L/kg/min [0.75–1] with a median [IQR] FiO_2 of 45% [31–55] (Table 2). NHF failed in only two children. One child required NIV because of worsening blood gas parameters in the first 24 h. NHF was discontinued in another patient because of the occurrence of pneumothorax. The pneumothorax occurred after 31 h with NHF (X-ray at admission without pneumothorax) and requiring chest tube for 24 h. The maximum NHF was 1 L/kg/min. NHF was discontinued and standard oxygen therapy was administered at 0.5 L/min for 22 h. No patient was intubated. The median [IQR] length of NHF treatment was 28 h [21–47], and the median PICU length of stay was 3 days [2.5–5].

Change of heart rate (HR) and respiratory rate (RR) during the first 24 h are presented in Fig. 3. The assumption of sphericity was violated for HR ($p = 0.016$), and a Greenhouse–Geisser correction was applied ($\varepsilon = 0.82$). HR decreased significantly over time $F(2.47, 91.41) = 22.77$, $p < 0.001$, partial $\eta 2 = 0.38$, as did RR $F(3, 111) = 8.65$, $p = 0.001$, partial $\eta 2 = 0.19$. Pairwise post hoc analysis found that mean ± SD HR and RR were significantly lower at hour 24 (141 ± 25 per min and 31 ± 8 per min, respectively) than at hour 0 (165 ± 21 per min, $p < 0.01$ and 40 ± 13 per min, $p < 0.01$). HR was also lower at hour 24 (141 ± 25 per min) than at hour 12 (155 ± 22 per min, $p < 0.01$) and at hour 6 (161 ± 22 per min, $p < 0.01$). For SpO_2/FiO_2 ratio the assumption of sphericity was also violated ($p < 0.01$) and a correction was applied ($\varepsilon = 0.33$). SpO_2/FiO_2 ratio changed significantly over time $F(2.1, 67.0) = 19.7$, $p < 0.001$, partial $\eta 2 = 0.38$. SpO_2/FiO_2 ratio was higher at hour 24 (359 ± 116) than at hour 12 (298 ± 104, $p < 0.01$), at hour 6 (277 ± 116, $p < 0.01$), and at hour 0 (225 ± 81, $p < 0.01$); it was also higher at hour 12 (298 ± 104) than at hour 0 (225 ± 81, $p < 0.01$; Fig. 3). Blood gas (pH and PCO_2) improved in the first 24 h for children treated with NHF (Table 3). Blood gas parameters were available at day 1 for only half of patients treated with standard oxygen ($n = 15$); the median [IQR] pH was 7.41 [7.38–7.42]; and pCO2 was 4.6 kPa [4.2–4.7].

Ten patients treated with NHF (6 boys and 4 girls), who had a median [IQR] age of 3.7 years [2.1–4.4], had at severe acidosis at admission (pH < 7.30). In this subgroup, median [IQR] pH increased significantly between hour 0 (7.25 [7.21–7.26]) and hour 2 (7.30 [7.27–7.33], $p = 0.009$), and pCO_2 decreased significantly (hour 0: 7.27 kPa [6.84–7.91], hour 2: 5.85 [5.56–6.11], $p = 0.007$; Fig. 4). In the patient who failed in the first 24 h (discontinuous line in Fig. 4), blood gases worsened from hour 0

Table 1 Baseline characteristics of children treated with nasal high flow and with standard oxygen therapy for status asthmaticus

	NHF $n = 39$	Standard oxygen $n = 30$	p*
Age (years), median [IQR]	3.6 [1.6–5.6]	3.6 [2.2–6.7]	0.72
Male/female ratio	20/19	21/9	0.11
Weight (kg), median [IQR]	15 [11–24]	15 [13–23]	0.64
PIM2 at admission, median [IQR]	1.5 [1.15–3.3]	1 [0.3–1.37]	<0.001
History of asthma or >2 bronchiolitis, *n* (%)	31 (80)	23 (77)	0.79
Previous admission for asthma, *n* (%)	19 (48)	11 (37)	0.31
In PICU, *n* (%)	4 (10)	2 (6)	0.66
Long-term control medicine, *n* (%)	17 (44)	14 (47)	0.80
Clinical parameters at admission, median [IQR]			
Respiratory rate (/min)	35 [31–47]	35 [30–43]	0.47
Heart rate (/min)	164 [154–185]	168 [153–180]	0.89
SpO_2 (%)	97 [95–98]	98 [97–100]	0.04
SpO_2/FiO_2	216 [175–303]	NA	
Venous blood gas at admission, median [IQR]			
pH	7.35 [7.28–7.39]	7.36 [7.34–7.39]	0.27
pCO_2 (kPa)	5.6 [4.7–7.7]	4.9 [4.4–5.6]	0.02
Bicarbonates (mmol/L)	22 [20–24]	20 [20–23]	0.35
Acidosis (pH < 7.30), *n* (%)	10 (26%)	2 (7%)	0.04
Associated medication, *n* (%)			
Salbutamol—nebulized	39 (100%)	30 (100%)	1.0
Corticosteroids—intravenous[a]	31 (79%)	19 (63%)	0.14
Salbutamol—intravenous	13 (33%)	5 (17%)	0.12
Magnesium sulphate	23 (59%)	8 (27%)	0.007
PICU LOS (days), median [IQR]	3 [2.5–5]	1.5 [1, 2]	<0.001

LOS length of stay, *PIM* Paediatric Index of Mortality, *PICU* paediatric intensive care unit, *NHF* nasal high flow

* Statistical analysis with Chi-square test for qualitative variables or Mann–Whitney *U* test for nonparametric independent sample

[a] All other children received oral corticosteroids

Table 2 Nasal high flow (NHF) parameters of 39 children treated for status asthmaticus

	$n = 39$
NHF settings, median [IQR]	
Initial FiO_2 (%)	45 [31–55]
Initial flow (L/kg/min)	0.9 [0.75–1]
Maximum flow (L/kg/min)	1.0 [0.8–1.1]
Length of NHF (h), median [IQR]	28 [21–47]
NHF failure, *n* (%)	2 (6)

PICU paediatric intensive care unit, *NHF* nasal high flow

to hour 2; the child was switched to non-invasive ventilation with success (Fig. 1).

Discussion

The present study is the largest report to have evaluated the use of NHF as a primary respiratory support for severe status asthmaticus. It showed the feasibility and the safety of management of children with status asthmaticus with NHF; NHF failed in only one patient, and blood gas and clinical parameters were significantly improved during the first 24 h.

During the study period, 39 children were treated with NHF and 30 with standard oxygen. The demographic data were similar in terms of age, weight, and medical history. However, NHF was used according to the physician's judgment (as was the use of additional therapy) and those who received standard oxygen seemed to be less severe at admission (lower PIM2 score, lower pCO_2 values, and less frequently had acidosis) although clinical parameters (heart and respiratory rate) were similar. Another marker of severity is the administration of magnesium sulphate that, in our PICU, is recommended as a second-line therapy before the use of intravenous salbutamol and this was used twice less frequently in the standard oxygen group. Furthermore, the length of PICU stay was also longer in the NHF group, but is of note that both NHF had to be discontinued and nebulization to be scheduled less than

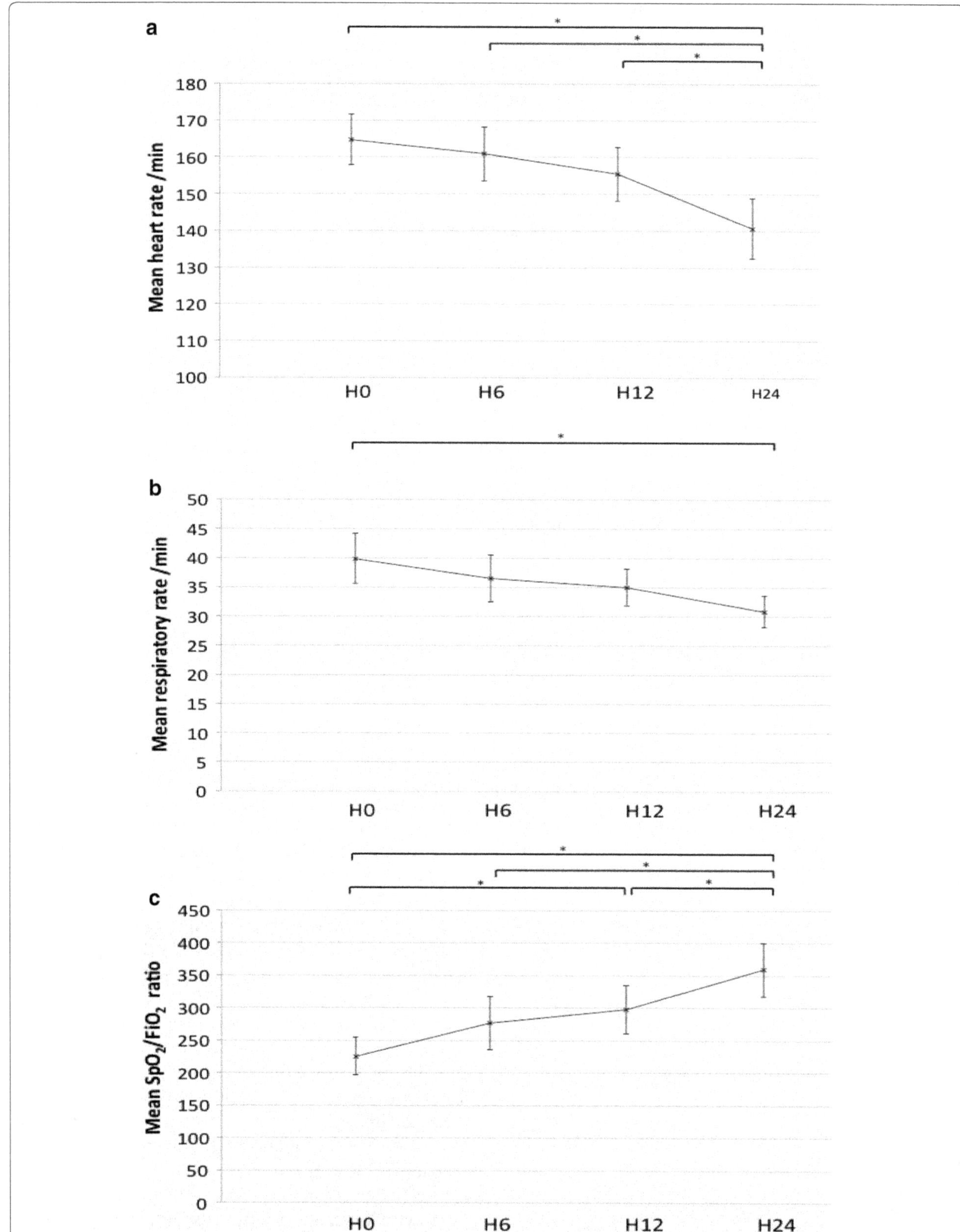

Fig. 3 Change of heart rate (**a**), respiratory rate (**b**), and SpO_2/FiO_2 ratio (**c**) during the first 24 h in 38 children with status asthmaticus treated by nasal high flow. Heart rate, respiratory rate, and SpO_2/FiO_2 ratio significantly change over time according to the repeated-measures analysis of variance (ANOVA). *Significant difference with pairwise post hoc analysis ($p < 0.01$). *Bars* indicate 95% confidence intervals. *H* hours

Table 3 Change of blood gas parameters between hour 0 and 24 in children treated with nasal high flow for status asthmaticus

	Hour 0 $n = 39$	Hour 24 $n = 37^a$	p
Venous blood gas, median [IQR]			
pH	7.35 [7.28–7.39]	7.42 [7.39–7.44]	$p < 0.001$
pCO_2 (kPa)	5.6 [4.7–7.7]	4.3 [4.0–4.8]	$p < 0.001$
Bicarbonates (mmol/L)	22 [20–24]	21 [19–22]	$p = 0.16$

[a] Nasal high flow failed for one patient during the first 24 h, and one patient had no blood gas at day 1

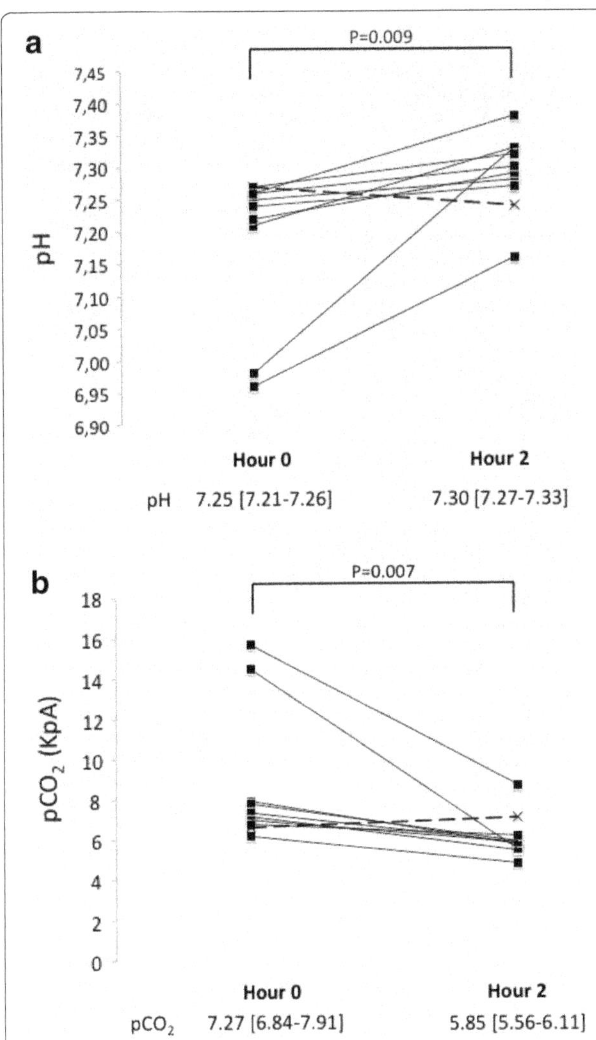

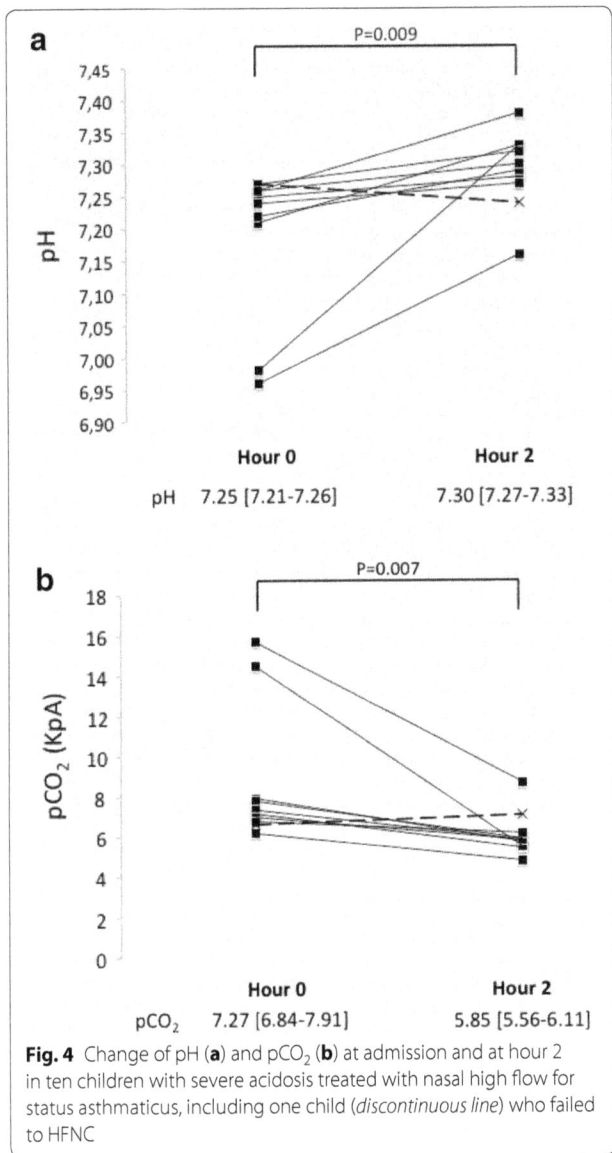

Fig. 4 Change of pH (**a**) and pCO_2 (**b**) at admission and at hour 2 in ten children with severe acidosis treated with nasal high flow for status asthmaticus, including one child (*discontinuous line*) who failed to HFNC

every 3 h for patients to be discharged. These differences preclude any strong conclusions as to the superiority of one technique over the other, which is coherent with the nature of this preliminary retrospective study. It is of note that no patient was intubated (in either group) and only one required NIV. Furthermore, clinical parameters (heart rate and respiratory rate) improved over time with NHF as did blood gas values, even in children with severe acidosis. These results are strengthened by the efforts made to reduce bias related to patient identification and missing data that affect many other retrospective studies. This was limited herein by the use of status asthmaticus and ARF associated with asthma diagnosis codes, and electronic medical records with automatic importation of clinical and biological parameters every 5 min. However, improvement of the physiological parameters may also be due to the normal change over time and more robust conclusions will be made from the results of the multicentre randomized controlled trial that will be implemented later this year.

The place of NHF in the management of ARF is controversial. Several physiological studies have supported that NIV relieves better work of breathing than continuous positive airway pressure [34, 35] and therefore that it is better than NHF [18]. However, the most recent studies in adults suggest either superiority of NHF over conventional oxygen [36], or equivalence [37] and even superiority over NIV [38]. Pulmonary function may be affected by emotion and stress [39, 40], and tolerance to NHF is better than NIV, both in adults [41, 42] and in children [18, 43], and may explain in part the benefit of NHF. It was not possible to assess comfort of children retrospectively. After analysis of nurse report forms, no notable discomfort was reported, and in particular no skin lesions. Clinical improvement observed with NHF in the present study was similar to that previously reported with NIV in children [7], and no patient was intubated. However, although the use of NIV for status asthmaticus in children [6, 7, 9, 44, 45] is common, the level of evidence remains limited [10]. Furthermore, in adults, the Cochrane review published in 2012 found that NIV did not provide additional benefit to medical treatment [46]. At this time, the use of NHF in the most severe asthmatic patients may not be recommended as current guidelines indicate that intubation should never be delayed [47], even though the benefit of NHF in this subgroup was particularly demonstrative and rapid herein. On the other hand, using NHF to treat all children with mild asthma would lead to increase costs but not the benefits. Therefore, it would be of great interest to define the population who would most benefit from NHF, for which the preschool respiratory assessment measure (PRAM) [48] could be of interest. In our PICU, NHF is currently used as the primary respiratory support for children with moderate-to-severe asthma, defined by an acidosis (pH < 7.35) or a PRAM score >7 after optimal care in the emergency department. For severe patients, a senior physician systematically evaluates children at 1 h and blood gases are measured after 2 h of use to ensure an early detection of patients who do not improve.

NHF allows the delivery of nebulized drugs (i.e. beta agonists) continuously and without changing the interface [30–32, 49, 50] as during NIV. Recent studies suggest greater efficacy of vibrating mesh nebulizers over jet nebulizers [30, 31]. The former was used in association with NHF, and a jet nebulizer was used for children treated with standard oxygen, which further complicates interpretation of the results. More generally, delivery of beta agonist with NHF is heterogeneous and depends on several aspects. According to the manufacturer recommendations and recent studies [30–32], the nebulization system was placed upstream from the active heated humidifier that seems to provide better effectiveness. The gas flow rate is probably the main parameter to take into account the delivery of nebulization drugs. A recent study showed that in infants and toddlers, increasing the flow rate by fourfold decreases tenfold the proportion of lung deposition [32]. For asthma patients, it is necessary to weigh the benefit/risk ratio of a higher flow with higher respiratory support but probably with a decrease of drug delivery. In the present study, the median flow rate was 0.9 L/kg/min [0.75–1] that remains relatively low for paediatric patient [14]. A lower flow rate may participate to a better nebulization drug delivery and a better tolerance in children, older than patient with bronchiolitis.

In conclusion, this study shows that NHF is feasible in children with status asthmaticus, may improve physiological parameters, and prevent the use of subsequent therapeutic steps. Based on these results, a multicentre randomized controlled study will start later this year to evaluate whether early management with NHF may prevent failure in comparison with conventional oxygen (and therefore escalation to NIV or IV) in patients with moderate-to-severe asthma defined as an acidosis (pH < 7.35) or a PRAM score >7 after optimal care in the emergency department.

Abbreviations

ANOVA: analysis of variance; ARF: acute respiratory failure; NHF: nasal high flow; HR: heart rate; ICD: International Classification of Diseases; IQR: interquartile range; IV: invasive ventilation; NIV: non-invasive ventilation; PEEP: positive end-expiratory pressure; PICU: paediatric intensive care unit; RR: respiratory rate; SD: standard deviation.

Authors' contributions

EJ, AB, RP, BM, and EJ participated in the design of the study. FB, AB, and BV collected and analysed the data. FB and EJ drafted the manuscript. BV, RP, and BM reviewed and improved the manuscript. All authors read and approved the final manuscript.

Author details

[1] Réanimation pédiatrique, Hôpital Femme Mère Enfant, Hospices Civils de Lyon, 69500 Bron, France. [2] UMRT_9405, UMRESTTE, Ifsttar, Université Claude Bernard Lyon1, Univ Lyon, 69373 Lyon, France.

Acknowledgements

We thank Philip Robinson for critical revision and correction of the manuscript.

Competing interests

Dr. Baudin has received speaking fees from Maquet Critical Care. The others authors have no competing interests.

References

1. Delmas MC, Fuhrman C, pour le groupe épidémiologie et recherche clinique de la SPLF. Asthma in France: a review of descriptive epidemiological data. Rev Mal Respir. 2010;27:151–9.
2. Asher I, Pearce N. Global burden of asthma among children. Int J Tuberc Lung Dis. 2014;18:1269–78.
3. Werner HA. Status asthmaticus in children: a review. Chest. 2001;119:1913–29.
4. Koninckx M, Buysse C, de Hoog M. Management of status asthmaticus in children. Paeditr Respir Rev. 2013;14:78–85.
5. Marguet C, Groupe de Recherche Sur Les Avancées En PneumoPédiatrie. Management of acute asthma in infants and children: recommendations from the French Pediatric Society of Pneumology and Allergy. Rev Mal Respir. 2007;24:427–39.
6. Basnet S, Mander G, Andoh J, Klaska H, Verhulst S, Koirala J. Safety, efficacy, and tolerability of early initiation of noninvasive positive pressure ventilation in pediatric patients admitted with status asthmaticus: a pilot study. Pediatr Crit Care Med. 2012;13:393–8.
7. Mayordomo-Colunga J, Medina A, Rey C, Concha A, Menéndez S, Arcos ML, et al. Non-invasive ventilation in pediatric status asthmaticus: a prospective observational study. Pediatr Pulmonol. 2011;46:949–55.
8. Thill PJ, McGuire JK, Baden HP, Green TP, Checchia PA. Noninvasive positive-pressure ventilation in children with lower airway obstruction. Pediatr Crit Care Med. 2004;5:337–42.
9. Needleman JP, Sykes JA, Schroeder SA, Singer LP. Noninvasive positive pressure ventilation in the treatment of pediatric status asthmaticus. Pediatr Asthma Allergy Immunol. 2004;17:272–7.
10. Silva PDS, Barreto SSM. Noninvasive ventilation in status asthmaticus in children: levels of evidence. Rev Bras Ter Intensiva. 2015;27:390–6.
11. Baudin F, Gagnon S, Crulli B, Proulx F, Jouvet PA, Emeriaud G. Modalities and complications associated with the use of high-flow nasal cannula: experience in a pediatric ICU. Respir Care. 2016;61:1305–10.
12. Ward JJ. High-flow oxygen administration by nasal cannula for adult and perinatal patients. Respir Care. 2013;58:98–122.
13. Lee JH, Rehder KJ, Williford L, Cheifetz IM, Turner DA. Use of high flow nasal cannula in critically ill infants, children, and adults: a critical review of the literature. Intensive Care Med. 2013;39:247–57.
14. Milési C, Boubal M, Jacquot A, Baleine J, Durand S, Odena MP, et al. High-flow nasal cannula: recommendations for daily practice in pediatrics. Ann Intensive Care. 2014;4:29.
15. Wraight TI, Ganu SS. High-flow nasal cannula use in a paediatric intensive care unit over 3 years. Crit Care Resusc. 2015;17:197–201.
16. Wing R, James C, Maranda LS, Armsby CC. Use of high-flow nasal cannula support in the emergency department reduces the need for intubation in pediatric acute respiratory insufficiency. Pediatr Emerg Care. 2012;28:1117–23.
17. McKiernan C, Chua LC, Visintainer PF, Allen H. High flow nasal cannulae therapy in infants with bronchiolitis. J Pediatr. 2010;156:634–8.
18. Milési C, Essouri S, Pouyau R, Liet J-M, Afanetti M, Portefaix A, et al. High flow nasal cannula (HFNC) versus nasal continuous positive airway pressure (nCPAP) for the initial respiratory management of acute viral bronchiolitis in young infants: a multicenter randomized controlled trial (TRAMONTANE study). Intensive Care Med. 2017;43:209–16.
19. Dysart K, Miller TL, Wolfson MR, Shaffer TH. Research in high flow therapy: mechanisms of action. Respir Med. 2009;103:1400–5.

20. Hasan RA, Habib RH. Effects of flow rate and airleak at the nares and mouth opening on positive distending pressure delivery using commercially available high-flow nasal cannula systems: a lung model study. Pediatr Crit Care Med. 2011;12:e29–33.
21. Volsko TA, Fedor K, Amadei J, Chatburn RL. High flow through a nasal cannula and CPAP effect in a simulated infant model. Respir Care. 2011;56:1893–900.
22. Kubicka ZJ, Limauro J, Darnall RA. Heated, humidified high-flow nasal cannula therapy: yet another way to deliver continuous positive airway pressure? Pediatrics. 2008;121:82–8.
23. Caramez MP, Borges JB, Tucci MR. Paradoxical responses to positive end-expiratory pressure in patients with airway obstruction during controlled ventilation. Crit Care Med. 2005;33:1519–28.
24. Tobin MJ, Lodato RF. PEEP, auto-PEEP, and waterfalls. Chest. 1989;96:449–51.
25. Milési C, Baleine J, Matecki S, Durand S, Combes C, Novais ARB, et al. Is treatment with a high flow nasal cannula effective in acute viral bronchiolitis? A physiologic study. Intensive Care Med. 2013;39:1088–94.
26. Mayfield S, Jauncey-Cooke J, Bogossian F. A case series of paediatric high flow nasal cannula therapy. Aust Crit Care. 2013;26:189–92.
27. Kelly GS, Simon HK, Sturm JJ. High-flow nasal cannula use in children with respiratory distress in the emergency department: predicting the need for subsequent intubation. Pediatr Emerg Care. 2013;29:888–92.
28. Sztrymf B, Messika J, Mayot T, Lenglet H, Dreyfuss D, Ricard J-D. Impact of high-flow nasal cannula oxygen therapy on intensive care unit patients with acute respiratory failure: a prospective observational study. J Crit Care. 2012;27(324):e9–13.
29. Lenglet H, Sztrymf B, Leroy C, Brun P, Dreyfuss D, Ricard J-D. Humidified high flow nasal oxygen during respiratory failure in the emergency department: feasibility and efficacy. Respir Care. 2012;57:1873–8.
30. Ari A, Atalay OT, Harwood R, Sheard MM, Aljamhan EA, Fink JB. Influence of nebulizer type, position, and bias flow on aerosol drug delivery in simulated pediatric and adult lung models during mechanical ventilation. Respir Care. 2010;55:845–51.
31. Réminiac F, Vecellio L, Heuzé-Vourc'h N, Petitcollin A, Respaud R, Cabrera M, et al. Aerosol therapy in adults receiving high flow nasal cannula oxygen therapy. J Aerosol Med Pulm Drug Deliv. 2016;29:134–41.
32. Réminiac F, Vecellio L, Loughlin RM, Le Pennec D, Cabrera M, Vourc'h NH, et al. Nasal high flow nebulization in infants and toddlers: an in vitro and in vivo scintigraphic study. Pediatr Pulmonol. 2016;52:337–44.
33. Greenhouse SW, Geisser S. On methods in the analysis of profile data. Psychometrika. 1959;24:95–112.
34. Vanpee D, el-Khawand C, Rousseau L, Jamart J, Delaunois L. Influence of respiratory behavior on ventilation, respiratory work and intrinsic PEEP during noninvasive nasal pressure support ventilation in normal subjects. Respiration. 2002;69:297–302.
35. L'her E, Deye N, Lellouche F, Taille S, Demoule A, Fraticelli A, et al. Physiologic effects of noninvasive ventilation during acute lung injury. Am J Respir Crit Care Med. 2005;172:1112–8.
36. Hernández G, Vaquero C, González P, Subira C, Frutos-Vivar F, Rialp G, et al. Effect of postextubation high-flow nasal cannula vs conventional oxygen therapy on reintubation in low-risk patients: a randomized clinical trial. JAMA. 2016;315:1354–61.
37. Stéphan F, Barrucand B, Petit P, Rézaiguia-Delclaux S, Médard A, Delannoy B, et al. High-flow nasal oxygen vs noninvasive positive airway pressure in hypoxemic patients after cardiothoracic surgery. JAMA. 2015;313:2331–9.
38. Frat J-P, Thille AW, Mercat A, Girault C, Ragot S, Perbet S, et al. High-flow oxygen through nasal cannula in acute hypoxemic respiratory failure. N Engl J Med. 2015;372:2185–96.
39. Miller BD, Wood BL. Influence of specific emotional states on autonomic reactivity and pulmonary function in asthmatic children. J Am Acad Child Adolesc Psychiatry. 1997;36:669–77.
40. Lehrer PM, Isenberg S, Hochron SM. Asthma and emotion: a review. J Asthma. 1993;30:5–21.
41. Sztrymf B, Messika J, Bertrand F, Hurel D, Leon R, Dreyfuss D, et al. Beneficial effects of humidified high flow nasal oxygen in critical care patients: a prospective pilot study. Intensive Care Med. 2011;37:1780–6.
42. Cuquemelle E, Pham T, Papon J-F, Louis B, Danin P-E, Brochard L. Heated and humidified high-flow oxygen therapy reduces discomfort during hypoxemic respiratory failure. Respir Care. 2012;57:1571–7.
43. Spentzas T, Minarik M, Patters AB, Vinson B, Stidham G. Children with respiratory distress treated with high-flow nasal cannula. J Intensive Care Med. 2009;24:323–8.
44. Akingbola OA, Simakajornboon N, Hadley EF Jr, Hopkins RL. Noninvasive positive-pressure ventilation in pediatric status asthmaticus. Pediatr Crit Care Med. 2002;3:181–4.
45. Carroll CL, Schramm CM. Noninvasive positive pressure ventilation for the treatment of status asthmaticus in children. Ann Allergy Asthma Immunol. 2006;96:454–9.
46. Lim WJ, Mohammed Akram R, Carson KV, Mysore S, Labiszewski NA, Wedzicha JA, et al. Non-invasive positive pressure ventilation for treatment of respiratory failure due to severe acute exacerbations of asthma. Cochrane Database Syst Rev. 2012;12:CD004360.
47. Organized jointly by the American Thoracic Society, the European Respiratory Society, the European Society of Intensive Care Medicine, and the Société de Réanimation de Langue Française, and approved by ATS Board of Directors. International consensus conferences in intensive care medicine: noninvasive positive pressure ventilation in acute respiratory failure. Am J Respir Crit Care Med. 2000;2001(163):283–91.
48. Chalut DS, Ducharme FM, Davis GM. The preschool respiratory assessment measure (PRAM): a responsive index of acute asthma severity. J Pediatr. 2000;137:762–8.
49. Hess DR. Aerosol therapy during noninvasive ventilation or high-flow nasal cannula. Respir Care. 2015;60:880–93.
50. Bhashyam AR, Wolf MT, Marcinkowski AL, Saville A, Thomas K, Carcillo JA, et al. Aerosol delivery through nasal cannulas: an in vitro study. J Aerosol Med Pulm Drug Deliv. 2008;21:181–8.

9

A new global and comprehensive model for ICU ventilator performances evaluation

Nicolas S. Marjanovic[1,2], Agathe De Simone[3], Guillaume Jegou[3] and Erwan L'Her[4,5*]

Abstract

Background: This study aimed to provide a new global and comprehensive evaluation of recent ICU ventilators taking into account both technical performances and ergonomics.

Methods: Six recent ICU ventilators were evaluated. Technical performances were assessed under two FIO_2 levels (100%, 50%), three respiratory mechanics combinations (*Normal*: compliance [*C*] = 70 mL cmH_2O^{-1}/resistance [*R*] = 5 $cmH_2O\ L^{-1}\ s^{-1}$; *Restrictive*: *C* = 30/*R* = 10; *Obstructive*: *C* = 120/*R* = 20), four exponential levels of leaks (from 0 to 12.5 L min^{-1}) and three levels of inspiratory effort (P0.1 = 2, 4 and 8 cmH_2O), using an automated test lung. Ergonomics were evaluated by 20 ICU physicians using a global and comprehensive model involving physiological response to stress measurements (heart rate, respiratory rate, tidal volume variability and eye tracking), psycho-cognitive scales (SUS and NASA-TLX) and objective tasks completion.

Results: Few differences in terms of technical performance were observed between devices. Non-invasive ventilation modes had a huge influence on asynchrony occurrence. Using our global model, either objective tasks completion, psycho-cognitive scales and/or physiological measurements were able to depict significant differences in terms of devices' usability. The level of failure that was observed with some devices depicted the lack of adaptation of device's development to end users' requests.

Conclusions: Despite similar technical performance, some ICU ventilators exhibit low ergonomics performance and a high risk of misusage.

Background

Mechanical ventilation is a fundamental part of critical care, and the accuracy of ventilatory settings is of utmost importance. When dealing with unstable patients, a bad technological performance may cause a patient harm, while low tidal volume (VT) and high positive expiratory pressure (PEEP) are key points for protective ventilation [1, 2]. Ineffective effort and asynchrony correction [3], along with effective triggering [4], may decrease inspiratory work and improve patients' outcome. Bench-test studies are essential to assess the technical characteristics of ventilators and determine their efficiency during critical care [5–9].

Besides technical performance, another major aspect of a device's reliability is its usability. Usability is defined as the extent to which a device can be used by specified users to achieve specific goals effectively, efficiently and satisfactorily, in a specified context of use. Usability is mainly related to the quality of the human–machine interface. Improved interface seems mandatory to limit human errors that could exacerbate morbidity and mortality [10–12]. There are few studies dedicated to ventilator ergonomics evaluation, and those that do exist are often limited to timed task and/or easy user-friendliness assessments [13–16].

The aims of this study were to provide a new global and comprehensive evaluation of recent ICU ventilators, taking into account both their technical performance and a comprehensive ergonomics evaluation (Fig. 1).

Methods

Tested devices

Six ICU ventilators were evaluated in a dedicated bench test. All ventilators were provided free of charge by

*Correspondence: erwan.lher@chu-brest.fr
[5] Médecine Intensive et Réanimation, CHRU de Brest, Boulevard Tanguy Prigent, 29200 Brest Cedex, France
Full list of author information is available at the end of the article

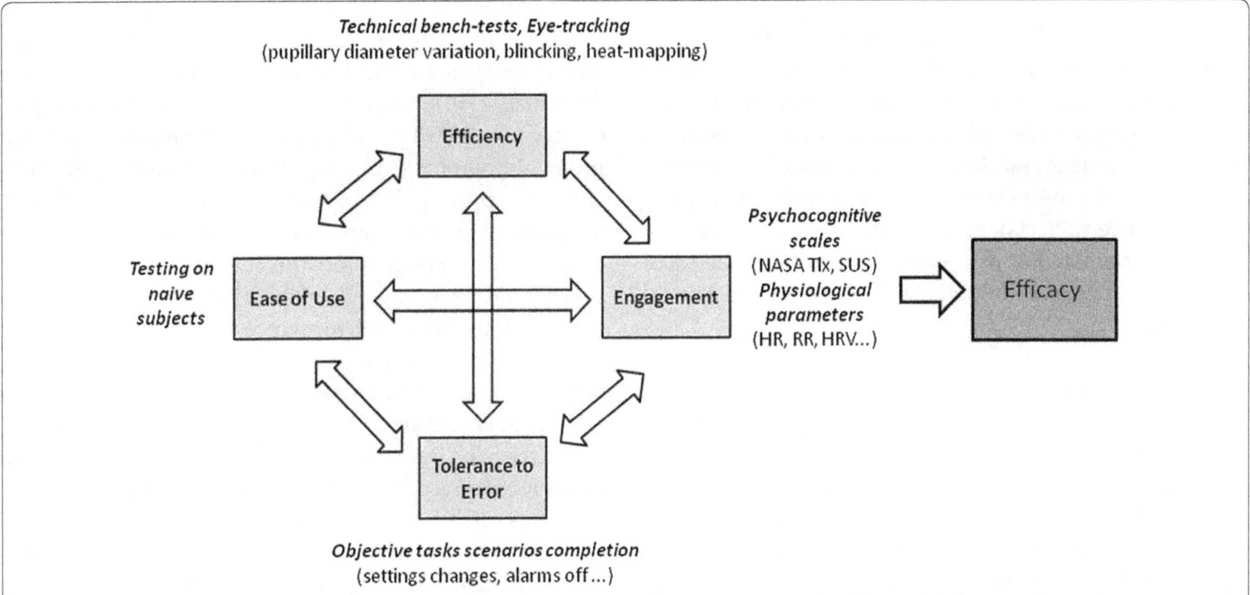

Fig. 1 The concept of devices' global evaluation. In order to assess *'efficacy'* of a device, we considered that a global ergonomics evaluation required evaluating concomitantly *'efficiency', 'engagement', 'ease of use'* and *'tolerance to error'*, as these four dimensions may be considered as interdependent. Tolerance to error was evaluated through the objective tasks completion scenarios. While considering that an easy-to-use device should be easily managed by a skilled physician, but not familiar to that specific device, we took particular attention to included naive subjects in the evaluation. Bench testings do explore the most important technical determinants of the efficiency of a device (tidal volume accuracy, triggering, etc.). Efficiency assessment might also include interfaces' performance evaluation. For such sake, we used pupillary diameter variation which can be considered as a determinant of stress. Other eye-tracking tools such as blinking measurements or heat mapping may also have been used. Engagement during use of the device was evaluated through the use of psycho-cognitive scales, combined with physiological parameters measurements. Heart rate variability (HRV) may also have been measured for such sake

manufacturers: (1) Dräger V500 (Lubeck, Germany); (2) Covidien PB980 (Mansfield, MA, USA); (3) Philips V680 (Murrysville, PA, USA); (4) Hamilton S1 (Bonaduz, Switzerland); (5) General Electrics R860 (Fairfield, CT, USA); and (6) Maquet Servo-U (Göteborg, Sweden). General characteristics of the devices are provided in the online repository (Additional file 1: Table S1).

Technical performance

Measurements were taken using an ASL5000™ lung simulator (Ingmar, Pittsburgh, PA, USA) under constant room temperature (22 °C), simulator temperature (37 °C), under dry ambient pressure (ATPD) conditions, and converted into body temperature and pressure, saturated (BTPS) as previously described [6, 17]. Technical performances were assessed under two FIO_2 levels (100%, 50%), three respiratory mechanics combinations (*Normal*: resistance [*R*] = 5 $cmH_2O\ L^{-1}\ s^{-1}$; compliance [*C*] = 70 mL cmH_2O^{-1}, *Restrictive*: $R = 10\ cmH_2O\ L^{-1}\ s^{-1}$; $C = 30$ mL cmH_2O^{-1} and *Obstructive*: $R = 20\ cmH_2O\ L^{-1}\ s^{-1}$; $C = 120$ mL cmH_2O^{-1}), three exponential levels of leaks (L1 = 3.5–4.0 L min^{-1}; L2 = 5.0–7.0 L min^{-1}; L3 = 9.0–12.5 L min^{-1}) and three levels of inspiratory effort (P0.1 = 2, 4 and 8 cmH_2O) in volume-controlled continuous mandatory ventilation (VC-CMV) and pressure-controlled continuous spontaneous ventilation (PC-CSV) [4]. Triggering capabilities, volume and pressurization accuracy were evaluated under the different respiratory mechanics at standardized respiratory settings. The asynchrony index [18] was defined as the number of asynchrony events divided by the total respiratory rate and expressed in percentage [3]. Asynchronies were evaluated under the different respiratory mechanics and the three exponential levels of leaks and inspiratory efforts.

Error was evaluated as the average difference between set and true dimension value (VT, PEEP, pressure support). Accuracy was a priori considered for an error value below 10% for all parameters. Precision of the dimension was defined as the range value of the dimension, considering that a narrow range was the more precise. An asynchrony index greater than 10% was also considered clinically significant [3, 19].

Details about the technical performance evaluation are provided in the online repository.

Ergonomics

For ergonomics evaluation, we included, as a reference, the use of a device that was familiar to all physicians (Avea, Carefusion, San Diego, CA, USA).

ICU physicians involved in ergonomics evaluation

Twenty senior ICU physicians from five different ICUs were included in the evaluation. Each physician tested 3–4 devices in a randomized order; each device was tested 11 or 12 times. All physicians used the Avea in their daily clinical practice; we paid particular attention to the fact that none of them were familiar with the tested devices (naive subjects), even though some of them were in some cases familiar with other devices from the same manufacturer (see Additional file 1: Table S2, Additional file 1: Table S3).

Objective task completion

The ICU physicians had to complete 11 specific tasks for each ventilator, four mainly dedicated to monitoring and seven to setting: (a) alarm control (users must shut down alarms, identify the reason and modify setting to stop alarms); (b) mode recognition (exact reading of the ventilator mode set by investigator); (c) identify humidification system on the screen and modify it; (d) ventilator setting reading (VT, ventilation rate, PEEP and trigger value); (e) power on the ventilator; (f) start ventilation; (g) set inspiratory flow to a value defined by the investigator (40–80 L min^{-1}); (h) ventilator mode modification; (i) set cycling to 60%; (j) non-invasive ventilation mode activation; and (k) ventilator extinction (complete ventilator powering down). In each group of tests (i.e. monitoring or setting), tasks were to be performed in a randomized order. The test was a priori considered as a failure if the correct response was given after more than 120 s, or if the physicians did not provide a correct response or abandoned the task. Due to technical constraints, we chose not to use a high-fidelity environment with a manikin, but to perform measurements with the ventilators connected solely to the test lung. Besides a task failure rate evaluation, these scenarios were also dedicated to enable usability and mental workload scoring using psycho-cognitive scales.

Psycho-cognitive scales evaluation

Psycho-cognitive scorings were performed immediately after all objective tasks completion.

System Usability Scale (SUS) The SUS is a reliability tool, developed to measure a device's usability [20]. It consists of a ten-item questionnaire and assesses usability by different aspects: effectiveness (ability of users to complete tasks); efficiency (level of resource used in performing tasks); and satisfaction (subjective reactions to using the system). The SUS score has a range of 0–100, the highest score being the best value ('simple to use').

Mental workload evaluation using the NASA-TLX Mental workload is a subjective ergonomic measurement and an indicator for interface development, assessment and comparison. NASA-TLX is a multidimensional tool that was developed by the National Aeronautics and Space Administration's Ames Research Center in 1986 for perceptual mental workload evaluations using the Task Load Index measurement through three dimensions, dependent on the user's perception of the task (mental workload, temporal workload and physical workload) and three dimensions dependent on the interaction between the subject and the task itself, which may be mostly related to the interface (effort, performance and frustration). Each dimension is rated using a Likert-type scale ranging from 0 to 100. The second part of Task Load Index calculation intends to create an individual weighting of these dimensions by letting the subjects compare them pairwise, based on their perceived importance. These 15 comparison pairings thus enable the inter-/intra-individual variability of the overall score to decrease. The overall workload score for each subject is composed by multiplying each rating by the weight given to that factor by that subject. The sum of the weighted ratings for each task is divided by 15 (the sum of the weights). The higher the Task Load Index, the higher the mental workload and the more difficult it is to use the device.

Physiological measurements

Several physiological parameters were recorded during the completion of the objective tasks. Pupil diameter modifications were assessed using an eye-tracking system (SMI ETG 1, SensoMotoric Instruments GmbH, Teltow, Germany) (Additional file 1: Fig. S1); heart and respiratory rate and thoracic volume variations were measured using a biometric belt (Hexoskin, Montréal, Canada). Analysis consisted of a data treatment by a systems' activation count, which corresponded to highly different values, as compared to baseline. Each of these activations is numerically integrated in order to evaluate the number of physiological variations in response to tasks. These activations are considered to be adequate stress indicators.

The concept of global ergonomics evaluation

A global and comprehensive model for a device's efficacy evaluation needs to either assess technical performances and ergonomics or thus to explore four different dimensions (Fig. 1). Each of these four dimensions can be explored separately, but they are all related one to the other. Tolerance to error was evaluated through the objective tasks completion scenarios. While considering that an easy-to-use device should be easily managed by a skilled physician, but not familiar to that specific device, we took particular attention to included naive subjects in the evaluation. Bench testings do explore the most important technical determinants of the efficiency of a device (tidal volume accuracy, triggering, etc.). Efficiency evaluation might also include interface's performance evaluation. For such sake, we used pupillary diameter variation which can be considered as a determinant of stress. Engagement during use of the device was evaluated through the use of psycho-cognitive scales, combined with physiological parameters measurements.

Statistical analysis

Parameters were calculated over 10–20 cycles after signal stabilization and are provided as mean ± SD to calculate error and as median ± interquartile to evaluate precision of the dimension, in response to respiratory mechanics changes. Data were compared using analysis of variance (ANOVA) and nonparametric Friedman and Wilcoxon signed-rank test. A p value <0.05 was considered statistically significant. Statistical analysis was performed using MedCalc 12.7.4 for Windows (MedCalc software, Ostend, Belgium).

Results

Technical performances

Tidal volume accuracy (Fig. 2)

There was a significant difference in terms of tidal volume delivery precision between devices (Fig. 2a; $p = 0.0498$). All devices except S1 depicted a median tidal volume value within the 10% error range (VT = 449 ± 2 mL; ΔDVT = −10.2%). PB980 had the lowest error in terms of tidal volume delivery, but Servo-U had the higher precision in response to respiratory mechanics modifications. V500 and V680 had relatively low error, but low precision in response to respiratory mechanics modifications.

Pressurization accuracy (Fig. 2)

Pressurization accuracy differed between devices. Mean PEEP accuracy was similar between devices, except for V500 in the obstructive condition (pressurization error = 18 ± 5%). Three ventilators delivered a mean pressure support over the 10% error range (Servo-U: 13 ± 6%; PB980: 11 ± 12%; S1: 17 ± 14.4%; $p < 0.001$). S1 had the lowest error, but with rather low precision. Servo-U, PB980 and R860 had low error and high precision. V500 and V680 had low precision.

Triggering evaluation (Fig. 3)

No differences were observed between devices in terms of inspiratory triggering. Triggering delay was below 150 ms among the different respiratory mechanics, but exceeded 200 ms in obstructive conditions, except for PB980. Triggering pressure presented a large difference among the devices ($p = 0.0004$) and was higher for S1 ($p = 0.0003$) and R860 ($p = 0.001$).

Asynchrony management (Fig. 4)

Mean asynchrony indexes were equal to 31 and 14.5% under standard or non-invasive ventilatory modes, respectively, for all devices. All ventilators presented an asynchrony index of over 10% without using the non-invasive ventilation mode. While using non-invasive ventilation algorithms, the asynchrony index was lower for R860 and Servo-U (9.6%) as compared to V500 (14.6%),

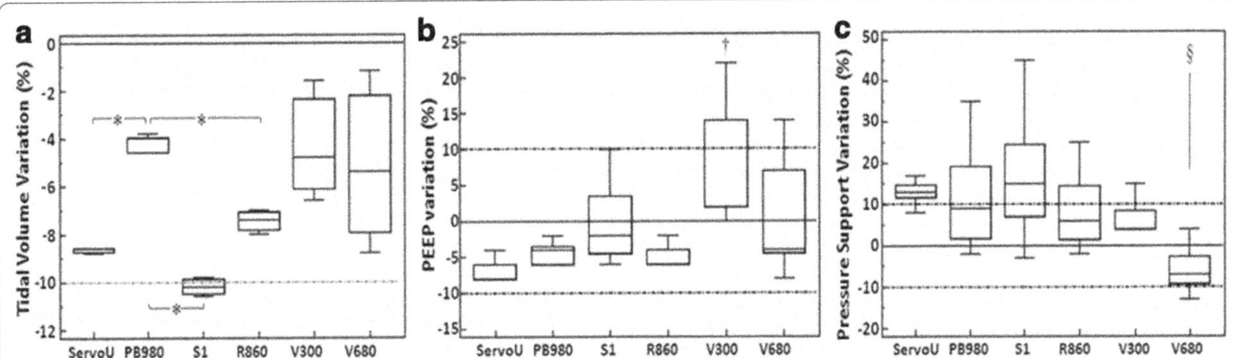

Fig. 2 *Box plot* of tidal volume (VT) (**a**), positive end-expiratory pressure (PEEP) (**b**) and pressure support (PS) (**c**). *Dotted lines* represent the 10% error range. *Black line* represents exact VT value delivery. Values are provided as median and interquartile. A p value equal or below 0.05 was considered significant. *$p < 0.05$; §$p < 0.05$ as compared to S1, PB980 and Servo-U. †$p < 0.005$ as compared to R860, PB980 and Servo-U. There was a significant difference in terms of VT delivery precision between devices (**a**; $p = 0.0498$). All devices except S1 depicted a median VT value within the 10% error range. PB980 had the lowest error in terms of VT delivery, but Servo-U had the highest precision in response to respiratory mechanics modifications. V500 and V680 had relatively low error, but low precision in response to respiratory mechanics modifications. While median PEEP delivery was within the reliability range for all devices (**b**), V500 was significantly different to the other devices in terms of precision. S1 had the lowest error, but with rather low precision. Servo-U, PB980 and R860 had low error and high precision. When considering mean values, three devices delivered PS values higher than the reliability range (Servo-U: 13 ± 6%; PB980: 11 ± 12%; S1: 17 ± 14.4%; $p < 0.001$). Pressure support delivery was higher than the 10% error range for two devices (Servo-U and S1). Precision in response to respiratory mechanics modifications was low for PB980, S1 and R860

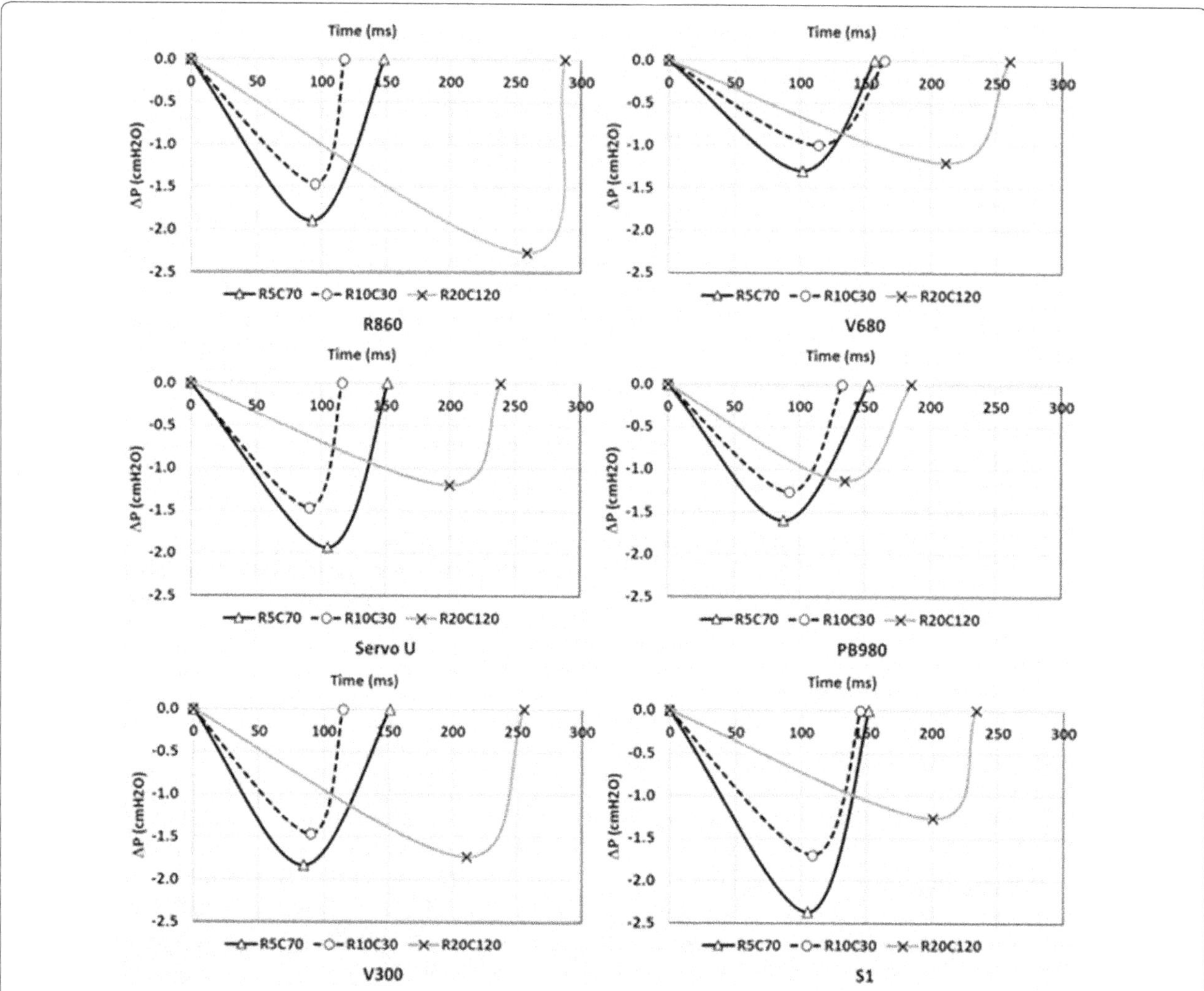

Fig. 3 Triggering evaluation according to respiratory mechanics combinations. R: resistance; C: compliance; ΔP: maximal pressure drop required to trigger inspiration; DT: triggering delay, from the onset of the airway pressure decay (beginning of the patient's effort) to flow delivery (beginning of ventilator pressurization); DP: pressurization delay, from the airway pressure signal rise to a return to positive pressure; DI: overall inspiratory delay (DT + DP). *Triangle* and *black line*: results for the 'Normal' respiratory mechanics; *circle* and *dotted line*: results for the 'Restrictive' respiratory mechanics; *cross* and *grey line*: results for the 'Obstructive' respiratory mechanics (*Normal*: resistance [*R*] = 5 $cmH_2O\ L^{-1}\ s^{-1}$; Compliance [*C*] = 70 $mL\ cmH_2O^{-1}$, *Restrictive*: R = 10 $cmH_2O\ L^{-1}\ s^{-1}$; C = 30 $mL\ cmH_2O^{-1}$ and *Obstructive*: R = 20 $cmH_2O\ L^{-1}\ s^{-1}$; C = 120 $mL\ cmH_2O^{-1}$). The *figure* presents individual results for each ventilator at the different respiratory mechanics combinations. *First point of each curve* represents inspiratory effort initiation; *second point* represents maximal depressurization (ΔP) before inspiratory pressure increase. There was no significant difference in terms of DT and DI between ventilators, nor in terms of maximal depressurization (ΔP). DI variability according to respiratory mechanics was higher for V500 and R860

V680 (17.5%) and PB980 (18.3%; $p < 0.05$) (Additional file 1: Fig. S2). Most frequent asynchronies were prolonged cycles and ineffective efforts, ineffective efforts being most of the time associated with prolonged cycles.

Ergonomics evaluation

Objective task completion (Table 1)

Of all ventilators, our reference device the Avea had the best success rate. In our comparison of the six ventilators, Covidien PB980 had the best results and the Servo-U the worst. A minority of users could power on Servo-U, but always took longer than the predefined 120 s time range. The V500 was the fastest ventilator to power on. Only 36% of the ICU physicians were able to power on Servo-U and always with over a 1-min delay. No users could set the inspiratory flow on Servo-U, and only 18% of them succeeded in the same task with S1. Difficulties in activating the non-invasive ventilation mode were frequent with Servo-U, V500 and V680. Servo-U had the worst global results (tasks failure rate = 42%) compared to our reference (Avea; tasks failure rate = 13%) ($p = 0.12$). The lack of sensitivity of the S1 touch screen proved to be a

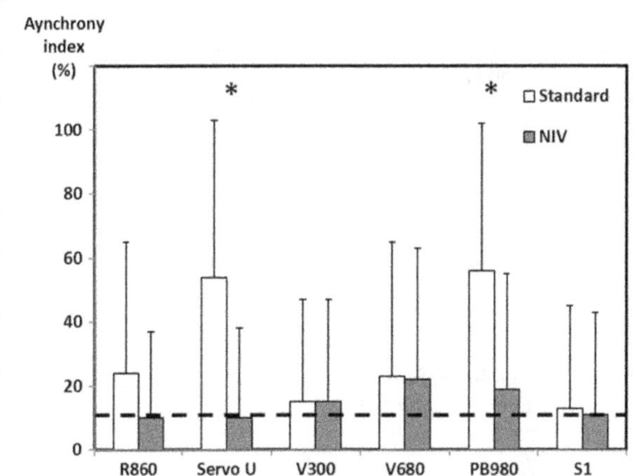

Fig. 4 Asynchrony index with or without the non-invasive ventilation mode. The asynchrony index (AI) is presented as mean ± SD and was measured under three different levels of exponential leaks (L1 = 3.5–4.0 L min^{-1}; L2 = 5.0–7.0 L min^{-1}; L3 = 9.0–12.5 L min^{-1}) and three levels of inspiratory effort (P0.1 = 2, 4, 8 cmH_2O). 'Standard' represents measurements performed under PC-CSV using unmodified manufacturers' settings in terms of inspiratory and expiratory triggering; 'NIV' represents the measurements performed under the same conditions, while switching the ventilator to the NIV mode. *Dotted line* represents the 10% AI clinical level of significance. *p value <0.001. All ventilators presented an AI over 10% without NIV mode ('standard' invasive PC-CSV setting). Under the same leaks conditions, switching the ventilator to the NIV mode enabled a decrease in the AI to below a 10% value for the R860 and Servo-U. V500 and S1 measurements did not depict a significant impact of the NIV mode, while 'standard' settings provided rather satisfactory results in terms of leak management

barrier for some task completion and a significant source of confusion. The settings reading represented one of the most difficult tasks, whatever the device. Sensitivity analysis while deleting powering on and switching off tasks did not significantly modify the overall results.

Psycho-cognitive scales measurements (Figs. 5, 6)

NASA-TLX and SUS scorings are presented in Fig. 5. V680 for NASA-TLX, V680 and S1 for SUS were the only devices to differ significantly from the reference (Avea). Except for the reference, not a single device reached an SUS score equal or higher than 68.

On the radar chart presentation of the NASA-TLX, except for our reference value (Avea, TLX = 41.6), the R860 had the lowest TLX value (TLX = 44.7) and V680 had the highest (TLX = 63.2; $p = 0.049$). The main dimensions involved in the higher mental workload were 'performance' and 'effort'.

Physiological measurements (Fig. 7)

For all parameters, our reference value depicted significantly less activation. Pupillary diameter, respiratory rate and tidal volume activations significantly differed between devices ($p < 0.05$). V500 caused the highest pupillary diameter activation and differed significantly from the reference ($p = 0.03$) and R860 ($p = 0.019$).

Discussion

Within this panel of recently available ICU ventilators, no technical features could be considered as differentiating between devices, while a contrario, ergonomics and interface features were considered inadequate, thus increasing the risks of misusage and adverse events.

Technical performances

While volume delivery and pressurization accuracy are critical issues, few differences were observed between devices. However, volume delivery and pressurization errors and precisions were important for some ventilators. In all cases, volume delivery was lower than that expected, as already observed [18].

Triggering performances depicted within our study are similar to those observed in a previous study concerning emergency transport ventilators [8] and tended to be higher than previously observed [9, 17]. These results may be explained by different respiratory mechanics and BTPS conditions [8]. No device enabled a triggering delay faster than 50 ms, and it exceeded 100 ms for two devices in normal respiratory mechanics conditions. As already described, flow or pressure triggering has not varied significantly over the last decade [7].

During non-invasive ventilation, patient–ventilator asynchronies are frequent [21, 22] and mainly related to leaks around the interfaces and/or overassistance. Our mean asynchrony index was close to that observed in other studies [8, 23]. Non-invasive ventilation algorithms that are implemented in most devices were able to decrease the asynchrony index significantly and might thus be systematically turned on during non-invasive ventilation, in an attempt to limit non-invasive ventilation failure.

Ergonomics assessment

While huge effort has been made by manufacturers to improve technical issues, increasing complexity of devices may in fact result in design errors. Not only are the devices' full capabilities underutilized, but also their main functions may often be handled improperly.

Human error has been demonstrated to be a leading cause of morbidity and death during medical care [10, 24–26]. Many devices have interfaces that are so poorly designed and difficult to use that they can increase the risks associated with the medical equipment and device-induced human error. Human error may be to some extent inevitable and equally caused by human performance and machine performance. In order to limit the

Table 1 Objective tasks completion rate

Device	Power on (%)	Start ventilation (%)	Inspiratory flow setting (%)	Ventilatory mode modification (%)	Cycling setting (%)	NIV mode activation (%)
Carefusion Avea	92	100	100	100	75	75
Dräger V500	100	92	100	100	92	50
Covidien PB980	100	100	100	91	100	100
Philips V680	100	100	50§	91	91	40†
Hamilton S1	91	91	18§	82	91	91
GE R860	100	100	100	91	100	91
Maquet Servo-U	36*	100	0¤	100	45‡	27†

Device	Ventilator offset (%)	Alarm shut down (%)	Mode recognition (%)	Humidification system recognition (%)	Settings reading (%)	Overall
Carefusion Avea	100	100	100	75	42	87%/85%
Dräger V500	100	75	100	42	25	80%/75%
Covidien PB980	73*	64	100	73	45	86%/86%
Philips V680	100	82	100	55	18	75%/70%
Hamilton S1	100	91	100	36	27	74%/70%
GE R860	100	64	100	9‖	27	80%/76%
Maquet Servo-U	100	82	100	0‖	45	58%#/55%‖

Results are presented as the different objective tasks success rate, expressed as the percentage of successful attempts. ICU's physicians with mechanical ventilation's knowledge had to complete 11 specific tasks of variable clinical importance for each ventilator, 4 mainly dedicated to monitoring and 7 to setting. Overall provides results of the entire bunch of test (first value), or after powering on/switching off tasks exclusion (second value)

Among all ventilators, our reference device the Avea had the better success rate. In between our comparison of the six ventilators, Covidien PB980 had the better results and the Servo-U the worst. A minority of users could power on Servo-U and always over the predefined 120 s time range. Settings reading represented the more difficult task, whatever the device, while their terminology was highly different from one device to the other

* $p < 0.01$ as compared to others. § $p < 0.001$ as compared to Avea, V500 and PB980. ¤ $p < 0.01$ as compared to V680. ‡ $p < 0.05$ as compared to others except Avea. † $p < 0.05$ as compared to PB980 S1 and R860. ‖ $p < 0.001$ as compared to Avea and PB980. # $p < 0.01$ as compared to others, except S1 and V680

number of errors, computing technology and human–machine interface development should be designed to correspond to human characteristics of reasoning and memory constraints [11]. It is also well known that the working memory of humans is limited and that the number of variables depicted on screens is excessive. This results in a large cognitive load (i.e. mental workload) on the user, which is also a determinant of human error [27]. An interface with a human-centred design increases efficiency and satisfaction and decreases the rate of medical error. While these data are integrated in the ventilators' interface development by manufacturers, and while ergonomics are as essential as technical performances, very few studies have assessed the ergonomics, and many were limited to timed tasks and subjective evaluation [13–15].

To the best of our knowledge, this is first time that such an innovative ergonomics evaluation of ICU mechanical ventilators has been performed, globally integrating the four main dimensions that enable a comprehensive approach to the problem: 1—tolerance to error; 2—ease of use; 3—efficiency; and 4—engagement. Tolerance to error may be directly linked to efficiency and ease of use to engagement. While all four dimensions may be considered independently, they are in fact related one to each other (Fig. 1). Most previous ergonomics evaluations have mainly focused on tolerance to error, while the three other dimensions were often missing data.

The integration of pupil diameter measurement, heart and respiratory rate or tidal volume activation to assess ergonomics are new data in the ICU field. Compared to subjective psychological measurements, these are objective data that allow the estimation of the physiological stress induced by a device's interface and an indirect assessment of the interface's usability.

The objective tasks results are often considered as the most representative of the devices' ergonomics' differences. Even if we entirely agree with the fact that not all scenarios may have the same importance, it is still surprising that some ventilators could not be powered on by a majority of physicians or that the NIV mode could not be easily activated. Excluding powering on/off tests from analysis, considering that these may be very different tasks that have been voluntarily been made difficult by the manufacturers for safety reasons, did not modify the overall results. While it may be one of the main tasks routinely performed, ventilator setting readings had the worst results of all tasks, probably because of the absence of a homogenized terminology among manufacturers. As already observed in another recent study, the lack of sensitivity of the S1 touch screen was specifically considered

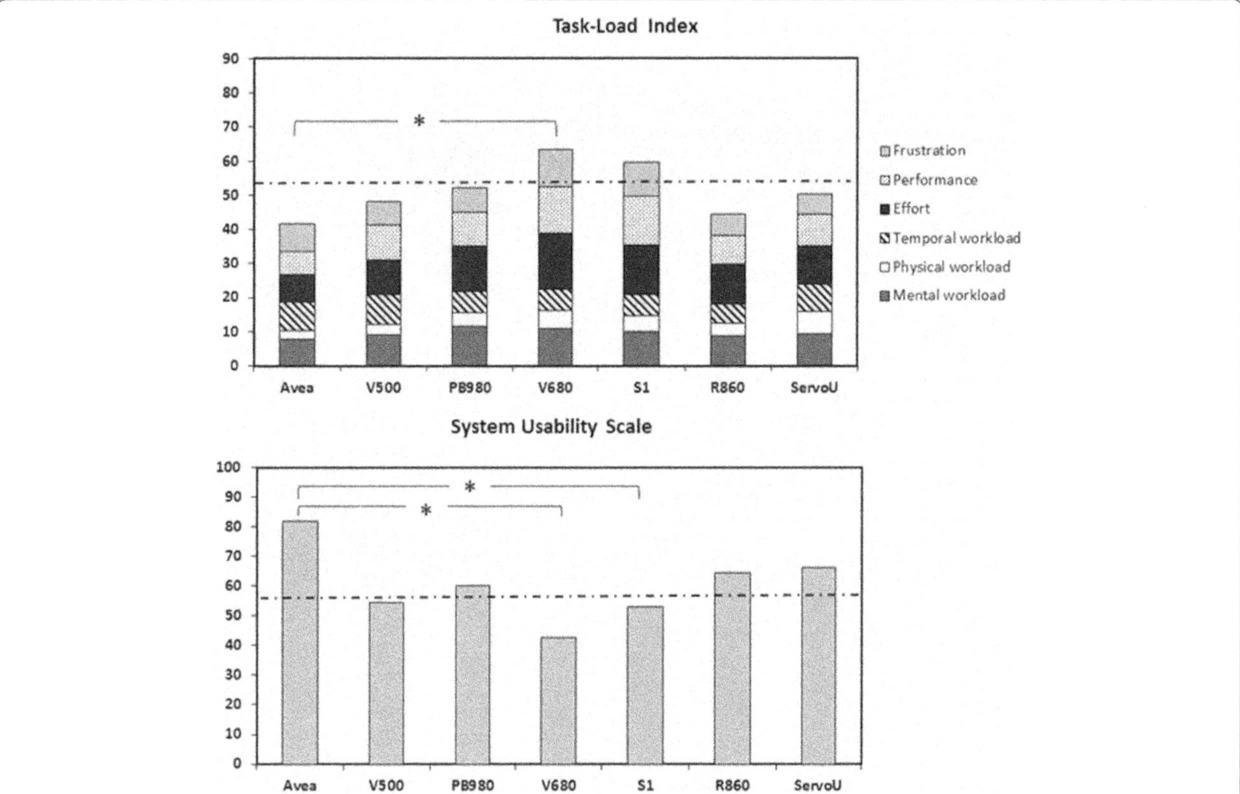

Fig. 5 Task Load Index and System Usability Scale scores. *Dotted line* represents the mean value across all scores (Avea excluded). SUS consists of a ten-item questionnaire and assesses usability from different aspects: effectiveness (ability of users to complete tasks); efficiency (level of resource used in performing tasks); and satisfaction (subjective reactions to using the system). SUS score has a range of 0–100, the highest score being the best value ('simple to use'). NASA-TLX is a multidimensional tool developed for mental workload evaluation. It explores three dimensions dependent on user perception of the task (mental workload, temporal workload and physical workload) and three dimensions dependent on the interaction between the subject and the task itself, which may be mostly related to the interface (effort, performance and frustration). An individual weighting of these dimensions by letting the subjects compare them pairwise enables a decrease in the inter-/intra-individual variability of the overall score. The higher the TLX, the lower the ergonomics. Our reference device (Avea) had the best TLX and SUS scores, and V680 the worst ($p = 0.049$). For usability (SUS), a difference between our reference device (Avea) and S1 was also observed. *p value <0.05

by the participants as responsible for an increased mental workload and higher rates of task failures [28]. The physicians praised the Servo-U interface, but the interface also tended to induce high mental workload during specific tasks, thus generating frustration and higher task failure rates.

The pupillary diameter variation is linked to mental workload and is used to assess cognitive skills [29, 30]. However, we must consider the variability related to the light reflex induced by the laboratory environment and the devices themselves [31]. To some extent, this could explain results from the V500 that has a screen luminosity that is higher than that of other devices. Heart and respiratory rates and/or tidal volume variations are linked to emotional behaviour [32–34]. The better results that were observed with the Avea can be explained by the fact that this device was well known to all participants. Our results on the other devices clearly enable the depiction of differences in terms of task completion perceptions among users while using these parameters. Importantly, while the evolution of physiological parameters may not provide comparable results to those obtained with the psycho-cognitive scores, they are consistent with the objective task completion rate results.

The System Usability Scale [20] and NASA Task Load Index [35, 36] are validated psycho-cognitive tools to assess devices' interface.

The SUS is a very easy scale to administer to participants. It can be used on small sample sizes with reliable results, and it can effectively differentiate between usable and unusable systems. A SUS score above 68 would be considered above average and anything below 68 is considered below average.

The NASA-TLX is a flexible, well-established and widely used multidimensional assessment tool that enables quick and easy workload estimation in order

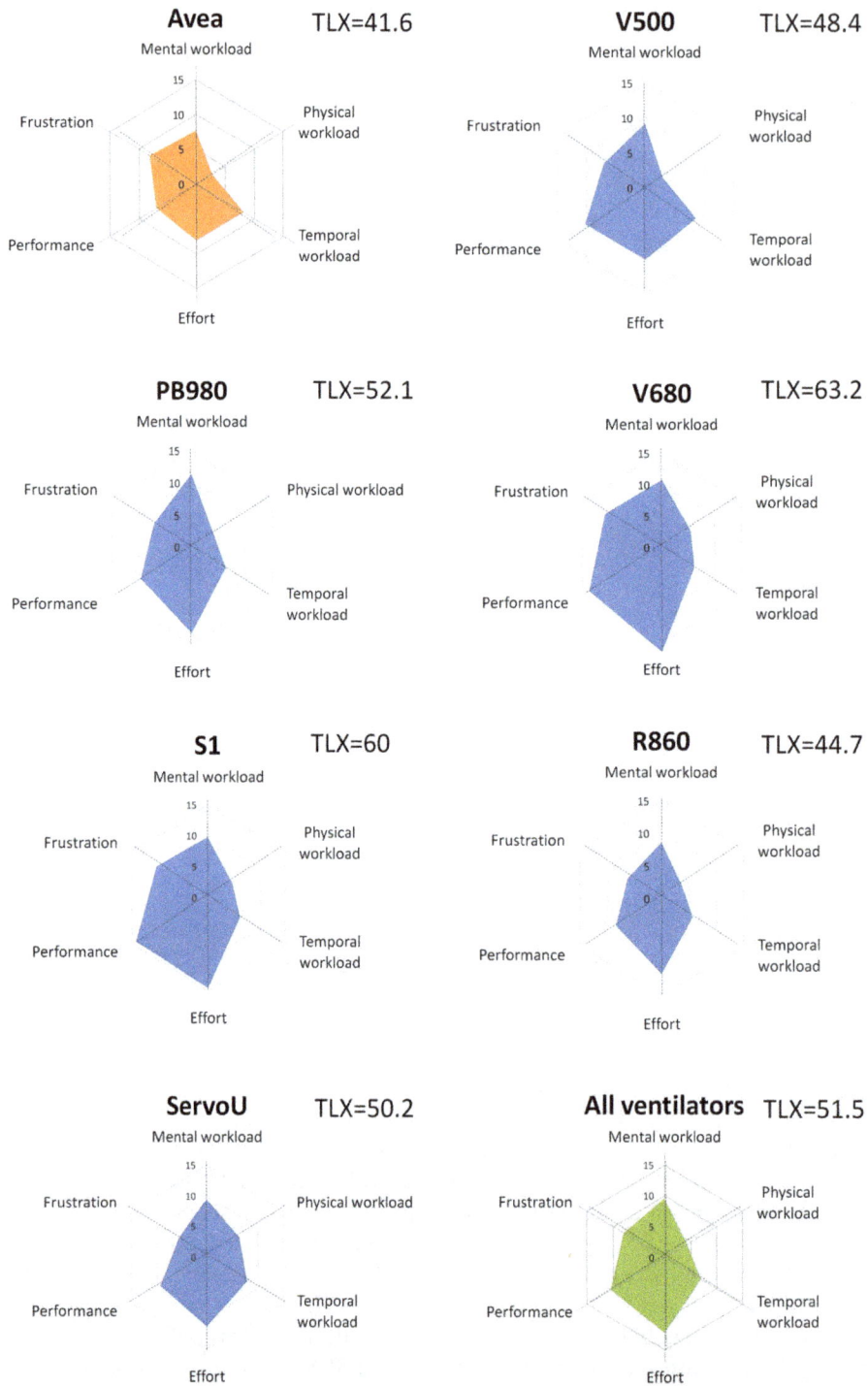

Fig. 6 Radar chart of National Aeronautics and Space Administration—Task Load Index for each ventilator. The *radar chart* of the NASA-TLX indicates both the overall mental workload evaluation (TLX value) and the different dimensions that are evaluated. Three dimensions are dependent on user perception of the task (mental workload, temporal workload and physical workload) and three dimensions dependent on the interaction between the subject and the task itself, which may be mostly related to the interface (effort, performance and frustration). The larger the area of the radar chart, the higher the TLX and thus the mental workload, and the lower the ergonomics. Values of the TLX score are indicated for each ventilator, our reference value being depicted in the upper left. Our reference value (Avea, in *orange*) had the lowest mental workload value (TLX = 41.6), thus depicting the potential influence of experience on mental workload. For this reason, it is strictly mandatory to compare measurements performed on naïve subjects. R860 had the lowest TLX value, and V680 had the highest ($*p = 0.049$). Dimensions of the mental workload that seemed to require the most important improvements were performance and efforts

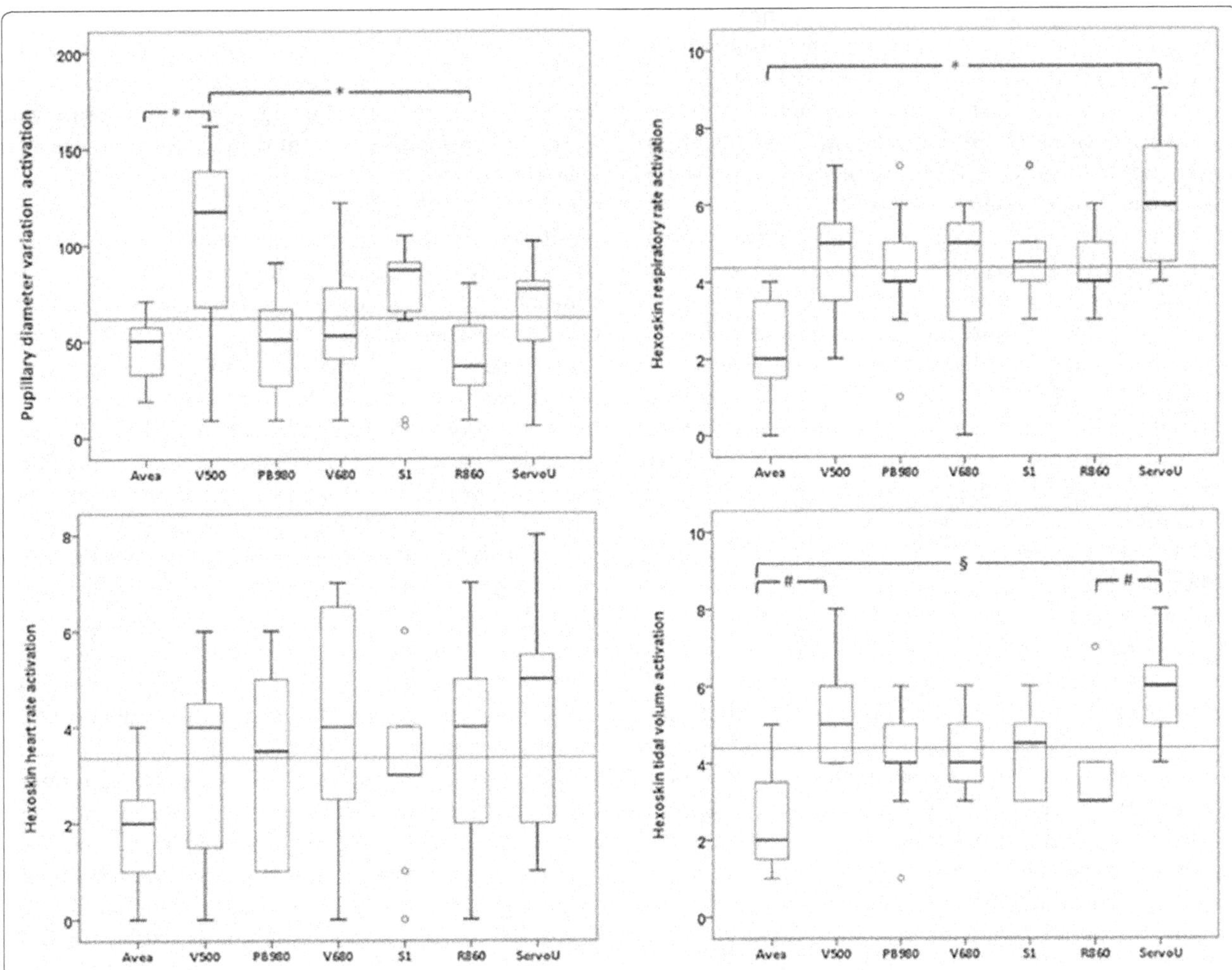

Fig. 7 *Box plot* of physiological measurements and eye-tracking activations. Several physiological parameters were recorded during objective tasks completion. These parameters were evaluated while detecting statistically different values, as compared to baseline. Each of these detections (*'activations'*) is numerically integrated in order to evaluate the number of physiological variations in response to tasks. These activations are considered to be adequate stress indicators. The *number of activations* is represented as median and interquartile. *Dotted line* is mean of activations for all ventilators, during all tests. For all parameters, our reference value depicted significantly fewer activations, thus validating our experimental concept. Significant papillary diameter, respiratory rate and tidal volume activations were observed for several devices (at least V500 and Servo-U). **p* value <0.05; #*p* value <0.005; §*p* value <0.0005

to assess a task or a system. It has been used in a great variety of domains and is considered as one of the most reliable questionnaires to measure workload in a healthcare setting. The higher the weighed TLX, the higher the mental workload and the more 'difficult to use' is the device. Each individual dimension can also be considered on its own, either those dependent on users' perception of the task (mental workload, temporal workload and physical workload) or those dependent on the interaction between the subject and the task itself, which may be mostly related to the interface (effort, performance and frustration). Mental demand describes how much mental and perceptual activity is required to perform the task (e.g. thinking, deciding, calculating). Physical demand describes how much physical activity is required (e.g. pushing, pulling, turning). Temporal demand describes how much time pressure is perceived to fulfil the task (was it slow and leisurely? Or rapid and frantic?). Effort describes how hard the task is to be fulfilled (mentally and physically) in order to accomplish the required level of performance. Performance describes how satisfied the subject feels or whether he/she thinks they were successful in accomplishing the goals. Frustration describes how insecure, discouraged or irritated the subject feels after accomplishing the task. The subscale rating enables inter-/intra-individual variability to be decreased, thus enabling the number of subjects in the experiment to be reduced.

Precedent studies have shown the influence of experience on SUS scores [37], and the better results of the Avea can clearly be related to the users' knowledge of and experience with this device and not specifically to a better interface. Given the overall expertise of all the physicians from the five ICUs with this device, it was used in the comparison as a reference value.

When considering both psycho-cognitive assessment tools, two devices (V680 and S1) could be considered as below our reference device in terms of usability and induced mental workload. In terms of usability, all devices except the R860 and the Servo-U were equal to or below a SUS value of 60, far below the acceptable average value of 68, which may enable us to consider that from an ergonomics point of view, a huge amount of work has to be done to improve the device's usability. With regard to the other ventilators, the SUS and NASA-TLX values did not differ, which corresponds with physiological analyses. If devices' interfaces are globally equivalent, the level of failure observed for some devices, combined with the high induced mental workload and the low usability score, clearly depicts a lack of adaptation of the device's development to end users. Considering our results and the impact of tasks on dimensions like performance and effort for some devices, manufacturers may primarily focus on interface simplification and rationalization, immediately providing the most important settings and alarms on a first screen, leaving expert settings to a second one. However, given individual physicians' heterogeneity, the perfect ventilator may be a difficult goal to achieve, and even with experience, some element of frustration and/or temporal workload may still occur, as with our reference device.

Limitations

As with other bench tests, the main limitations of our study may concern the inability to extrapolate our results to the real clinical situation. First, our technical evaluation was performed on a model, which cannot mimic the complexity of all interactions between a patient and a ventilator. The ASL5000 is a simulator and it remains different from patients, mainly because the spontaneous inspiratory profile is not modified by pressurization during the inspiratory phase. However, the bench simulates most other situations and combinations that can be encountered in the clinical field. Second, the objective and subjective ergonomics measurements were assessed during standardized conditions that may be considered as different from real-life conditions. In order to be able to use various physiological sensors during the ergonomics evaluation, we chose not to use a high-fidelity environment with a manikin. We do agree with the fact that human behaviour under test may be significantly affected by the context and set-up of the experiment. However, while we only included experts, it would have been difficult to reach our experimental goals while also trying to run after a more important degree of immersion that may not be necessary with these types of physicians. A simulated condition may never reproduce all the complexities of the interactions between a patient, a clinician and a ventilator, especially if the tester is an experienced clinician [39]. There are many techniques available for usability evaluation, such as cognitive walk-through, expert reviews, focus groups, Delphi technique, heuristic evaluation or objective timed tasks completion, all of them providing different information [38]. To the best of our knowledge, our study is the only one to provide a global and complete ergonomics evaluation, taking into account different techniques. Third, we may also consider that the small number of senior ICU physicians that were included in our study does not enable firm conclusions to be drawn. Considering the design of the ergonomics evaluation, it required a huge amount of dedicated time from the physicians to undergo the different scenarios and various measurements for the experimental team. Moreover, none of them were familiar with the six tested devices, which exacerbated the difficulty in recruitment. It was therefore unrealistic to use more testers, and such a drawback also tended to be limited by the use of a device that was known to everyone as a comparison and by the fact that we included physicians from five different ICUs. The pairwise comparison that is performed while using the NASA-TLX also limits inter-/intra-individual variability. Finally, the use of the Avea as a 'reference' also depicts a specific limitation about the use of subjective psycho-cognitive scales. The better results of the Avea, with both the SUS and the NASA-TLX, clearly indicate that these values may be highly influenced by previous experience. Such a bias was limited within our evaluation by the fact that, in an attempt to assess the ease of use, we only included naive subjects in order to limit the impact of such experience on the evaluation.

Conclusions

The choice of an '*ideal*' ventilatory device is a difficult task that may concomitantly consider technical performances and ergonomics. While technical bench tests are essential to assess technical performances and a ventilator's accuracy, a global ergonomics evaluation, taking into account different variables and dimensions, is crucial to enable physicians to focus on their patients, rather than on technological problems. Despite significant technological improvements, several ICU ventilators do exhibit low ergonomics performance and a high risk of misusage.

Abbreviations

ICU: intensive care unit; NIV: non-invasive ventilation; C: compliance; R: resistance; VT: tidal volume; PEEP: positive end-expiratory pressure; VC-CMV: volume-controlled continuous mandatory ventilation; PC-CSV: pressure-controlled continuous spontaneous ventilation; BTPS: body temperature, pressure and saturated; SUS: System Usability Scale; NASA-TLX: National Aeronautics and Space Administration—Task Load Index.

Authors' contributions

ELH designed the study. ELH, NM, ADS and GJ acquired data. ELH and NM wrote the manuscript. All authors read and approved the final manuscript.

Author details

[1] Urgences Adultes/SAMU 86, CHU de Poitiers, 86000 Poitiers Cedex, France. [2] ABS-Lab, Laboratoire d'Anatomie, Biomécanique et Simulation, Université de Poitiers, Rue de la Milétrie, 86000 Poitiers Cedex, France. [3] B-Com Technical Research Institute, 29200 Brest Cedex, France. [4] CeSim/LaTIM INSERM UMR 1101, Université de Bretagne Occidentale, Rue Camille Desmoulins, 29200 Brest Cedex, France. [5] Médecine Intensive et Réanimation, CHRU de Brest, Boulevard Tanguy Prigent, 29200 Brest Cedex, France.

Acknowledgements

The authors would like to acknowledge the help of all ICU Physicians from Brest, Morlaix and Quimper who made this study possible.

Competing interests

Erwan L'Her has been a consultant for Air Liquide Medical Systems, Novartis and Smiths Medical. He is the co-founder of Oxy'nov Inc., a spin-off company from the Universite Laval, Quebec, dedicated to automation in critical care. Nicolas Marjanovic has received honorarium from Weinmann Emergency and Air Liquide Medical Systems for lectures.

References

1. The Acute Respiratory Distress Syndrome Network. Ventilation with lower tidal volumes as compared with traditional tidal volumes for acute lung injury and the acute respiratory distress syndrome. NEJM. 2000;342:1301–8.
2. Mercat A, Richard JC, Vielle B, Jaber S, Osman D, Diehl JL, et al. Positive end-expiratory pressure setting in adults with acute lung injury and acute respiratory distress syndrome: a randomized controlled trial. JAMA. 2008;299:646–55.
3. Thille AW, Rodriguez P, Cabello B, Lellouche F, Brochard L. Patient-ventilator asynchrony during assisted mechanical ventilation. Intensive Care Med. 2000;32:1515–22.
4. Chatburn RL, El-Khatib M, Mireles-Cabodevila E. A taxonomy for mechanical ventilation: 10 fundamental maxims. Respir Care. 2014;59:1747–63.
5. Richard JC, Carlucci A, Breton L, Langlais N, Jaber S, Maggiore S, et al. Bench testing of pressure support ventilation with three different generations of ventilators. Intensive Care Med. 2002;28:1049–57.
6. Lyazidi A, Thille AW, Carteaux G, Galia F, Brochard L, Richard JC. Bench test evaluation of volume delivered by modern ICU ventilators during volume-controlled ventilation. Intensive Care Med. 2010;36:2074–80.
7. Thille AW, Lyazidi A, Richard JC, Galia F, Brochard L. A bench study of intensive-care-unit ventilators: new versus old and turbine-based versus compressed gas-based ventilators. Intensive Care Med. 2009;35:1368–76.
8. L'Her E, Roy A, Marjanovic N. Bench-test comparison of 26 emergency and transport ventilators. Crit Care. 2014;18:506.
9. Boussen S, Gainnier M, Michelet P. Evaluation of ventilators used during transport of critically Ill patients: a bench study. Respir Care. 2013;58:1911–22.
10. Institute of Medicine. To err is human: building a safer health system. Washington: The National Academies Press; 1999.
11. Horsky J, Zhang J, Patel VL. To err is not entirely human: complex technology and user cognition. J Biomed Inform. 2005;38:264–6.
12. Richard JC, Kacmarek RM. ICU mechanical ventilators, technological advances vs. user friendliness: the right picture is worth a thousand numbers. Intensive Care Med. 2009;35:1662–3.
13. Templier F, Miroux P, Dolveck F, Descatha A, Goddet NS, Jeleff C, et al. Evaluation of the ventilator-user interface of 2 new advanced compact transport ventilators. Respir Care. 2007;52:1701–9.
14. Uzawa Y, Yamada Y, Suzukawa M. Evaluation of the user interface simplicity in the modern generation of mechanical ventilators. Respir Care. 2008;53:329–37.
15. Vignaux L, Tassaux D, Jolliet P. Evaluation of the user-friendliness of seven new generation intensive care ventilators. Intensive Care Med. 2009;35:1687–91.
16. Gonzalez-Bermejo J, Laplanche V, Husseini FE, Duguet A, Derenne JP, Similowski T. Evaluation of the user-friendliness of 11 home mechanical ventilators. Eur Respir J. 2006;27:1236–43.
17. Garnier M, Quesnel C, Fulgencio JP, Degrain M, Carteaux G, Bonnet F, et al. Multifaceted bench comparative evaluation of latest intensive care unit ventilators. Br J Anaesth. 2015;115:89–98.
18. Chao DC, Scheinhorn DJ, Stearn-Hassenpflug M. Patient-ventilator trigger asynchrony in prolonged mechanical ventilation. Chest. 1997;112:1592–9.
19. Vitacca M, Bianchi L, Zanotti E, Vianello A, Barbano L, Porta R, et al. Assessment of physiologic variables and subjective comfort under different levels of pressure support ventilation. Chest. 2004;126:851–9.
20. Brooke J. SUS: A quick and dirty usability scale. In: Jordan PW, Weerdmeester B, Thomas A, McLelland IL, editors. Usability evaluation in industry. London: Taylor and Francis; 1996.
21. Vignaux L, Vargas F, Roeseler J, Tassaux D, Thille AW, Kossowsky MP, et al. Patient-ventilator asynchrony during non-invasive ventilation for acute respiratory failure: a multicenter study. Intensive Care Med. 2009;35:840–6.
22. Vignaux L, Tassaux D, Jolliet P. Performance of noninvasive ventilation modes on ICU ventilators during pressure support: a bench model study. Intensive Care Med. 2007;33:1444–51.
23. Carteaux G, Lyazidi A, Cordoba-Izquierdo A, Vignaux L, Jolliet P, Thille AW, et al. Patient-ventilator asynchrony during noninvasive ventilation: a bench and clinical study. Chest. 2012;142:367–76.
24. Giraud T, Dhainaut JF, Vaxelaire JF, Joseph T, Journois D. Bleichner G Iatrogenic complications in adult intensive care units: a prospective two-center study. CCM. 1993;21:40–51.
25. Bracco D, Favre JB, Bissonnette B, Wasserfallen JB, Revelly JP, Ravussin P, et al. Human errors in a multidisciplinary intensive care unit: a 1-year prospective study. Intensive Care Med. 2001;27:137–45.
26. Garrouste-Orgeas M, Philippart F, Bruel C, Max A, Lau N, Misset B. Overview of medical errors and adverse events. Ann Intensive Care. 2012;2:2.
27. Cowan N. The magical number 4 in short-term memory: a reconsideration of mental storage capacity. Behav Brain Sci. 2001;24:87–114 **(discussion 114–185)**.
28. Morita PP, Weinstein PB, Flewwelling CJ, Banez CA, Chiu TA, Iannuzzi M, et al. The usability of ventilators: a comparative evaluation of use safety and user experience. Crit Care. 2016;20:263.
29. Hess EH, Polt JM. Pupil size in relation to mental activity during simple problem-solving. Science. 1964;143:1190–2.
30. Beatty J, Kahneman D. Pupillary changes in two memory tasks. Psychon Sci. 2013;5:371–2.
31. Chen S, Epps J, Chen F. An investigation of pupil-based cognitive load measurement with low cost infrared webcam under light reflex interference. In: Conference proceedings: annual international conference of the IEEE engineering in medicine and biology society IEEE engineering in medicine and biology society annual conference. 2013. p. 3202–05.
32. Boiten FA. The effects of emotional behaviour on components of the respiratory cycle. Biol Psychol. 1998;49:29–51.
33. Boiten FA, Frijda NH, Wientjes CJ. Emotions and respiratory patterns: review and critical analysis. Int J Psychophysiol. 1994;17:103–28.

34. Anttonen J, Surakka V. Emotions and heart rate while sitting on a chair. In: Anttonen J, Surakka V, editors. Book emotions and heart rate while sitting on a chair. New York: ACM; 2005. p. 491–9.
35. Hart SG, Staveland LE. Development of NASA-TLX (Task Load Index): results of empirical and theoretical research. In: Peter AH, Najmedin M, editors. Advances in psychology. Amsterdam: North-Holland; 1988. p. 139–83.
36. Hart S. Nasa-Task Load Index (Nasa-TLX); 20 years later. In: Hart S (ed) Book Nasa-Task Load Index (Nasa-TLX); 20 years later. City;2006.
37. McLellan S, Muddimer A, Peres SC. The effect of experience on System Usability Scale ratings. J Usability Stud. 2012;7:56–67.
38. Martin JL, Norris BJ, Murphy E, Crowe JA. Medical device development: the challenge for ergonomics. Appl Ergon. 2008;39:271–83.
39. Alessi SM. Fidelity in the design of instructional simulations. J Comput Based Instruct. 1988;15:40–7.

10

Systemic antibiotics for preventing ventilator-associated pneumonia in comatose patients

Cássia Righy[1,2*], Pedro Emmanuel Americano do Brasil[1], Jordi Vallés[3,4], Fernando A. Bozza[1,5] and Ignacio Martin-Loeches[3,6,7]

Abstract

Background: Early-onset ventilator-associated pneumonia (EO-VAP) is the leading cause of morbidity and mortality in comatose patients. However, VAP prevention bundles focus mainly on late-onset VAP and may be less effective in preventing EO-VAP in comatose patients. Systemic antibiotic administration at the time of intubation may have a role in preventing EO-VAP. Therefore, we evaluated the effectiveness of systemic antibiotic administration in VAP prevention in comatose patients through a systematic review and meta-analysis.

Methods: We searched for studies published through December 2015 that evaluated systemic antibiotic prophylaxis in comatose patients. Two authors independently selected and evaluated full-length reports of randomized clinical trials or prospective cohorts in patients aged >16 years that evaluated the impact of systemic antibiotics at the time of intubation on EO-VAP compared to placebo or no prophylaxis. The outcome variables were the incidence of EO-VAP, the duration of mechanical ventilation, ICU length of stay, and ICU mortality.

Results: We identified 10,988 citations, yielding 26 articles for further analysis; three studies with 267 patients were finally analyzed. Most patients ($n = 135$) were comatose due to head trauma. Systemic antibiotic administration was associated with decreased incidence of EO-VAP (RR 0.32; 95% CI 0.19–0.54) and shorter ICU LOS (standardized mean difference −0.32; 95% CI −0.56 to −0.08), but had no effect on mortality (RR 1.03; 95% CI 0.7–1.53) or duration of mechanical ventilation (standardized mean difference −0.16; 95% CI −0.41 to 0.08).

Conclusions: Antibiotic prophylaxis in comatose patients reduced the incidence of EO-VAP and decreased the ICU stay slightly. Future trials are needed to confirm these results.

Keywords: Systematic review, Meta-analysis, Ventilator-associated pneumonia, Coma

Background

Ventilator-associated pneumonia (VAP) is a frequent cause of morbidity and mortality in comatose patients. In this population, pneumonia usually occurs within the first four days of mechanical ventilation and is termed early-onset pneumonia (EO-VAP) [1]. The incidence of EO-VAP ranges from 21 to 60% [2, 3] in critically ill patients with traumatic brain injury (TBI) and is about 48% in those with subarachnoid hemorrhage. In a mixed population of patients in coma due to various causes, EO-VAP accounted for 70% of all cases of pneumonia [4]. In neurosurgical patients, the incidence of VAP peaks in the first three days after admission [5]. Pneumonia is associated with higher mortality in acute neurological patients [6]; a recent meta-analysis by the Cochrane Group found that pneumonia in stroke patients is associated with mortality (OR 3.62) [7]. Jovanovic et al. [8] found that VAP was associated with higher and earlier mortality in comatose patients with TBI.

The predominance of EO-VAP in comatose patients is in striking contrast to general critical care patients,

*Correspondence: cassiarighy@gmail.com
[1] National Institute of Infectious Disease Evandro Chagas, Oswaldo Cruz Foundation (FIOCRUZ), Rio de Janeiro, Brazil
Full list of author information is available at the end of the article

in whom accounts for 62–73% of all cases of VAP are late onset [9, 10]. Many risk factors are related to the increased incidence of EO-VAP in brain-injured patients. Massive or microbronchoaspiration, leakage of colonized subglottic secretions around the cuff of the endotracheal tube, and brain injury-induced immunosuppression may all play significant roles [11]. Moreover, it is not always feasible to implement VAP prevention bundles in brain-injured patients [12], and preventive measures that are effective for late-onset VAP might not be effective for EO-VAP [13]. Thus, alternative prophylactic measures should be explored in comatose patients.

Among other measures, antibiotic administration at the time of intubation seems a reasonable alternative. Systemic antibiotics have been reported to protect against EO-VAP [14]. However, the role of antibiotic prophylaxis in comatose patients remains unclear. Therefore, we performed a systematic review and meta-analysis of prospective studies to answer the following question: Is the administration of systemic antibiotics at the time of intubation superior to placebo or no prophylaxis in preventing VAP and decreasing all-cause mortality reduction in comatose patients?

Methods

Data sources and study selection

Following the methodological recommendations of the Cochrane Collaboration and the PRISMA statement [15], two authors (CR and IML) independently searched PubMed and the Cochrane Library (2015) for the terms aspiration pneumonia, pneumonia, ventilator-associated pneumonia (VAP), coma, altered level of consciousness, and depressed level of consciousness, cross-referenced to the terms antibiotic prophylaxis, and preemptive antibiotic therapy. The search strategy performed was the following:

First Search: #1

Search (((((((((aspiration pneumonia[MeSH Terms]) OR "pneumonia"[MeSH Terms]) OR "pneumonia, ventilator associated"[MeSHTerms]) OR respiratory infections[MeSH Terms]) AND coma[MeSH Terms]) OR altered level of consciousness[MeSH Terms]) OR depressed level of consciousness[MeSH Terms]) OR consciousness disorder[MeSH Terms]) OR consciousness, loss of[MeSH Terms]) AND antibiotic prophylaxis[MeSHTerms]) OR antibiotic premedication[MeSH Terms].

Second Search: #2

Search ((((((((("aspiration pneumonia"[Title/Abstract]) OR"pneumonia"[Title/Abstract]) OR "ventilator associated pneumonia"[Title/Abstract]) OR "respiratory infection"[Title/Abstract])AND "coma"[Title/Abstract]) OR "depressed level of consciousness"[Title/Abstract]) AND "antibiotic prophylaxis"[Title/Abstract]) OR "antibiotic premedication"[Title/Abstract]) OR "preemptive antibiotic treatment"[Title/Abstract]) OR "preemptive antibiotic therapy"[Title/Abstract].

Third Search:

#1 OR #2

Then, we manually searched personal files for full-length articles published in peer-reviewed journals by May 12 (2017). We selected the inclusion criteria for articles using the PICO approach. The inclusion criteria were: (1) clinical trials or prospective cohorts; (2) population analyzed—adult (>18 years) comatose patients; (3) intervention—systemic antibiotic prophylaxis at the time, or just before orotracheal intubation; (4) control group—patients who did not receive antibiotics for intubation; and (5) outcome—studies that evaluated VAP incidence, ICU and hospital mortality, as well as length of hospital stay and length of mechanical ventilation. We excluded studies that did not report enough data to estimate the odds ratio (OR) or relative risk (RR) and their variance.

Two authors (CR and IML) screened citations and articles identified by the initial search, selecting potentially relevant titles, reviewing their abstracts, and determining whether the articles met the inclusion criteria. We also searched the reference lists in the selected articles to look for any study that was not identified in the original search. The protocol was published in the International Prospective Register of Systematic Reviews (PROSPERO identifier: CRD42016033698).

Data extraction and study quality assessment

Two authors (CR and IML) independently abstracted data from the selected articles, recording the following information, when available:

- Study characteristics (study location, period of enrollment, criteria for patient enrollment, number of patients enrolled, duration of follow-up);
- Study design;
- Patients' characteristics (age, sex, mechanical ventilation, disease severity, cause of coma, and Glasgow Outcome Scale);
- VAP definition (early and late onset);
- Antibiotic therapy and controls;
- Outcomes (incidence of VAP (early and late); ICU and hospital mortality; duration of mechanical ventilation; ICU and hospital length of stay).

Any discrepancies were resolved by discussion among authors (CRS, IML, FAB). If data were not reported, we planned to contact first or senior authors by email.

To assess the methodological quality of the studies included, we used the Cochrane Risk of Bias Tool (for

RCT) [16] and the Newcastle-Ottawa Score, for observational studies.

Outcomes

The main outcomes of interest were incidence of VAP (early and late) and ICU and hospital mortality. The secondary outcomes were ICU and hospital length of stay as well as duration of mechanical ventilation.

Patient involvement

This review and meta-analysis did not involve patients directly.

Statistical analysis

We compared patients' characteristics and outcomes between the group of patients who received antibiotic prophylaxis and those who did not (control group). Primary outcome variables were the incidence of EO-VAP and ICU mortality; secondary outcome variables were ICU length of stay and duration of mechanical ventilation.

Primary outcome variables are reported as relative risks (RR) with their corresponding 95% confidence intervals (CI), analyzed with the Mantel–Haenszel fixed-effects method. Secondary outcome variables are reported as standardized mean differences (SMD) with their respective 95% CI. To assess the impact of heterogeneity across studies on the meta-analysis, we used the I^2 statistic, which reflects the amount of heterogeneity between studies over and above the sampling variation and is robust to the number of studies and choice of effect measure. We used the R statistical package for all analyses.

Results

The literature search produced 11,340 citation titles, yielding 26 articles for detailed analysis; three studies including a total of 267 patients met the inclusion criteria and were included in the systematic review (Fig. 1).

Definitions

All studies defined EO-VAP as pneumonia developed within the first four days of mechanical ventilation. Clinical criteria for VAP definition varied among the studies; however, all studies required a microbiological confirmation of pneumonia—either by bronchoalveolar lavage (BAL) or by protected brush sampling or by tracheal

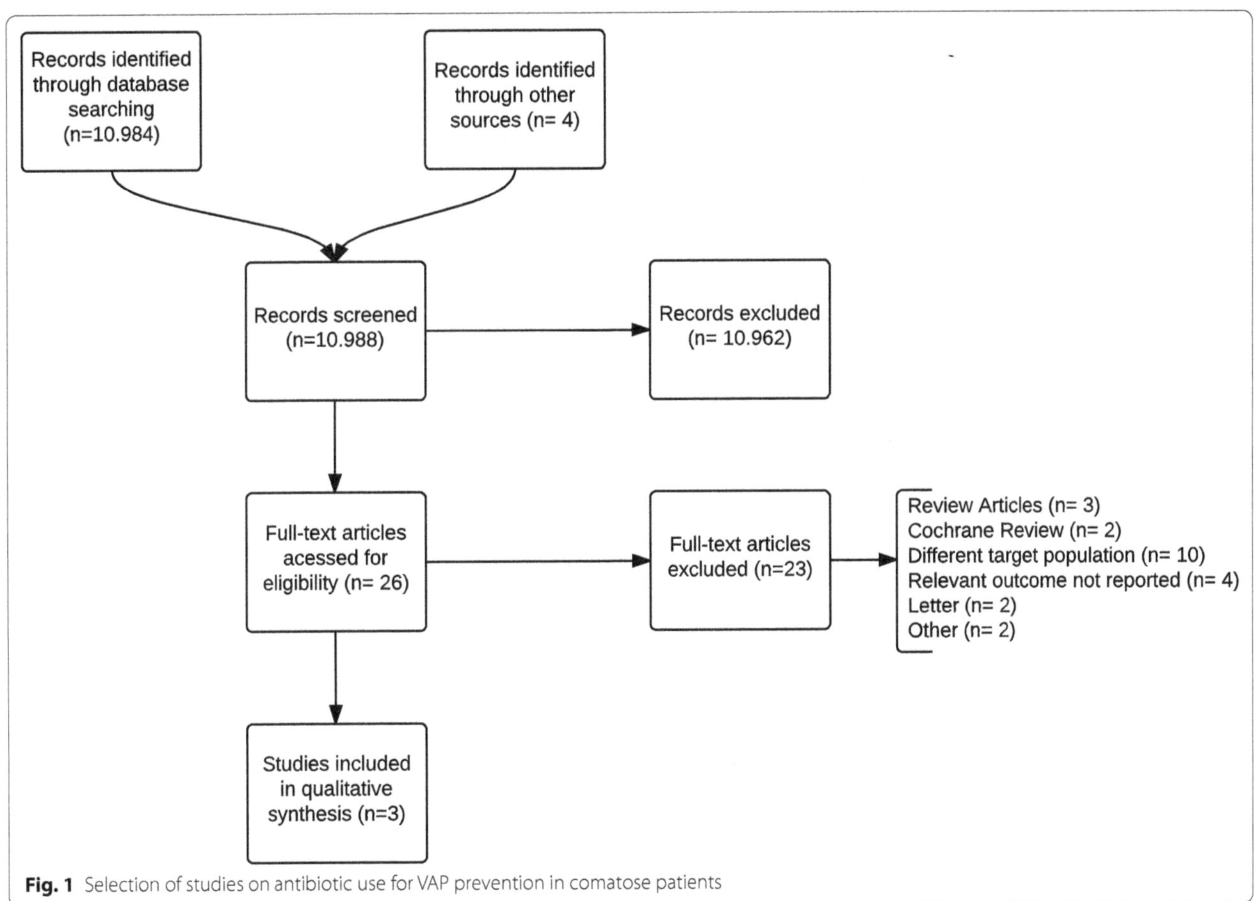

Fig. 1 Selection of studies on antibiotic use for VAP prevention in comatose patients

aspirate. The definition of coma also varied—Vallés et al. [17] and Acquarolo et al. [18] defined as a Glasgow Coma Scale (GCS) ≤ 8 and Sirvent et al. [4] defined it as a GCS ≤ 12. The definitions are summarized in Table 1.

Characteristics of the studies included

The meta-analysis included two randomized clinical trials and one prospective observational cohort with a non-randomized historical control group. Table 2 provides

Table 1 Studies' characteristics

	Sirvent JM et al.		Acquarolo A et al.		Vallés J et al.	
Year published	**1997**		**2007**		**2013**	
Country	**Spain**		**Italy**		**Spain**	
Study design	**RCT**		**RCT**		**Prospective study with historical control or non-randomized control**	
Inclusion criteria	**Head injury or coma due to stroke or surgery for space occupying lesions with Glasgow ≤ 12**		**Adults, comatose patients (GCS ≤ 8) in mechanical ventilation**		**Adults, comatose patients (GCS ≤ 8) in mechanical ventilation**	
Tested antibiotic	**Cefuroxime**		**Ampicillin–sulbactam**		**Ceftriaxone or ertapenem or levofloxacin**	
Antibiotics used in control group?[b]	**Yes**		**Yes**		**No**	
	Intervention group	**Control group**	**Intervention group**	**Control group**	**Intervention group**	**Control group**
Number of subjects	50	50	19	19	71	58
Age (mean ± SD), years	42 ± 20	37 ± 21	54.8 (18.0)[a]	54.6 (17.7)[a]	56 ± 19	59 ± 16
Male gender, *n* (%)	34 (68%)	40 (80%)	13 (68.4%)	12 (63.2%)	48 (67.6%)	43 (74.1%)
Glasgow Coma Scale (mean ± SD)	7.5 ± 2.4	8.0 ± 1.8	5 (3–7)[a]	5 (4–7)[a]	5 ± 2	5 ± 2
APACHE II (mean ± SD)	14 ± 5	13 ± 5	20 (17–24)[a]	22 (18–23)[a]	17 ± 7	18 ± 7
Early VAP, *n* (%)	8 (16%)	18 (36%)	4 (21%)	11 (57.8%)	2 (2.8%)	13 (22.4%)
Late VAP, *n* (%)	4 (8%)	7 (14%)	10 (episodes)	9 (episodes)	6.5 (incidence/1000 days MV)	5.3 (incidence/1000 days MV)
Total VAP, *n* (%)	12 (24%)	25 (50%)	14 (episodes)	20 (episodes)	10.8 (incidence/1000 days MV)	28.4 (incidence/1000 days MV)
Duration of mechanical ventilation (mean ± SD), days	4.6 ± 1.5	4.4 ± 2.1	9.9 (6.9)[a]	10.6 (9.4)[a]	6.4 ± 6.5	9.7 ± 9.6
ICU LOS (mean ± SD), days	13 ± 8	16 ± 11	12.8 (8.7)[a]	12.6 (9.7)[a]	9.7 ± 9.8	14.9 ± 13.9
Hospital LOS (mean ± SD), days	27 ± 16	28 ± 13	Not informed	Not informed	17.5 ± 17.7	23.5 ± 24.3
ICU mortality, *n* (%)	10 (20%)	7 (14%)	7 (36.8%)	8 (42.1%)	21 (29.6%)	18 (31%)

RCT randomized controlled trial, *VAP* ventilator-associated pneumonia, *LOS* length of stay, *APACHE II* Acute Physiology and Chronic Health Evaluation II, *MV* mechanical ventilation

[a] Median (interquartile range)

[b] Antibiotics used mainly as surgical prophylaxis

Table 2 Summary of the quality evaluation by Jadad Scale of clinical trials of antibiotic prophylaxis in comatose patients

	Randomization	Blinding	Description of withdrawals and dropout	Score
Sirvent JM	2	0	1	3
Acquarolo A	2	2	1	5
Vallés J	0	0	1	1

detailed information about the three studies. Study populations ranged from 38 to 129 patients. The most common cause of coma was head trauma ($n = 135$), followed by stroke ($n = 49$) and cardiac arrest ($n = 37$). All studies evaluated EO-VAP, defined as VAP acquired within four days after intubation for mechanical ventilation. All studies reported short-term outcomes (ICU mortality, duration of mechanical ventilation, and ICU LOS). Two studies also evaluated hospital mortality. Table 3 provides details about the Jadad Scale evaluation of the methodological quality of the studies. There was no heterogeneity among the studies in the main outcomes.

Main outcomes

Figure 2 shows the association between systemic antibiotic administration and the outcomes of interest. The RR of EO-VAP was 0.32 (95% CI 0.19–0.54, $p < 0.01$), favoring the intervention group, which suggests a protective effect, and the RR of ICU mortality was 1.03 (95% CI 0.7–1.53, $p = 0.88$), showing no protective effect.

Antibiotic administration did not affect the duration of mechanical ventilation (SMD: −0.16; 95% CI −0.41–0.08, $p = 0.18$), but decreased ICU LOS slightly (SMD: −0.32; 95% CI −0.56 to −0.08, $p < 0.01$), indicating that antibiotic prophylaxis reduced the ICU stay by 9 h on average.

Table 3 VAP microbiology

	Early VAP	Late VAP
Sirvent et al.	*S. aureus*—14	Enterobacter—1
	H. influenzae—11	Serratia—2
	Strep pneumoniae—1	Proteus—1
		P. aeruginosa—4
		Acinetobacter sp—3
Vallés et al.	*S. aureus*—3	E cloacae—3
	Anaerobes—1	*S. aureus*—1
	Mixed flora—1	*P. aeruginosa*—3
		Streptococcus sp—1
Total	*S. aureus*—17	*P. aeruginosa*—7
	H. influenza—11	E cloacae/Acinetobacter sp—3 each
	S. pneumoniae/Anaerobes/ mixed flora—1 each	Serratia—2
		Enterobacter/Proteus/*S. aureus*/*Streptococcus* sp—1 each

Discussion

Antibiotic prophylaxis seems effective in preventing EO-VAP in a mixed cohort of comatose patients and may also decrease the ICU LOS slightly; however, it had no effect on the length of mechanical ventilation or ICU mortality.

One explanation for the decrease in the incidence of EO-VAP in comatose patients receiving antibiotic prophylaxis is the reduction of bacterial inoculum in the lungs. After brain injury, many concurrent phenomena act to increase the bacterial burden within the alveolar space: micro- or macroaspiration, brain-induced immunosuppression, or even increased capillary leakage from sympathetic overstimulation [19]. Antibiotic administration may prevent the propagation of bacteria into the lung, thereby preventing EO-VAP, whereas many traditional prophylactic measures included in the VAP bundle may be less effective in brain-injured patients.

EO-VAP is frequent in critically ill acute neurological patients. Although we found no impact of antibiotic prophylaxis on ICU mortality, preventing EO-VAP may reduce overall antibiotic use and costs, improve functional prognosis, and indirectly decrease long-term mortality. Finlayson et al. [20] showed that, in patients with ischemic stroke, pneumonia is associated with higher 30-day and 1-year mortality, as well as with a poorer functional outcome. While mortality from infection is estimated to account for up to 30% of stroke deaths and infection is an independent predictor of neurological deterioration, patients that have a decrease in EO-VAP did not show significantly different mortality [21]; this kind of cases are specially complex and might present some complications especially common in this subset of patients. In addition, while the mortality represents a very robust outcome, we consider that mortality could be analyzed cautiously just because of the impact of this intervention. Moreover, infection is the primary cause of readmission after stroke [22]. Hospital-acquired pneumonia is independently associated with poor functional outcome up to 5 years after TBI [23].

Our meta-analysis also found that antibiotic prophylaxis decreased ICU LOS slightly, possibly due to the decrease in EO-VAP. Just as treating tracheobronchitis can lead to a reduction in VAP and consequent reduction in ICU LOS [24, 25], prophylaxis against EO-VAP may have an impact in reducing ICU LOS and may also affect functional outcomes. However, none of the studies included in the meta-analysis was designed to evaluate functional outcome, so we could not assess the effect of antibiotic prophylaxis on long-term prognosis.

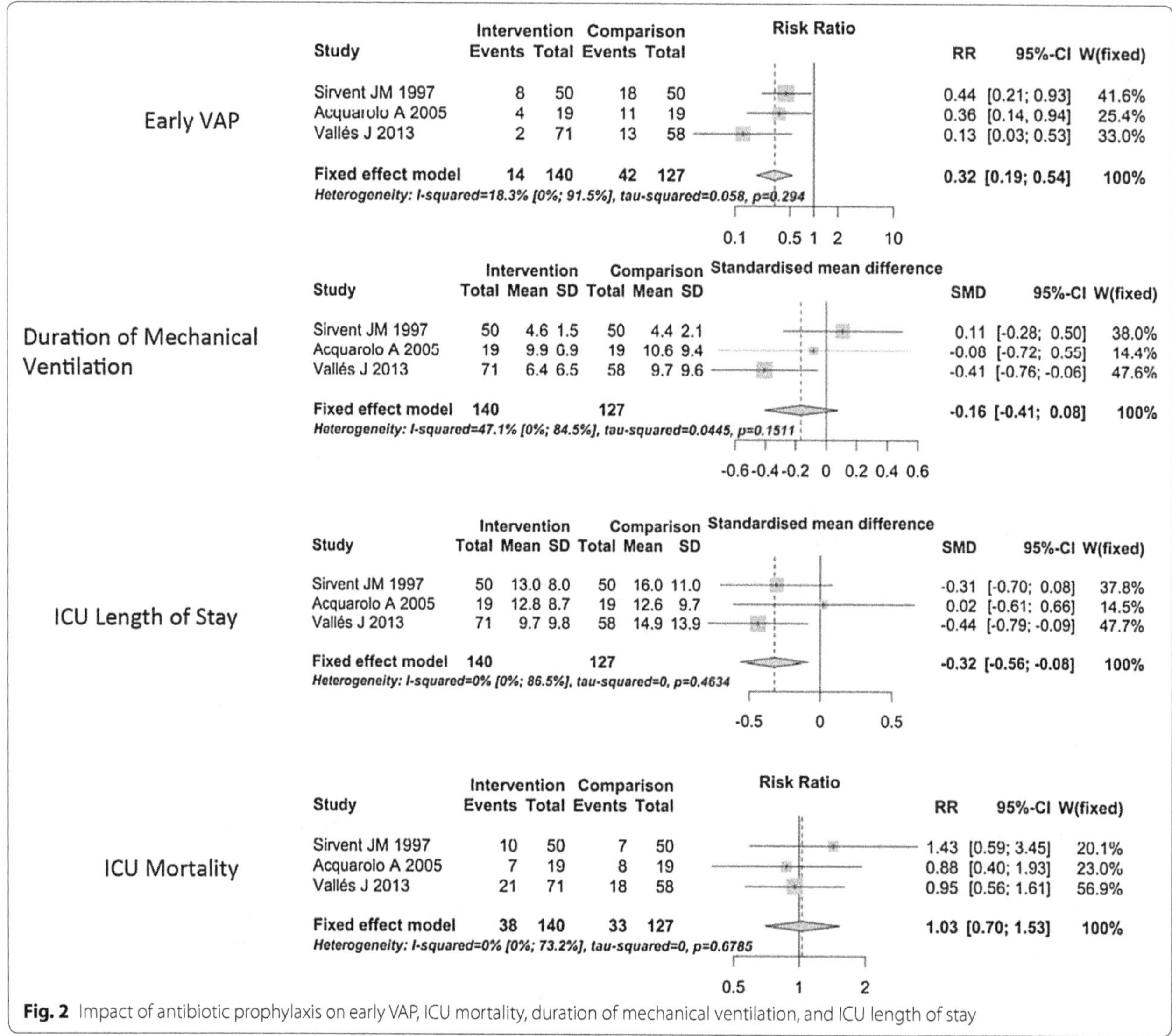

Fig. 2 Impact of antibiotic prophylaxis on early VAP, ICU mortality, duration of mechanical ventilation, and ICU length of stay

Whether antibiotic prophylaxis induces bacterial resistance is a well-founded concern. An association between broad-spectrum systemic antibiotics and the development of antibiotic resistance was pointed out a decade ago [26]. Depuydt et al. [27] showed VAP involving multidrug-resistant pathogens was associated with higher mortality and that the risk of developing VAP involving multiresistant bacteria was associated with previous antibiotic use. These findings have led to the development of antibiotic stewardship programs that minimize antibiotic exposure to diminish resistance to antibiotics and improve outcomes [28].

However, the use of one- or two-dose prophylactic antibiotic regimens may not be as deleterious to the patient and ICU ecology as prolonged, inadequate antibiotic administration. In a landmark randomized controlled trial, Chastre et al. [29] showed that multidrug-resistant pathogens emerged less frequently in recurrent infections developing in patients assigned to an 8-day course of antibiotic than in those developing in patients assigned to a 15-day course (42.1 vs. 62.3%). In neutropenic patients, quinolone prophylaxis was not associated with increased antimicrobial resistance [30], and in cardiac surgery patients, antibiotic resistance was associated only with antibiotic prophylaxis for more than 48 h [31]. Although our meta-analysis was not planned to analyze this issue, none of the studies included reported any increase in multidrug-resistant pathogens. This finding suggests that very short antibiotic regimens may not lead to greater resistance, but this hypothesis must be confirmed in future trials.

Antibiotic prophylaxis is a simple and cheap measure that can be easily reproduced all around the world. Other prophylactic measures have not proven effective. Corticosteroid administration was not effective in preventing nosocomial pneumonia in TBI patients, although the overall incidence of pneumonia in this study was lower than expected [32]. The effectiveness of beta-blockers [33, 34], or statins [35, 36], in preventing pneumonia in stroke patients is controversial and must be tested in future trials.

This meta-analysis has some limitations. First and most importantly, numbers of studies are low, which has consequences for the interpretation of the data and may amplify a hypothetically minor impact on pneumonia prevention. We would, however, highlight our surprise in such an easy intervention and the low number of studies conducted when compared to the literature of more complex interventions [37, 38]. Based on the low number of patients in each subgroup and the lack of individual information, we considered that more exploratory analyses such as: (1) dose of antibiotic; (2) time of initiation; and (3) type of antibiotic would increase the heterogeneity and would not allow robust conclusions. Moreover, most patients were admitted to intensive care for TBI, and this patient mix might limit the generalizability of our results. Finally, the broad-spectrum antibiotic regimens tested varied among the different studies. Despite the common goal of preventing EO-VAP, these differences in antibiotic use, dosage, and timing of administration may preclude the analysis of their impact as a single group. However, the results of this meta-analysis support the hypothesis that antibiotic prophylaxis reduces EO-VAP without increasing antimicrobial resistance.

Conclusion

This meta-analysis found that antibiotic prophylaxis in comatose patients reduced the incidence of EO-VAP and decreased ICU LOS slightly. However, a larger randomized trial focusing on measuring both the decrease in the incidence of EO-VAP and possible improvements in long-term functional outcomes is needed to confirm these findings. The 2005 ATS guidelines on hospital-acquired pneumonia concluded that although administering antibiotics at the time of intubation may prevent EO-VAP, its routine use could not be recommended until more evidence was available [39]. The current IDSA/ATS guidelines do not make any recommendation regarding antibiotic prophylaxis against EO-VAP [40]. We were surprised that a non-complex intervention has been not widely studied. We think that the results of this meta-analysis strongly support undertaking new clinical trials in the incidence of EO-VAP in other subsets of critically ill patients and possible improvements in long-term functional.

Authors' contributions

IML had full access to the data in the study and takes responsibility for the integrity of the data and the accuracy of the data analysis. CR and IML independently searched and assisted in collection of the data. PA assisted in analysis and interpretation of the results. JV, IML, CR, PA, FB contributed substantially to the study design, interpretation of the data, and writing and critical revision of the manuscript. All authors read and approved the final manuscript.

Author details

[1] National Institute of Infectious Disease Evandro Chagas, Oswaldo Cruz Foundation (FIOCRUZ), Rio de Janeiro, Brazil. [2] ICU, Paulo Niemeyer Brain Institute, Rio de Janeiro, Brazil. [3] CIBER Enfermedades Respiratorias (CIBERES), Barcelona, Spain. [4] Critical Care Center, CIBER Enfermedades Respiratorias, Hospital Sabadell, Sabadell, Spain. [5] IDOR, D'Or Institute for Research and Education, Rio de Janeiro, Brazil. [6] Department of Clinical Medicine, Trinity Centre for Health Sciences, Multidisciplinary Intensive Care Research Organization (MICRO), Wellcome Trust, HRB Clinical Research, St James's University Hospital Dublin, Dublin, Ireland. [7] Irish Centre for Vascular Biology (ICVB), Dublin, Ireland.

Competing interests

The authors declare that they have no competing interests.

Funding

Clinical Research Collaboration (CRC) by European Respiratory Society.

References

1. Zilahi G, Artigas A, Martin-Loeches I. What's new in multidrug-resistant pathogens in the ICU? Ann Intensive Care. 2016;6:96. doi:10.1186/s13613-016-0199-4.
2. Bronchard R, Albaladejo P, Brezac G, et al. Early onset pneumonia: risk factors and consequences in head trauma patients. Anesthesiology. 2004;100:234–9.
3. Lepelletier D, Roquilly A, Demeure dit latte D, et al. Retrospective analysis of the risk factors and pathogens associated with early-onset ventilator-associated pneumonia in surgical-ICU head-trauma patients. J Neurosurg Anesthesiol. 2010;22:32–7. doi:10.1097/ANA.0b013e3181bdf52f.
4. Sirvent JM, Torres A, El-Ebiary M, et al. Protective effect of intravenously administered cefuroxime against nosocomial pneumonia in patients with structural coma. Am J Respir Crit Care Med. 1997;155:1729–34.
5. Berrouane Y, Daudenthun I, Riegel B, et al. Early onset pneumonia in neurosurgical intensive care unit patients. J Hosp Infect. 1998;40:275–80.
6. Ruhnke AM, Paiva J, Meersseman W, et al. Online Supplementary Appendix Article title: Anidulafungin for the treatment of candidaemia/invasive candidiasis in selected critically ill patients.
7. Westendorp WF, Vermeij J-D, Vermeij F, et al. Antibiotic therapy for preventing infections in patients with acute stroke. Cochrane Database Syst Rev. 2012;1:CD008530. doi:10.1002/14651858.CD008530.pub2.
8. Jovanovic B, Milan Z, Djuric O, et al. Twenty-eight-day mortality of blunt traumatic brain injury and co-injuries requiring mechanical ventilation. Med Princ Pract Int J Kuwait Univ Health Sci Cent. 2016;25:435–41. doi:10.1159/000447566.
9. Giard M, Lepape A, Allaouchiche B, et al. Early- and late-onset ventilator-associated pneumonia acquired in the intensive care unit: comparison of risk factors. J Crit Care. 2008;23:27–33. doi:10.1016/j.jcrc.2007.08.005.
10. Vallés J, Pobo A, García-Esquirol O, et al. Excess ICU mortality attributable to ventilator-associated pneumonia: the role of early vs late onset. Intensive Care Med. 2007;33:1363–8. doi:10.1007/s00134-007-0721-0.
11. Winklewski PJ, Radkowski M, Demkow U. Cross-talk between the inflammatory response, sympathetic activation and pulmonary infection in the ischemic stroke. J Neuroinflamm. 2014;11:213. doi:10.1186/s12974-014-0213-4.
12. Croce MA, Brasel KJ, Coimbra R, et al. National Trauma Institute prospective evaluation of the ventilator bundle in trauma patients: Does it really work? J Trauma Acute Care Surg. 2013;74:354–60. doi:10.1097/TA.0b013e31827a0c65 **(discussion 360–362)**.
13. Seguin P, Laviolle B, Dahyot-Fizelier C, et al. Effect of oropharyngeal povidone-iodine preventive oral care on ventilator-associated pneumonia

in severely brain-injured or cerebral hemorrhage patients: a multicenter, randomized controlled trial. Crit Care Med. 2014;42:1–8. doi:10.1097/CCM.0b013e3182a2770f.
14. Bornstain C, Azoulay E, De Lassence A, et al. Sedation, sucralfate, and antibiotic use are potential means for protection against early-onset ventilator-associated pneumonia. Clin Infect Dis Off Publ Infect Dis Soc Am. 2004;38:1401–8. doi:10.1086/386321.
15. Moher D, Liberati A, Tetzlaff J, et al. Preferred reporting items for systematic reviews and meta-analyses: the PRISMA statement. PLoS Med. 2009;6:e1000097. doi:10.1371/journal.pmed.1000097.
16. Higgins JPT, Altman DG, Gøtzsche PC, et al. The Cochrane Collaboration's tool for assessing risk of bias in randomised trials. BMJ. 2011;343:d5928.
17. Vallés J, Peredo R, Burgueño MJ, et al. Efficacy of single-dose antibiotic against early-onset pneumonia in comatose patients who are ventilated. Chest. 2013;143:1219–25. doi:10.1378/chest.12-1361.
18. Acquarolo A, Urli T, Perone G, et al. Antibiotic prophylaxis of early onset pneumonia in critically ill comatose patients. A randomized study. Intensive Care Med. 2005;31:510–6. doi:10.1007/s00134-005-2585-5.
19. Mascia L. Acute lung injury in patients with severe brain injury: a double hit model. Neurocrit Care. 2009;11:417–26. doi:10.1007/s12028-009-9242-8.
20. Finlayson O, Kapral M, Hall R, et al. Risk factors, inpatient care, and outcomes of pneumonia after ischemic stroke. Neurology. 2011;77:1338–45. doi:10.1212/WNL.0b013e31823152b1.
21. Boehme AK, Kumar AD, Dorsey AM, et al. Infections present on admission compared with hospital-acquired infections in acute ischemic stroke patients. J Stroke Cerebrovasc Dis Off J Natl Stroke Assoc. 2013;22:e582–9. doi:10.1016/j.jstrokecerebrovasdis.2013.07.020.
22. Shah SV, Corado C, Bergman D, et al. Impact of poststroke medical complications on 30-day readmission rate. J Stroke Cerebrovasc Dis Off J Natl Stroke Assoc. 2015;24:1969–77. doi:10.1016/j.jstrokecerebrovasdis.2015.04.037.
23. Kesinger MR, Kumar RG, Wagner AK, et al. Hospital-acquired pneumonia is an independent predictor of poor global outcome in severe traumatic brain injury up to 5 years after discharge. J Trauma Acute Care Surg. 2015;78:396–402. doi:10.1097/TA.0000000000000526.
24. Martin-Loeches I, Povoa P, Rodríguez A, et al. Incidence and prognosis of ventilator-associated tracheobronchitis (TAVeM): a multicentre, prospective, observational study. Lancet Respir Med. 2015;3:859–68. doi:10.1016/S2213-2600(15)00326-4.
25. Nseir S, Martin-Loeches I, Makris D, et al. Impact of appropriate antimicrobial treatment on transition from ventilator-associated tracheobronchitis to ventilator-associated pneumonia. Crit Care Lond Engl. 2014;18:R129. doi:10.1186/cc13940.
26. Gould CV, Rothenberg R, Steinberg JP. Antibiotic resistance in long-term acute care hospitals: the perfect storm. Infect Control Hosp Epidemiol Off J Soc Hosp Epidemiol Am. 2006;27:920–5. doi:10.1086/507280.
27. Depuydt PO, Vandijck DM, Bekaert MA, et al. Determinants and impact of multidrug antibiotic resistance in pathogens causing ventilator-associated-pneumonia. Crit Care Lond Engl. 2008;12:R142. doi:10.1186/cc7119.
28. Schuts EC, Hulscher MEJL, Mouton JW, et al. Current evidence on hospital antimicrobial stewardship objectives: a systematic review and meta-analysis. Lancet Infect Dis. 2016;16:847–56. doi:10.1016/S1473-3099(16)00065-7.
29. Chastre J, Wolff M, Fagon J-Y, et al. Comparison of 8 vs 15 days of antibiotic therapy for ventilator-associated pneumonia in adults: a randomized trial. JAMA. 2003;290:2588–98. doi:10.1001/jama.290.19.2588.
30. Imran H, Tleyjeh IM, Arndt CAS, et al. Fluoroquinolone prophylaxis in patients with neutropenia: a meta-analysis of randomized placebo-controlled trials. Eur J Clin Microbiol Infect Dis Off Publ Eur Soc Clin Microbiol. 2008;27:53–63. doi:10.1007/s10096-007-0397-y.
31. Harbarth S, Samore MH, Lichtenberg D, Carmeli Y. Prolonged antibiotic prophylaxis after cardiovascular surgery and its effect on surgical site infections and antimicrobial resistance. Circulation. 2000;101:2916–21.
32. Asehnoune K, Seguin P, Allary J, et al. Hydrocortisone and fludrocortisone for prevention of hospital-acquired pneumonia in patients with severe traumatic brain injury (Corti-TC): a double-blind, multicentre phase 3, randomised placebo-controlled trial. Lancet Respir Med. 2014;2:706–16. doi:10.1016/S2213-2600(14)70144-4.
33. Maier IL, Karch A, Mikolajczyk R, et al. Effect of beta-blocker therapy on the risk of infections and death after acute stroke—a historical cohort study. PLoS ONE. 2015;10:e0116836. doi:10.1371/journal.pone.0116836.
34. Sykora M, Siarnik P, Diedler J, Acute Collaborators VISTA. β-Blockers, pneumonia, and outcome after ischemic stroke: evidence from virtual international stroke trials archive. Stroke J Cereb Circ. 2015;46:1269–74. doi:10.1161/STROKEAHA.114.008260.
35. Scheitz JF, Endres M, Heuschmann PU, et al. Reduced risk of post-stroke pneumonia in thrombolyzed stroke patients with continued statin treatment. Int J Stroke Off J Int Stroke Soc. 2015;10:61–6. doi:10.1111/j.1747-4949.2012.00864.x.
36. Rodríguez de Antonio LA, Martínez-Sánchez P, Martínez-Martínez MM, et al. Previous statins treatment and risk of post-stroke infections. Neurol Barc Spain. 2011;26:150–6. doi:10.1016/j.nrl.2010.07.030.
37. Pileggi C, Bianco A, Flotta D, et al. Prevention of ventilator-associated pneumonia, mortality and all intensive care unit acquired infections by topically applied antimicrobial or antiseptic agents: a meta-analysis of randomized controlled trials in intensive care units. Crit Care Lond Engl. 2011;15:R155. doi:10.1186/cc10285.
38. Bo L, Li J, Tao T, et al. Probiotics for preventing ventilator-associated pneumonia. Cochrane Database Syst Rev. 2014;. doi:10.1002/14651858.CD009066.pub2.
39. American Thoracic Society, Infectious Diseases Society of America. Guidelines for the management of adults with hospital-acquired, ventilator-associated, and healthcare-associated pneumonia. Am J Respir Crit Care Med. 2005;171:388–416. doi:10.1164/rccm.200405-644ST.
40. Kalil AC, Metersky ML, Klompas M, et al. Executive summary: management of adults with hospital-acquired and ventilator-associated pneumonia: 2016 clinical practice guidelines by the Infectious Diseases Society of America and the American Thoracic Society. Clin Infect Dis Off Publ Infect Dis Soc Am. 2016;63:575–82. doi:10.1093/cid/ciw504.

Bedside selection of positive end-expiratory pressure by electrical impedance tomography in hypoxemic patients

Nilde Eronia[1], Tommaso Mauri[2,3], Elisabetta Maffezzini[4], Stefano Gatti[4], Alfio Bronco[4], Laura Alban[2,3], Filippo Binda[3], Tommaso Sasso[2,3], Cristina Marenghi[3], Giacomo Grasselli[3], Giuseppe Foti[1,4], Antonio Pesenti[2,3] and Giacomo Bellani[1,4*]

Abstract

Background: Positive end-expiratory pressure (PEEP) is a key element of mechanical ventilation. It should optimize recruitment, without causing excessive overdistension, but controversy exists on the best method to set it. The purpose of the study was to test the feasibility of setting PEEP with electrical impedance tomography in order to prevent lung de-recruitment following a recruitment maneuver. We enrolled 16 patients undergoing mechanical ventilation with PaO_2/FiO_2 <300 mmHg. In all patients, under constant tidal volume (6–8 ml/kg) PEEP was set based on the PEEP/FiO_2 table proposed by the ARDS network ($PEEP_{ARDSnet}$). We performed a recruitment maneuver and monitored the end-expiratory lung impedance (EELI) over 10 min. If the EELI signal decreased during this period, the recruitment maneuver was repeated and PEEP increased by 2 cmH_2O. This procedure was repeated until the EELI maintained a stability over time ($PEEP_{EIT}$).

Results: The procedure was feasible in 87% patients. $PEEP_{EIT}$ was higher than $PEEP_{ARDSnet}$ (13 ± 3 vs. 9 ± 2 cmH_2O, $p < 0.001$). PaO_2/FiO_2 improved during $PEEP_{EIT}$ and driving pressure decreased. Recruited volume correlated with the decrease in driving pressure but not with oxygenation improvement. Finally, regional alveolar hyperdistention and collapse was reduced in dependent lung layers and increased in non-dependent lung layers.

Conclusions: In hypoxemic patients, a PEEP selection strategy aimed at stabilizing alveolar recruitment guided by EIT at the bedside was feasible and safe. This strategy led, in comparison with the ARDSnet table, to higher PEEP, improved oxygenation and reduced driving pressure, allowing to estimate the relative weight of overdistension and recruitment.

Keywords: EIT, PEEP, Overdistension, Recruitment

Background

Acute respiratory distress syndrome (ARDS) is a relatively common and severe form of respiratory failure, characterized by massive non-cardiogenic pulmonary edema, with consequent loss of aeration in the alveolar spaces [1]. ARDS patients require intubation and mechanical ventilation as lifesaving procedures, and positive end-expiratory pressure (PEEP) is a key element of mechanical ventilation settings. Since both lower and higher PEEP levels may be associated with significant adverse consequences [2], personalized PEEP setting might be of cornerstone importance. Ideally, PEEP should optimize recruitment to improve oxygenation and reduce lung strain, without causing excessive overdistension, but

*Correspondence: giacomo.bellani1@unimib.it
[4] Department of Medicine, School of Medicine and Surgery, University of Milan-Bicocca, Via Cadore 48, Monza, Italy
Full list of author information is available at the end of the article

controversy exists on the best bedside method to select PEEP. A common clinical approach is based on the severity of hypoxemia, relying on the use of PaO_2/FiO_2 tables [3]. Other approaches to select "personalized PEEP" are based on its effect on respiratory mechanics, focusing on plateau pressure [4], on stress index [5] or on transpulmonary pressure [6, 7]. These methods, however, do not provide consistent finding [8] and share the limitation of "lumping" into one measurement heterogeneous processes within the lung (i.e., recruitment, tidal opening–closing and overdistension [9, 10]) and of using surrogate rather than direct measures for lung recruitment induced by PEEP. In summary, bedside personalization of PEEP is still quite far from clinical practice. Randomized clinical trials have not shown clear benefit by indiscriminate application of high PEEP levels: Although a meta-analysis suggested that "higher" PEEP might be beneficial in moderate–severe ARDS [11], in everyday clinical practice clinicians still tend to apply relatively low PEEP levels even in severe ARDS patients [12].

In the present study, we hypothesized that the optimal PEEP level for each patient may be selected by assessing its efficacy in maintaining alveolar recruitment induced by a recruitment maneuver (RM). RMs are transient and voluntary increases in transpulmonary pressure that could reopen previously collapsed alveoli; they typically consist of application of continuous positive airway pressure of 30–50 cmH_2O for 20–40 s, or transient increases in PEEP and/or inspiratory pressure, with a consequent increase in end-expiratory lung volume (EELV), decrease in lung strain and improvement in patient's oxygenation [13, 14].

However, if RM is not followed by the application of adequate PEEP, EELV will progressively decrease over time (alveolar de-recruitment). At the opposite, RM plus adequate PEEP level will minimize de-recruitment and maintain sustained recruitment.

Electrical impedance tomography (EIT) is a noninvasive, radiation-free, bedside lung monitoring technique [15], that tracks real-time changes in regional lung ventilation and end-expiratory lung impedance (EELI), which closely correlate with EELV changes [16]. While several studies demonstrated the ability of EIT in assessing alveolar recruitment [17, 18], only a few used this method to guide therapy in humans [19]. The aim of the present study was to assess the feasibility of personalized PEEP selection based on its efficacy in stabilizing the EELV increase induced by a RM, using EIT as tool to monitor EELV changes. Moreover, we compared the effects of the selected PEEP on gas exchange, respiratory mechanics, hemodynamics and tidal recruitment/de-recruitment and overdistension with those induced by the application of PEEP levels selected according to $PEEP/FiO_2$ tables. This comparator was chosen because of its large acceptance in the clinical practice and the frequent use of this approach as a control in other studies aimed at testing physiological-based methods to titrate PEEP [4, 6].

Methods

The study was conducted in the general intensive care units of the university-affiliated hospitals San Gerardo, Monza and Fondazione IRCCS Ca' Granda Ospedale Maggiore Policlinico, Milan, both in Italy. Institutional ethical committees of each institution approved the study, and informed consent was obtained according to local recommendations. Inclusion criteria were as follows: patient with acute hypoxemic respiratory failure (PaO_2/FiO_2 ratio $\leq$300 mmHg) of non-cardiogenic origin undergoing controlled mechanical ventilation with PEEP $\geq$ 5 cmH_2O. Exclusion criteria were as follows: age <18 years, pregnancy, hemodynamic instability (requiring vasoactive drugs), presence of pneumothorax or lung emphysema, previous history of severe chronic obstructive pulmonary disease (GOLD III or IV), contraindications to the use of EIT (e.g., presence of pacemaker or automatic implantable cardioverter–defibrillator) and impossibility to place the EIT belt in the right position (e.g., presence of surgical wounds dressing). At enrollment, the following variables were collected: sex, age, predicted body weight (PBW), body mass index, Simplified Acute Physiology Score II (SAPS II) value at ICU admission, etiology of acute respiratory failure, diagnosis of ARDS and duration of intubation before enrollment. Vital status was recorded for all patients at ICU discharge.

EIT monitoring

An EIT-dedicated belt equipped with 16 electrodes was placed around each patient's chest at the fifth or sixth intercostal space and connected to a commercial EIT monitor (PulmoVista® 500, Dräger Medical GmbH, Lübeck, Germany). EIT data were generated by application of small alternate electrical currents rotating around patient's thorax, registered at 20 Hz and stored for offline analysis. When patients were ventilated with a ventilator able to communicate by serial protocol with the EIT device, airway pressure, flow and volume tracings were continuously recorded by EIT machine.

Study protocol

Patients were deeply sedated (Richmond sedation scale −4 or −5) and paralyzed and mechanical ventilation was set in volume controlled according to the ARDSnet guidelines, as follows: Vt = 6–8 mL/kg of PBW; plateau pressure lower than 30 cmH_2O; respiratory rate was targeted to a pH value of 7.30–7.45; PEEP and FiO_2 were set according to the lower PEEP/higher FiO_2 table [3], targeting a partial arterial oxygen tension = 55–80 mmHg or SpO_2 = 88–95%.

Then, study protocol, shown in Fig. 1A, consisted of three consecutive steps:

1. Baseline phase (20 min): volume-controlled ventilation set as previously described ($PEEP_{ARDSnet}$)
2. $PEEP_{EIT}$ selection phase, which included:

   2.1. Application of a RM, with a positive pressure of 40 cmH_2O for 40 s.
   2.2. Measure of EELI variation (ΔEELI) 30 s (ΔEELIstart) and 10 min (ΔEELIend) after the RM.
   2.3. Calculation of ΔEELI change: If ΔEELIend decreased more than 10% of ΔEELIstart (Fig. 1B-a), a new RM was performed, and PEEP increased by 2 cmH_2O
   2.4. If ΔEELI decreased less than 10% of ΔEELIstart (Fig. 1B-b), PEEP was left unchanged.
   If, after the first RM, ΔEELI increased less than 10% of ΔEELIstart, PEEP was reduced by 2 cmH_2O, every 10 min, until a decrease in ΔEELI of 10% or more was observed.
   2.5. The first three points of STEP 2 were repeated until ΔEELI change fulfilled point 2.4 requirement, up to a maximum PEEP level of 18 cmH_2O. ($PEEP_{EIT}$).

3. $PEEP_{EIT+2}$ phase, lasting 10 min: A new RM was performed and PEEP increased by 2 cmH_2O from $PEEP_{EIT}$ (Fig. 1A).

The reliability of bedside-derived calculation of relative changes in ΔEELIstart and ΔEELIend was also verified offline (Additional file 1: Figure E2).

At the end of each phase (i.e., $PEEP_{ARDSnet}$, $PEEP_{EIT}$, $PEEP_{EIT+2}$), arterial blood gases were collected, mean arterial pressure, central venous pressure and heart rate were recorded and end-inspiratory and end-expiratory occlusions performed, lasting about 3 s. Then, from offline analysis of ventilation tracings, plateau pressure and total PEEP (including intrinsic PEEP) were measured. Driving pressure was calculated as plateau pressure – total PEEP and respiratory system compliance as Vt/driving pressure.

Tidal volume was held constant during the protocol. PEEP was increased up to a maximum level of 18 cmH_2O; the protocol foresaw a decrease in Vt if a plateau pressure higher than 30 was reached. This was, however, never the case in our patients. Clinically set FiO_2 was left unchanged throughout the study. However, from the value of PaO_2 measured at $PEEP_{EIT}$, we calculated the "predicted FiO_2" value at which the PaO_2 in $PEEP_{EIT}$ step would have been equal to ARDSnet step: "predicted FiO_2" = [PaO_2/FiO_2ARDSnet/PaO_2/FiO_2EIT × FiO_2 ARDSnet]. Since PaO_2 is not linearly related to FiO_2, this calculation, not previously validated, should be interpreted with caution [20].

We also calculated the PEEP level that would have resulted from the Express protocol [4] as 30 cmH_2O minus driving pressure (at $PEEP_{EIT}$).

EIT data

Besides the previously described bedside evaluation of EIT tracings used to titrate PEEP, EIT data were also analyzed offline to derive further parameters. The whole PEEP titration protocol was acquired as sequential EIT files lasting 5 min with the same baseline reference. EIT data analyses were performed after identification of a sequence of breaths deemed as representative (i.e., stable Vt and EELI) at the end of each phase. We defined four horizontal same-size contiguous layers [ventral (V), middle-ventral (MV), middle-dorsal (MD), dorsal (D)], encompassing the entire field of view (Additional file 1: Figure E1), and from offline analyses (performed by EIT Data Analysis Tool 6.0, Dräger Medical GmbH, Lübeck, Germany) of average raw EIT data of the selected breaths, the following variables were obtained for each study phase:

- Regional compliance: We obtained regional distribution of Vt during inspiratory occlusion ($Vt_{\%}$) expressed as percentage of its global value, and then we calculated regional compliance as $Vt_{\%}/100$ * compliance.
- Alveolar hyperdistension and collapse: As Vt correlates well with local impedance lung changes [21–24], pixel-by-pixel compliance was calculated as Δimpedance/(plateau pressure—PEEP). Alveolar overdistension and collapse was then computed as previously described by Costa et al. [25]. Finally, alveolar hyperdistension and collapse was calculated as the sum of alveolar hyperdistension and collapse expressed as percentage value.
- The amount of recruited volume was calculated as the difference between actual EELV change (measured by EIT) minus the product of compliance at lower PEEP and the PEEP change, as previously described: Recruited volume = ΔEELV – [$compliance_{ARDSnet}$ * ($PEEP_{EIT}$ – $PEEP_{ARDSnet}$)] [16].

Statistical analysis

In the study population, we expected a PaO_2/FiO_2 ratio = 199 ± 57 [16]. In order to detect an increase in PaO2/FiO2 ratio of 25%, in a crossover design, we

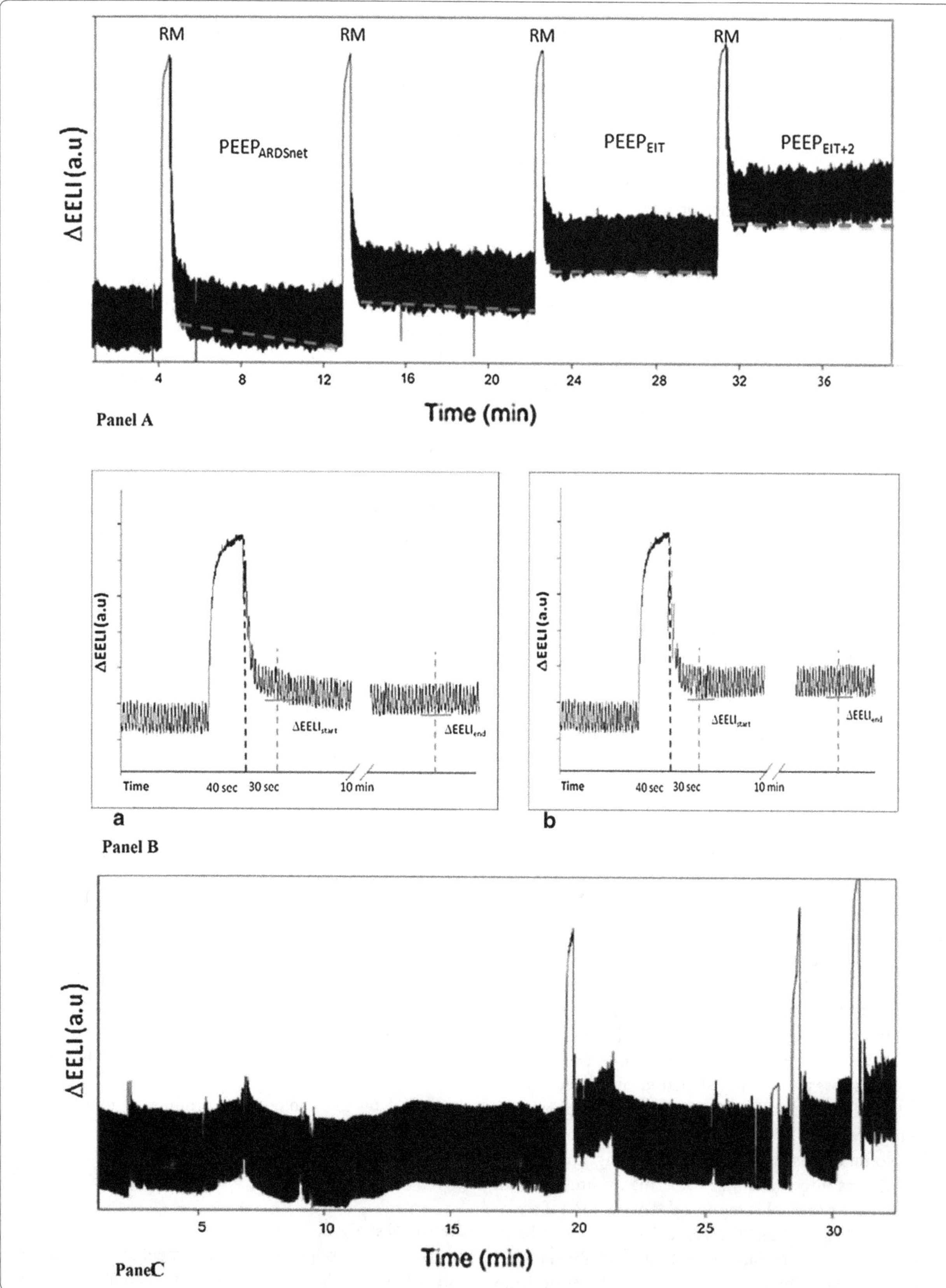
RM
RM
RM
RM
PEEPARDSnet
PEEPEIT
PEEPEIT+2
ΔEELI (a.u)
4
8
12
16
20
24
28
32
36
Time (min)
Panel A
ΔEELI (a.u)
Time
40 sec
30 sec
10 min
ΔEELIstart
ΔEELIend
a
ΔEELI (a.u)
Time
40 sec
30 sec
10 min
ΔEELIstart
ΔEELIend
b
Panel B
ΔEELI (a.u)
5
10
15
20
25
30
Time (min)
PaneC

(See figure on previous page.)
Fig. 1 PEEP selection by EIT (*Panel A* and *B*): After a baseline phase lasting 20 min ($PEEP_{ARDSnet}$), a RM was performed (whose duration is shortened in the image for clarity purposes); end-expiratory lung impedance variation (ΔEELI) was measured after 30 s (ΔEELIstart) and after 10 min (ΔEELIend); if ΔEELIend decreased more than 10% of ΔEELIstart, a new RM was performed, and PEEP increased by 2 cmH_2O. This was repeated until ΔEELIend decreased less than 10% of ΔEELIstart, or up to maximum PEEP level of 18 cmH_2O ($PEEP_{EIT}$). A new RM was performed and PEEP increased by 2 cmH_2O from $PEEP_{EIT}$ ($PEEP_{EIT+2}$). Unstable EELI track (*Panel C*): an example of unstable EELI track

estimated that 12 patients would be necessary. Since the feasibility of the technique was unknown, we increased this by 30%, obtaining a final sample size of 16 patients. Differences between variables obtained during each study phase were tested by one-way analysis of variance (ANOVA) for repeated measures, or by one-way repeated measures ANOVA on ranks for non-normally distributed variables; post hoc comparisons were made by the Bonferroni's method. Comparisons between two groups of normally distributed variables were made by independent samples *t* test, while non-normally distributed variables were compared by Mann–Whitney *U* test. A level of $p < 0.05$ (two-tailed) was considered as statistically significant. Normally distributed data are indicated as mean ± standard deviation, while median and interquartile range [IQR] are used to report non-normally distributed variables. Statistical analyses were performed by SigmaPlot 11.0 (Systat Software Inc., San Jose, CA).

Results

Patients' characteristics

Patients' main characteristics are summarized in Table 1. Patients were 66 ± 11 years old and 14 (87%) were men. On the day of the study, 12 patients (75%) fulfilled ARDS criteria. Fourteen patients (87%) were enrolled within a week from intubation. The diagnosis at ICU admission was pneumonia in ten patients (62%), thoracic trauma in three patients (19%) and septic shock in three patients (19%). Three patients (19%) died during their hospital stay.

Feasibility of setting PEEP by EIT-based evidence of sustained recruitment

We enrolled 16 patients: Clinical PEEP level at study enrollment was 11 ± 3 cmH_2O; EELI tracing could successfully detect the PEEP level associated with sustained recruitment in 14 (87%) patients; of these 14 patients, 11 (78%) fulfilled ARDS; the distribution of tidal volume during $PEEP_{ARDSnet}$ phase was 52 ± 11% in right lung and 48 ± 10% in left lung ($p = 0.557$).

In two patients (13%), EIT tracings could not be used due to the lack of stability of the EELI signal (Fig. 1C), and thus, their data were excluded from further analysis.

$PEEP_{EIT}$ was significantly higher than $PEEP_{ARDSnet}$ (13 ± 3 vs. 9 ± 2 cmH_2O, $p < 0.001$), and the correlation between them was significant, but loose ($R^2 = 0.36$,

Table 1 Patients' main characteristics

Patient #	Age (years)	Sex	Body mass index (Kg/m^2)	SAPS II score	PaO_2/FiO_2 (mmHg)	Diagnosis at admission	ARDS	Days of intubation before enrollment	ICU outcome
1	59	M	26	39	121	Thoracic trauma	Y	1	Survive
2	67	M	29	33	114	Pneumonia	Y	3	Survive
3	67	M	24	34	236	Pneumonia	Y	4	Survive
4	55	M	26	46	170	Pneumonia	Y	15	Survive
5	75	F	31	47	84	Pneumonia	Y	2	Survive
6	80	F	28	78	145	Pneumonia	Y	1	Dead
7	63	M	29	45	140	Pneumonia	N	2	Survive
8	41	M	34	33	209	Pneumonia	Y	3	Survive
9	79	M	24	44	97	Pneumonia	Y	1	Survive
10	69	M	25	35	279	Thoracic trauma	Y	3	Survive
11	64	M	26	48	238	Thoracic trauma	N	3	Dead
12	63	M	28	42	104	Pneumonia	Y	3	Dead
13	56	M	37	39	86	Pneumonia	Y	2	Survive
14	88	M	26	38	210	Septic shock	Y	1	Survive
15	68	M	26	51	196	Septic shock	N	19	Survive
16	59	M	29	31	132	Septic shock	N	6	Survive
Mean ± SD	66 ± 11	2 F	28 ± 4	43 ± 11	160 ± 60	10 pneumonia, 3 thoracic trauma, 3 septic shock	12 Y	4 ± 5	3 dead

SAPS, Simplified Acute Physiologic Score; ARDS, acute respiratory distress syndrome; ICU, intensive care unit

$p = 0.022$). The mean number of stepwise changes in PEEP performed between $PEEP_{ARDSnet}$ and $PEEP_{EIT}$ phases was 2 ± 1, and the total duration of time required to arrive at the $PEEP_{EIT}$ was 48 ± 12 min. The largest PEEP variations performed were 6 cmH2O in two patients and 10 cmH_2O in one patient.

Effects of PEEP selection on oxygenation, respiratory mechanics and hemodynamics

Ventilation tracings were continuously recorded by EIT in 9/14 patients; FiO_2 during all study phases was kept stable at 0.5 ± 0.1; PaO_2/FiO_2 ratio improved during both $PEEP_{EIT}$ and $PEEP_{EIT+2}$ phases compared with $PEEP_{ARDSnet}$ (Fig. 2), but no significant changes occurred between $PEEP_{EIT}$ and $PEEP_{EIT+2}$ phases ($p = 0.121$). The predicted FiO_2 at $PEEP_{EIT}$ would have been significantly lower compared with the ARDSnet table (0.44 ± 0.1 vs. 0.53 ± 0.1, $p \leq 0.001$). Moreover, while (as expected) there was a strong correlation between $PEEP_{ARDSnet}$ and FiO_2 ARDSnet, no significant association was observed between $PEEP_{EIT}$ and predicted FiO_2 (Fig. 3). At $PEEP_{EIT}$ levels, compliance did not significantly change ($p = 0.097$), whereas the driving pressure was significantly reduced in $PEEP_{EIT}$ phase compared with ARDSnet phase (Table 2), albeit with a probably modest clinical relevance (range between −2 and 0 cmH_2O). The PEEP level theoretically achieved with Express trial approach was significantly higher than $PEEP_{EIT}$ (20.6 ± 1.9 vs. 13.1 2.9 cmH_2O, $p < 0.001$), without any significant association ($R_2 = 0.002$).

No significant hemodynamic changes were observed during all study phases (Table 3); $PaCO_2$ remained stable over all study phases (45 ± 7, vs. 46 ± 9, vs. 47 ± 9 mmHg, $p = 0.1$).

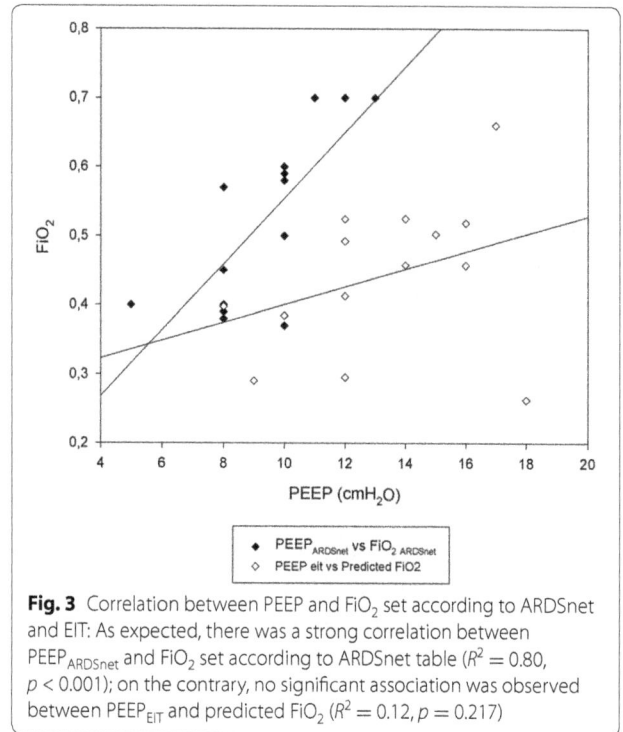

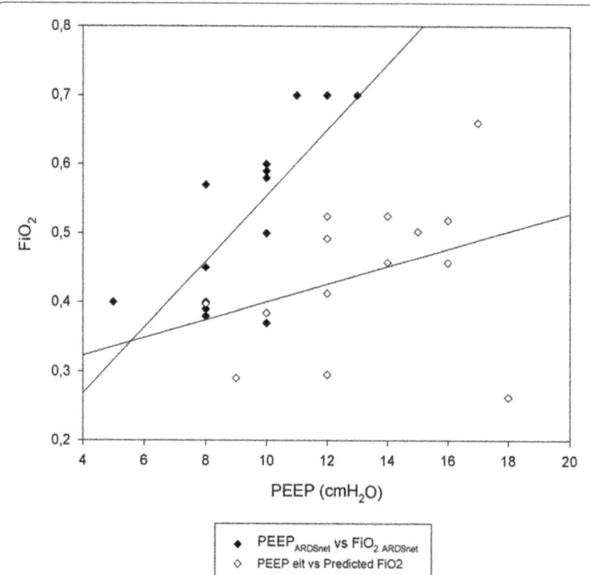

Fig. 3 Correlation between PEEP and FiO_2 set according to ARDSnet and EIT: As expected, there was a strong correlation between $PEEP_{ARDSnet}$ and FiO_2 set according to ARDSnet table ($R^2 = 0.80$, $p < 0.001$); on the contrary, no significant association was observed between $PEEP_{EIT}$ and predicted FiO_2 ($R^2 = 0.12, p = 0.217$)

Homogeneity and regional mechanics

Regional compliance was reduced in ventral lung layer, and it improved in middle-dorsal lung layers, during both $PEEP_{EIT}$ and $PEEP_{EIT+2}$ phases compared with $PEEP_{ARDSnet}$. In dorsal layer, compliance improved in $PEEP_{EIT+2}$ phase, while no significant changes in middle-ventral layer were observed (Table 2). Interestingly, regional alveolar hyperdistension and collapse was significantly reduced in dependent lung layers and significantly increased in non-dependent lung layers during both $PEEP_{EIT}$ and $PEEP_{EIT+2}$ compared with $PEEP_{ARDSnet}$.

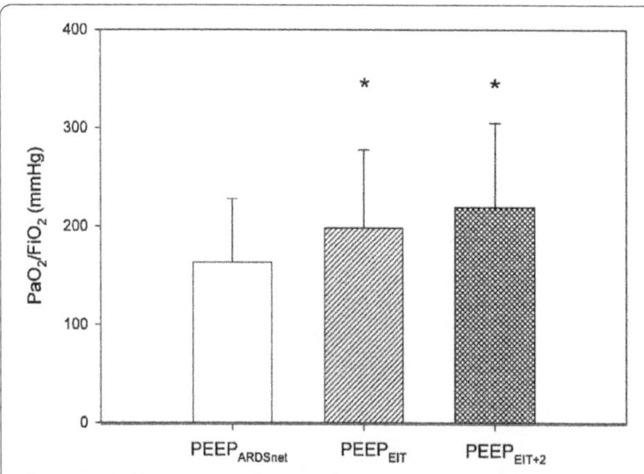

Fig. 2 PaO_2/FiO_2 ratio in all study phases. It significantly improved in both $PEEP_{EIT}$ and $PEEP_{EIT+2}$ phases compared with $PEEP_{ARDSnet}$. *$p < 0.05$ compared with $PEEP_{ARDSnet}$ phase

Table 2 Global and regional respiratory system compliance in all study phases

	$PEEP_{ARDSnet}$	$PEEP_{EIT}$	$PEEP_{EIT+2}$	*p* value
Driving pressure (cmH_2O)	10.2 ± 1.9	9.3 ± 1.9*	9.7 ± 2.5	0.035
Compliance (ml/cmH_2O)	44.6 ± 11	49.5 ± 12	49.5 ± 17	0.097
$Compliance_V$ (ml/cmH_2O)	6.9 ± 3	5.0 ± 2*	4.1 ± 2*	<0.01
$Compliance_{MV}$ (ml/cmH_2O)	24.3 ± 9	24.9 ± 10	23.8 ± 12	0.873
$Compliance_{MD}$ (ml/cmH_2O)	6.9 ± 6	14.6 ± 6*	16.1 ± 7*	<0.001
$Compliance_D$ (ml/cmH_2O)	3.2 ± 2	4.8 ± 5	5.1 ± 5*	<0.05

V, ventral; MV, middle-ventral; MD, middle-dorsal; D, dorsal

* $p < 0.05$ compared with $PEEP_{ARDSnet}$ phase

Table 3 Hemodynamics during all study phases

	$PEEP_{ARDSnet}$	$PEEP_{EIT}$	$PEEP_{EIT+2}$	*p* value
Mean arterial pressure (mmHg)	77 ± 10	73 ± 7	75 ± 11	0.079
Heart rate (bpm)	86 ± 16	83 ± 18	87 ± 18	0.066
Central venous pressure (mmHg)	12 ± 5	13 ± 6	13 ± 6	0.214

Furthermore, in middle-ventral lung layers alveolar hyperdistension and collapse was significantly higher in $PEEP_{EIT+2}$ phase than in $PEEP_{ARDSnet}$, but did not change in $PEEP_{EIT}$ step (Fig. 4). The recruited volume at $PEEP_{EIT}$ was 306 (159–522) ml. The amount of recruited volume did not correlate with oxygenation improvement (Fig. 5), whereas it correlated with changes in respiratory system compliance ($R^2 = 0.50$, $p < 0.01$, Fig. 5) and with the decrease in driving pressure ($R^2 = 0.36$, $p < 0.05$). No significant correlation was observed between oxygenation improvement and driving pressure reduction ($R = 0.26$, $p = 0.36$).

Discussion

The main findings of this study can be summarized as follows: Bedside PEEP setting based on sustained recruitment following a RM as visualized by EIT was feasible in the majority of patients with acute hypoxemic respiratory failure (most of whom fulfilled ARDS criteria). This method invariably led to the application of higher PEEP levels in comparison with the commonly used ARDSnet table and was associated with improved oxygenation. Furthermore, EIT allowed to disclose and quantitate the presence of regional overdistension associated with PEEP increase. PEEP setting in hypoxemic respiratory failure and ARDS remains controversial. A meta-analysis on three large randomized trials [3] showed that higher PEEP could be beneficial in more severe ARDS patients, but no indication was provided on how to titrate this higher PEEP: Indeed, while in two studies an oxygenation-based criterion was used, in the third trial a respiratory mechanics-based method was used. Later, a secondary analysis by Goligher et al. [26] showed that the benefit of higher PEEP on mortality was limited to the patients who had an oxygenation improvement, likely indicating the presence of recruitment. Even if the aforementioned paper does not necessarily proof a cause relationship effect (i.e., that higher PEEP prevented death in recruiters), we reasoned that it would have been desirable to have a method to set PEEP directly targeting alveolar recruitment combined with prevention of de-recruitment, and we focused on EIT as a bedside non-invasive tool. While the ability of EIT in assessing lung recruitment has been previously shown, most studies

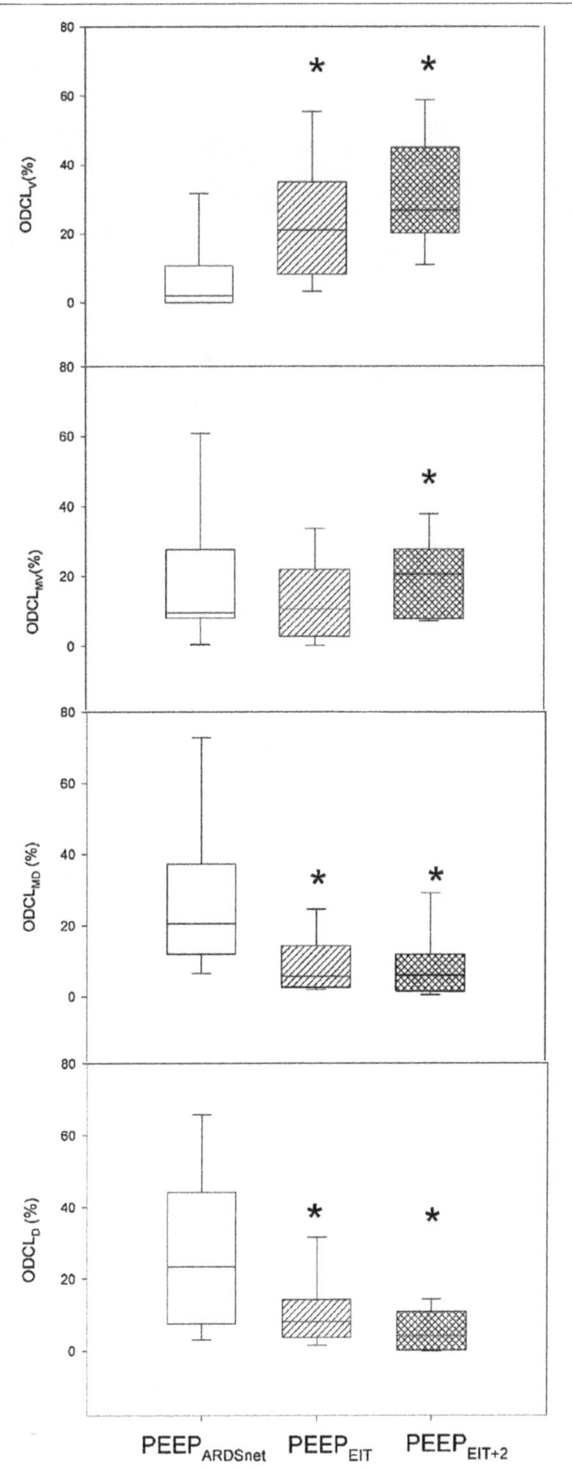

Fig. 4 Regional alveolar hyperdistension and collapse distribution in all study phases. Alveolar hyperdistension and collapse was significantly reduced in dependent lung layers and significantly increased in non-dependent lung layers compared with $PEEP_{ARDSnet}$ in both $PEEP_{EIT}$ and $PEEP_{EIT+2}$ phases. Furthermore, in middle-ventral lung layers alveolar hyperdistension and collapse was significantly higher in $PEEP_{EIT+2}$ phase compared with $PEEP_{ARDSnet}$, but did not change in $PEEP_{EIT}$ step. *$p < 0.05$ compared with $PEEP_{ARDSnet}$ phase

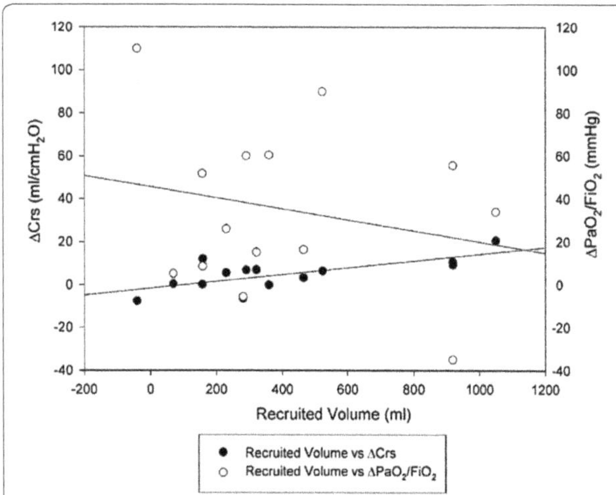

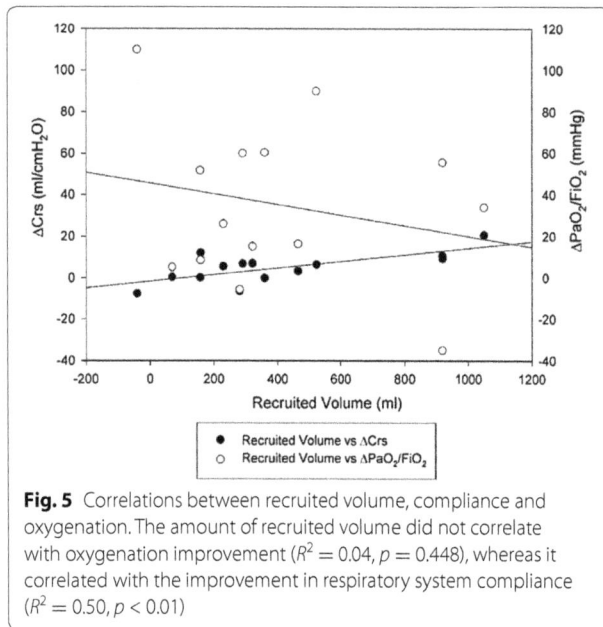

Fig. 5 Correlations between recruited volume, compliance and oxygenation. The amount of recruited volume did not correlate with oxygenation improvement ($R^2 = 0.04$, $p = 0.448$), whereas it correlated with the improvement in respiratory system compliance ($R^2 = 0.50$, $p < 0.01$)

were conducted on animal models and/or explored the effects of relatively high PEEP changes (in the order of 10 cmH_2O) [27, 28]. On the contrary, we aimed to test the feasibility of a specific protocol, with a "fine tuning" of PEEP in steps of 2 cmH_2O. Since we expected that in most patients the EIT-based approach would have led to increase in PEEP from the NIH table, we added $PEEP_{EIT+2}$ phase, in order to establish the effects on oxygenation and respiratory mechanics of a further increase in PEEP above the level set by EIT. The method proposed appeared feasible in most patients: This is encouraging in prospect of future evaluation of the protocol in a clinical setting. A PEEP increase will always be associated with an increment of EELV, even if no recruitment occurs, simply because of the expansion of ventilated alveoli. Hence, to dissect these two phenomena, we took advantage of RM. Although available literature shows that RM does not impact outcome, it also shows that it is safe and devoid of major complications [29]. Grasso et al. [30] showed how RMs are unlikely to benefit patients with more than 5 days of ARDS; plus, Borges et al. [31, 32] obtained best results in terms of recruitability with RMs involving stepwise increases in PEEP compared with sustained inflation methods; however, we included in the algorithm RMs more as "diagnostic" tools to exploit potential for lung recruitment, rather than therapeutic measures; for this reason, we did not focus on a specific category of patients and we chose the most simple and immediate method of recruitment, usually used in our clinical practice.

As a reference method, we used the ARDSnet table, one of the most frequently applied methods. Not surprisingly, EIT led to an increase in PEEP in all subjects: This finding is not surprising, since the ARDSnet table has been used to set PEEP in the control group of all studies testing "higher" PEEP strategies.

In the majority of patients, we found that the protocol was feasible: It led to the univocal identification of a PEEP level associated with sustained recruitment after a RM, without exceeding the upper safety limit set to 18 cmH_2O. In the majority of patients, the PEEP changes were within a relatively narrow range (mean 4 cmH_2O) and hence safe to apply. Despite relatively small, however, these changes were clinically relevant, leading to improvement in oxygenation. It was likely due to lung recruitment and increased lung size (as indicated also by the positive correlation between these two variables), and this might possibly lead to a decreased injury from mechanical ventilation. Interestingly, these improvements were not due to the increase in PEEP per se, since a further increase in PEEP above $PEEP_{EIT}$ was not associated with further improvement in gas exchange and respiratory mechanics.

The global change in compliance between $PEEP_{ARDSnet}$ and $PEEP_{EIT}$ phases was the net result of two opposed changes in regional compliance: increasing in the dorsal layers (likely due to recruitment) and decreasing in the ventral layers (likely due to overdistension). We cannot exclude that part of the improvement in the compliance of dorsal layers might be due to the presence of intratidal recruitment; however, this effect was unlikely since previus studies showed that increasing PEEP leads to a decrease in intratidal recruitment [2]. FiO_2 was kept stable in all study phases (0.5 ± 0.1); in this way, we avoided erroneous estimation of alveolar collapse and recruitment due to low alveolar oxygen concentration [31, 33]. We believe that this result further underlines the need for a regional real-time monitoring of the distribution of ventilation, which could prompt a decrease in tidal volume until overdistension of ventral regions drops back to baseline.

This study has some limitations that need to be acknowledged. EIT measurement encompasses only a cross-sectional slice of 5–10 cm of the thorax, and we assumed that other lung regions behave similarly. However, previous studies on similar patient populations showed that ΔEELV measured by EIT well represents the entire lung [34]. The study population was relatively small, but large enough to test the feasibility, safety and efficacy on selected physiological endpoints. Our results do not provide any evidence that a strategy aimed at obtaining stable recruitment leads to a decreased lung injury, but show that such aim can be achieved and that the overdistension also induced by PEEP can be simultaneously monitored and could be used to further adjust ventilation (e.g., reducing tidal volume). Therefore, these results pave the way to a larger study, aimed at assessing whether this approach to PEEP setting leads to benefit in outcome.

Finally, we have not limited our population to ARDS patients: This choice was on one the hand pragmatic, facilitating the enrollment of patients, but on the other hand it also acknowledges the fact that alveolar de-recruitment is not unique of ARDS and that mechanical ventilation can be a challenge also in acutely hypoxemic patients. As this study aimed to test the feasibility of the method, we exclude that the inclusion of non-ARDS patient introduced a significant bias, while we are uncertain of what would be the best approach in an outcome study.

Conclusions

This study shows that, in a cohort of patients with acute hypoxemic respiratory failure undergoing lung protective ventilation, a PEEP selection strategy aimed at maximizing alveolar recruitment and preventing de-recruitment, guided by EIT at the bedside, is feasible, simple and safe, leading to systematically higher PEEP values than the ARDSnet table, with positive effects on gas exchange and respiratory system mechanical properties. This strategy also allows estimating the relative weight of overdistension and recruitment following a PEEP change. These results do not necessarily imply that benefits of recruitment achieved out weight the negative effects induced by overdistension and larger study are required to elucidate if this strategy could also lead to improved clinical outcome.

Abbreviations

ARDS: acute respiratory distress syndrome; EELI: end-expiratory lung impedance; EELV: end-expiratory lung volume; EIT: electrical impedance tomography; ICU: intensive care unit; PBW: predicted body weight; PEEP: positive end-expiratory pressure; RM: recruitment maneuver; SAPS II: Simplified Acute Physiology Score II.

Authors' contributions

NE, GB and AP planned the study design, TM and GF were the principal investigators; EM, SG, AB and TS acquired data, LA, FB and CM undertook the statistical analysis; NE, GG and GB wrote the manuscript. All authors made substantial contributions to conception and design, or acquisition of data, or analysis and interpretation of data, have been involved in drafting the manuscript and revising it critically for important intellectual content and have given final approval of the version to be published. Each author has participated sufficiently in the work to take public responsibility for appropriate portions of the content and agreed to be accountable for all aspects of the work in ensuring that questions related to the accuracy or integrity of any part of the work are appropriately investigated and resolved. All authors read and approved the final manuscript

Author details

[1] Department of Emergency and Intensive Care, San Gerardo Hospital, Via Pergolesi 33, Monza, Italy. [2] Department of Pathophysiology and Transplantation, University of Milan, Via Festa del Perdono 7, Milan, Italy. [3] Department of Anesthesia, Critical Care and Emergency, Fondazione IRCCS Ca' Granda Ospedale Maggiore Policlinico, Via Francesco Sforza 28, Milan, Italy. [4] Department of Medicine, School of Medicine and Surgery, University of Milan-Bicocca, Via Cadore 48, Monza, Italy.

Acknowledgements

None.

Competing interests

GB received fees from Dreager Medical for lecturing and consulting outside the scope of this work.

Funding

The present study was supported by departmental funding.

References

1. Matthay MA, Ware LB, Zimmerman GA. The acute respiratory distress syndrome. J Clin Invest. 2012;122(8):2731–40.
2. Caironi P, Cressoni M, Chiumello D, Ranieri M, Quintel M, Russo SG, Cornejo R, Bugedo G, Carlesso E, Russo R, Caspani L, Gattinoni L. Lung opening and closing during ventilation of acute respiratory distress syndrome. Am J Respir Crit Care Med. 2010;181(6):578–86.
3. The National Heart, Lung, and Blood Institute ARDS Clinical Trials Network. Higher versus lower positive end-expiratory pressures in patients with the acute respiratory distress syndrome. N Engl J Med. 2004;351(4):327–36.
4. Mercat A, Richard JC, Vielle B, Expiratory Pressure (Express) Study Group, et al. Positive end-expiratory pressure setting in adults with acute lung injury and acute respiratory distress syndrome: a randomized controlled trial. JAMA. 2008;299:646–55.
5. Grasso S, Terragni P, Mascia L, et al. Airway pressure-time curve profile (stress index) detects tidal recruitment/hyperinflation in experimental acute lung injury. Crit Care Med. 2004;32:1018–27.
6. Talmor D, Sarge T, Malhotra A, et al. Mechanical ventilation guided by esophageal pressure in acute lung injury. N Engl J Med. 2008;359:2095–104.
7. Mauri T, Yoshida T, Bellani G, et al. Esophageal and transpulmonary pressure in the clinical setting: meaning, usefulness and perspectives. Intensive Care Med. 2016;42(9):1360–73.
8. Chiumello D, Cressoni M, Carlesso E, et al. Bedside selection of positive end-expiratory pressure in mild, moderate, and severe acute respiratory distress syndrome. Crit Care Med. 2014;42(2):252–64.
9. Pelosi P, Goldner M, McKibben A, et al. Recruitment and derecruitment during acute respiratory failure: an experimental study. Am J Respir Crit Care Med. 2001;164(1):122–30.
10. Hickling KG. Best compliance during a decremental, but not incremental, positive endexpiratory pressure trial is related to open-lung positive end-expiratory pressure: a mathematical model of acute respiratory distress syndrome lungs. Am J Respir Crit Care Med. 2001;163:69–78.
11. Briel M, Meade M, Mercat A, et al. Higher vs lower positive end-expiratory pressure in patients with acute lung injury and acute respiratory distress syndrome: systematic review and meta-analysis. JAMA. 2010;303(9):865–73.
12. Bellani G, Laffey JG, Pham T, et al. Epidemiology, patterns of care, and mortality for patients with acute respiratory distress syndrome in intensive care units in 50 countries. JAMA. 2016;315(8):788–800.
13. Keenan JC, Formenti P, Marini JJ. Lung recruitment in acute respiratory distress syndrome: what is the best strategy? Curr Opin Crit Care. 2014;20:63–8.
14. Fan E, Wilcox ME, Brower RG, et al. Recruitment maneuvers for acute lung injury. A systematic review. Am J Respir Crit Care Med. 2008;178(11):1156–63.
15. Frerichs I, Amato MB, van Kaam AH, et al. Chest electrical impedance tomography examination, data analysis, terminology, clinical use and recommendations: consensus statement of the TRanslational EIT development stuDy group. Thorax. 2016;0:1–11.
16. Mauri T, Eronia N, Turrini C, et al. Bedside assessment of the effects of

positive end expiratory pressure on lung inflation and recruitment by the helium dilution technique and electrical impedance tomography. Intensive Care Med. 2016;42(10):1576–87.
17. Bikker IG, Leonhardt S, Miranda DR, et al. Bedside measurement of changes in lung impedance to monitor alveolar ventilation in dependent and nondependent parts by electrical impedance tomography during a positive end-expiratory pressure trial in mechanically ventilated intensive care unit patients. Crit Care. 2010;14(3):R100.
18. Liu S, Tan L, Möller K, et al. Identification of regional overdistension, recruitment and cyclic alveolar collapse with electrical impedance tomography in an experimental ARDS model. Crit Care. 2016;20(1):119.
19. Bellani G, Laffey JG, Pham T, et al. Noninvasive ventilation of patients with acute respiratory distress syndrome. insights from the LUNG SAFE study. Am J Respir Crit Care Med. 2017;195(1):67–77.
20. Aboab J, Louis B, Jonson B, Brochard L. Relation between PaO_2/FIO_2 ratio and FIO_2: a mathematical description. Intensive Care Med. 2006;32(10):1494–7.
21. Victorino JA, Borges JB, Okamoto VN, et al. Imbalances in regional lung ventilation: a validation study on electrical impedance tomography. Am J Respir Crit Care Med. 2004;169(7):791–800.
22. Frerichs I, Hinz J, Herrmann P, et al. Detection of local lung air content by electrical impedance tomography compared with electron beam CT. J Appl Physiol. 2002;93(2):660–6.
23. Frerichs I, Hahn G, Schiffmann H, et al. Monitoring regional lung ventilation by functional electrical impedance tomography during assisted ventilation. Ann N Y Acad Sci. 1999;873:493–505.
24. Adler A, Amyot R, Guardo R, et al. Monitoring changes in lung air and liquid volumes with electrical impedance tomography. J Appl Physiol. 1997;83(5):1762–7.
25. Costa EL, Borges JB, Melo A, et al. Bedside estimation of recruitable alveolar collapse and hyperdistension by electrical impedance tomography. Intensive Care Med. 2009;35(6):1132–7.
26. Goligher EC, Kavanagh BP, Rubenfeld GD, et al. Oxygenation response to positive endexpiratory pressure predicts mortality in acute respiratory distress syndrome. A secondary analysis of the LOVS and ExPress trials. Am J Respir Crit Care Med. 2014;190(1):70–6.
27. Meier T, Luepschen H, Karsten J, et al. Assessment of regional lung recruitment and derecruitment during a PEEP trial based on electrical impedance tomography. Intensive Care Med. 2008;34(3):543–50.
28. Fagerberg A, Stenqvist O, Aneman A. Electrical impedance tomography applied to assess matching of pulmonary ventilation and perfusion in a porcine experimental model. Crit Care. 2009;13(2):R34.
29. Hodgson C, Carteaux G, Tuxen D, et al. Hypoxaemic rescue therapies in acute respiratory distress syndrome: why, when, what and which one? Injury. 2013;44(12):1700–9.
30. Grasso S, Mascia L, Del Turco M, et al. Effects of recruiting maneuvers in patients with acute respiratory distress syndrome ventilated with protective ventilatory strategy. Anesthesiology. 2002;96:795–802.
31. Borges JB, Costa ELV, Suarez-Sipmann F, Widström C, Larsson A, Amato M, et al. Early inflammation mainly affects normally and poorly aerated lung in experimental ventilator-induced lung injury. Crit Care Med. 2014;42:e279–87.
32. Borges JB, Costa ELV, Bergquist M, et al. Lung inflammation persists after 27 hours of protective acute respiratory distress syndrome network strategy and is concentrated in the nondependent lung. Crit Care Med. 2015;43:e123–32.
33. Derosa S, Borges JB, Segelsjö M, Tannoia A, Pellegrini M, Larsson A, et al. Reabsorption atelectasis in a porcine model of ARDS: regional and temporal effects of airway closure, oxygen, and distending pressure. J Appl Physiol. 2013;115:1464–73.
34. Van der Burg PS, Miedema M, de Jongh FH, et al. Cross-sectional changes in lung volume measured by electrical impedance tomography are representative for the whole lung in ventilated preterm infants. Crit Care Med. 2014;42(6):1524–30.

12

Endocan as an early biomarker of severity in patients with acute respiratory distress syndrome

Diego Orbegozo[†], Lokmane Rahmania[†], Marian Irazabal, Manuel Mendoza, Filippo Annoni, Daniel De Backer, Jacques Creteur and Jean-Louis Vincent[*]

Abstract

Background: Plasma concentrations of endocan, a proteoglycan preferentially expressed in the pulmonary vasculature, may represent a biomarker of lung (dys)function. We sought to determine whether the measurement of plasma endocan levels early in the course of acute respiratory distress syndrome (ARDS) could help predict risk of death or of prolonged ventilation.

Methods: All patients present in the department of intensive care during a 150-day period were screened for ARDS (using the Berlin definition). Endocan concentrations were measured at the moment of ARDS diagnosis (T0) and the following morning (T1). We compared data from survivors and non-survivors and data from survivors with less than 10 days of ventilator support (good evolution) and those who died or needed more than 10 days of mechanical ventilation (poor evolution). Results are presented as numbers (percentages), mean ± standard deviation or medians (percentile 25–75).

Results: Ninety-six consecutive patients were included [median APACHE II score of 21 (17–27) and SOFA score of 9 (6–12), PaO_2/FiO_2 ratio 155 (113–206)]; 64 (67%) had sepsis and 51 (53%) were receiving norepinephrine. Non-survivors were older (66 ± 15 vs. 59 ± 18 years, $p = 0.045$) and had higher APACHE II scores [27 (22–30) vs. 20 (15–24), $p < 0.001$] and blood lactate concentrations at study inclusion [2.1 (1.3–4.0) vs. 1.5 (0.9–2.6) mmol/L, $p = 0.024$] than survivors, but PaO_2/FiO_2 ratios [150 (116–207) vs. 158 (110–206), $p = 0.95$] were similar in the two groups. Endocan concentrations on the day after ARDS diagnosis were significantly higher in patients with poor evolution than in those with good evolution [12.0 (6.8–18.6) vs. 7.2 (5.4–12.5), $p < 0.01$].

Conclusion: Blood endocan concentrations early in the evolution of ARDS may be a useful marker of disease severity.

Keywords: Proteoglycan, Glycocalyx, Pulmonary vasculature, Risk stratification, Acute respiratory failure, Multiple organ failure

Background

Acute respiratory distress syndrome (ARDS) remains a major concern, with mortality rates around 30–45% [1, 2]. The severity of disease is often assessed using the PaO_2/FiO_2 ratio (mainly to optimize treatment strategies), even though the prognostic power of this variable remains low to moderate, with an area under the receiver operating characteristic curve (AUC) of only 0.58 (95% CI 0.56–0.59) in a recent large study [3]. New, early biomarkers of the severity of ARDS are needed, because early optimization of treatment in patients at greatest risk of a poor outcome could improve survival.

ARDS is characterized by important functional and morphological alterations in the pulmonary endothelium that are directly related to mortality [4–8]. Endocan

*Correspondence: jlvincent@intensive.org
[†]Diego Orbegozo and Lokmane Rahmania contributed equally to this work
Department of Intensive Care, Erasme University Hospital, Université Libre de Bruxelles, Route de Lennik 808, 1070 Brussels, Belgium

[previously called endothelial cell-specific molecule 1 (ESM-1)] is a proteoglycan that is mainly expressed in the pulmonary microcirculation, where it plays an important role in endothelial homeostasis [9, 10], able to modulate cell adhesion, endothelial permeability and leukocyte migration from the circulation into the tissues [11, 12]. The preferential expression of endocan in the lung microvasculature and repeated observations suggesting the presence of endothelial dysfunction and upregulation of different inflammatory pathways in the pathogenesis of ARDS [7, 13, 14] support a possible role for endocan in the pathophysiology of ARDS.

During experimental endotoxemia, plasma endocan concentrations increase together with concentrations of inflammatory cytokines and concentrations are correlated with the degree of endothelial dysfunction [15]. Moreover, specific endocan blockade with neutralizing antibodies improved survival in a mouse model of peritonitis [16]. Human studies have indicated that plasma endocan concentrations are increased in patients with sepsis and are correlated with the degree of organ dysfunction and mortality [17, 18]. There are few data on endocan concentrations in patients with ARDS. In one prospective cohort of 42 patients with ARDS, endocan concentrations (1 day after the diagnosis of ARDS) were higher in non-survivors than in survivors [19].

We hypothesized that plasma endocan concentrations would be increased in ARDS patients with poor outcomes and could represent a potential early biomarker of ARDS severity.

Methods

This study was conducted in our 35-bed Department of Intensive Care, which has more than 3200 admissions per year. The Institutional Ethics Committee approved the study (protocol number 2013/269), and written informed consent was obtained from the patient or the patient's representative or next of kin.

During a 150-day period, a medical team not involved in patient care prospectively screened on a daily basis all patients with an ICU stay of more than 24 h. All adult (>18 years) patients with ARDS as defined by the Berlin definition [3] [PaO_2/FiO_2 ratio <300 while receiving mechanical ventilation with a positive end-expiratory pressure (PEEP) of at least 5 cmH_2O, who had a known risk factor for ARDS and bilateral infiltrates on the chest X ray] were included in the study. If a patient was admitted several times to the ICU during the screening period, only the first admission was considered.

Endocan concentrations

When a patient met the criteria for ARDS, the closest residual blood sample taken on the same day was obtained from the central hospital laboratory (T0). A second residual blood sample taken at 8 am the next morning (T1) was also obtained. Retrieved tubes were immediately centrifuged and plasma separated and frozen at −80 °C degrees for future analysis. Endocan concentrations were measured using a human specific quantitative sandwich enzyme-linked immunosorbent assay (ELISA) technique (Lunginnov, Lille, France). All measurements were performed in the central immunochemistry laboratory of the hospital. Data provided from Lunginnov (Lille, France) have shown that concentrations of endocan remain stable over time in EDTA tubes stored for less than 72 h at room temperature and support repeated freeze thaw cycles; use of citrate, heparin or plasma tubes leads to underestimation of endocan concentrations.

Demographic, hemodynamic and clinical data

We collected data on demographics, diagnosis, comorbidities and the presence of infection. All available hemodynamic and respiratory data from patient monitoring systems, including respiratory rate, mean arterial pressure, heart rate, PEEP, and FiO_2, were recorded at the two study time points (T0 and T1); laboratory data from the same time points were also noted. ARDS was defined as mild when the PaO_2/FiO_2 ratio was between 201 and 300, moderate when it was between 101 and 200 and severe when it was ≤100 [3]. The APACHE II score [20] was calculated using the worst data during the first 24 h in the ICU, and the SOFA score [21] was calculated at T0 and T1.

Outcome measures

We recorded the duration of mechanical ventilation until definitive weaning (able to breath spontaneously for more than 72 h) from respiratory support (including non-invasive ventilation). We also recorded the length of ICU stay and the survival status at the end of the ICU stay. We compared endocan concentrations in ICU survivors and non-survivors but also used a composite outcome measure of mortality and prolonged mechanical ventilation (analogous to the concept of ventilator-free days): survivors who needed <10 days of mechanical ventilation (arbitrarily selected) were classified as having a good evolution and non-survivors or survivors who required >10 days of mechanical ventilation were classified as having a poor evolution.

We also compared plasma endocan concentrations in subgroups of septic and non-septic patients, and trauma and non-trauma patients. Because of the known preferential expression of endocan in the lungs, we evaluated the correlation between endocan plasma concentrations and the PaO_2/FiO_2 as an index of lung function at T0. We also explored the role of possible confounding factors, including the degree of organ dysfunction (SOFA score ≥10 vs. <10 [cut-off selected because the median value for the whole population was 9]), the presence of renal failure (SOFA renal score of 0 vs. 1–4), the presence of comorbidities (patients with and without chronic lung disease, comorbid diabetes, hypertension and cardiovascular disease) and the etiology of ARDS [pulmonary (primary) vs. extra-pulmonary (secondary)].

Statistical analysis

Continuous variables were explored for normality of distribution by looking at the Q-Q plots and using Skewness and Kurtosis tests. Values are presented as means ± standard deviations when normality was confirmed and as medians with percentiles (25–75%) when the distribution was not normal. Categorical data are presented as numbers of events and percentages. Comparisons between groups were performed using *t* tests or Mann–Whitney *U* tests as appropriate. Proportions were compared using a Chi-square test or Fisher's exact test as appropriate. Correlations between different variables were examined using the Pearson coefficient (r). We plotted sensitivity and specificity on a ROC graph and the area under the curve (AUC) was calculated for the different variables to predict mortality or poor evolution. A post hoc analysis was performed to determine cut-off values with high specificity and/or sensitivity for predicting poor outcome or mortality by exploring the data at different points on the ROC curves. A post hoc binary logistic regression (univariate and multivariate analysis) was performed to identify the role of T1 endocan and other variables to predict poor evolution, calculating the odds ratio (OR) and its respective 95% confidence interval (CI). A two-sided p value less than 0.05 was considered as significant for all analyses. Statistical analysis was performed using SPSS 22.0 (IBM, New York, NY) software.

Results

Ninety-six patients met ARDS criteria during the screening period and were included in the study (Fig. 1). The median time between ICU admission and inclusion in the study (confirmed diagnosis of ARDS = T0) was 3 (0–12) h. The median time between T0 and T1 samples was 24 (16–24) h.

The main baseline characteristics of the patients at T0 are shown in Table 1. Non-survivors were older (66 ± 15 vs. 59 ± 18 years, $p = 0.045$) and had higher APACHE II scores [27 (22–30) vs. 20 (15–24), $p < 0.001$] and blood lactate concentrations [2.1 (1.3–4.0) vs. 1.5 (0.9–2.6), $p = 0.024$] than survivors but similar PaO_2/FiO_2 ratios [150 (116–207) vs. 158 (110–206), $p = 0.95$].

Plasma endocan concentrations were statistically significantly higher in patients with poor evolution than in those

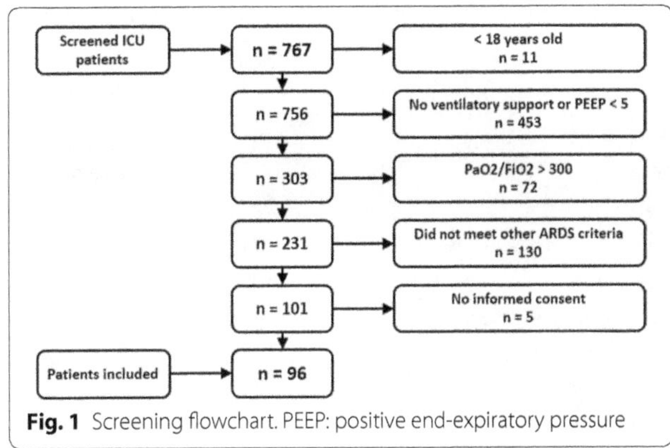

Fig. 1 Screening flowchart. PEEP: positive end-expiratory pressure

with good evolution at T1, but not at T0 (Fig. 2). This pattern was similar, but differences were not statistically significant, in the comparison of endocan concentrations in non-survivors and survivors. The change in endocan concentrations between T0 and T1 was not significantly different in patients with poor and good evolution ($p = 0.127$) or in non-survivors and survivors ($p = 0.476$). The AUC of T1 endocan concentrations for prediction of poor evolution is shown in Fig. 3. The AUCs for the APACHE II score, the T0 SOFA score and the T0 PaO_2/FiO_2 ratio are shown in Additional file 1: Table S1. In the multivariate analysis, APACHE II score (but not endocan at T1) was retained as the best predictor of poor evolution (OR 1.149 [1.067–1.237], $p < 0.01$). A cut-off value of endocan of 6 ng/mL at T0 and T1 had good sensitivity to exclude poor outcome or death, and a cut-off value of 14 ng/mL at T0 and T1 had good specificity for poor outcome or death, with acceptable negative predictive values at T1, but modest positive predictive values (Additional file 1: Table S2).

Endocan concentrations at T0 and T1 were higher in patients with higher SOFA scores than in those with lower SOFA scores (using a cut-off of 10 points) (Additional file 1: Fig. S1). At T0, they were also higher in patients with sepsis than in those without, but were no different in trauma and non-trauma patients, patients with or without chronic lung comorbidities, patients with primary versus secondary ARDS (Additional file 1: Fig S2), patients with or without diabetes ($p = 0.198$), patients with or without arterial hypertension ($p = 0.407$), and patients with or without coronary heart disease ($p = 0.473$). At T1, patients with higher renal SOFA scores had higher endocan concentrations than did patients with a SOFA renal score of 0 (Fig. 4).

At T0, there was a modest correlation between endocan concentrations and the renal ($r = 0.235$, $p = 0.001$) and the total ($r = 0.332$, $p < 0.001$) SOFA scores. Endocan concentrations at T0 were not correlated with the PaO_2/FiO_2 ratio at T0 (Fig. 5) ($r = 0.137$, $p = 0.18$), with

Table 1 Main characteristics (at time of inclusion) and outcomes of the patients with ARDS

	Total $n = 96$	Survivors $n = 64$	Non-survivors $n = 32$	*p*	Good evolution $n = 54$	Poor evolution $n = 42$	*p*
Age (years)	61 ± 17	59 ± 18	66 ± 15	*0.045*	59 ± 18	64 ± 15	0.219
Male *n* (%)	64 (67)	44 (69)	20 (63)	0.647	39 (72)	25 (60)	0.275
Trauma *n* (%)	8 (8)	7 (11)	1 (3)	0.262	5 (9)	3 (7)	1.000
Primary ARDS *n* (%)	45 (47)	31 (48)	14 (44)	0.828	25 (46)	20 (48)	1.000
Sepsis *n* (%)	64 (67)	39 (61)	25 (78)	0.111	33 (61)	31 (74)	0.275
Chronic lung disease *n* (%)	16 (17)	7 (11)	9 (28)	*0.044*	6 (11)	10 (24)	0.166
Chronic kidney disease *n* (%)	15 (16)	9 (14)	6 (19)	0.767	7 (13)	8 (19)	0.572
Active cancer *n* (%)	4 (4)	4 (6)	0 (0)	0.298	3 (6)	1 (2)	0.629
APACHE II score	21 (17–27)	20 (15–24)	27 (22–30)	*<0.001*	20 (15–22)	27 (22–31)	*<0.001*
SOFA score	9 (6–12)	8 (5–11)	9 (7–13)	0.070	8 (4–10)	10 (7–13)	*0.004*
Respiratory rate (bpm)	24 ± 7	24 ± 7	23 ± 6	0.773	24 ± 7	24 ± 6	0.992
FiO_2 (%)	50 (40–60)	50 (50–60)	50 (40–61)	0.913	50 (50–60)	50 (40–60)	0.794
PEEP (cmH_20)	8 (5–8)	8 (5–8)	6 (5–10)	0.264	8 (5–8)	6 (5–10)	0.574
Arterial pH	7.38 ± 0.09	7.40 ± 0.08	7.33 ± 0.10	0.002	7.40 ± 0.07	7.35 ± 0.11	0.009
PaO_2 (mmHg)	79 (67–98)	79 (65–97)	79 (68–107)	0.724	80 (65–98)	77 (68–97)	0.631
$PaCO_2$ (mmHg)	38 (35–44)	39 (36–44)	38 (32–45)	0.508	40 (36–45)	38 (34–44)	0.252
PaO_2/FiO_2 ratio	155 (113–206)	158 (110–206)	150 (116–207)	0.946	164 (108–214)	143 (115–198)	0.413
ARDS				0.870			0.600
Severe ARDS *n* (%)	15 (16)	11 (17)	4 (12)		9 (17)	6 (14)	
Moderate ARDS *n* (%)	56 (58)	36 (56)	20 (63)		29 (54)	27 (64)	
Mild ARDS *n* (%)	25 (26)	17 (27)	8 (25)		16 (29)	9 (22)	
MAP (mmHg)	81 ± 13	80 ± 13	83 ± 13	0.379	81 ± 13	82 ± 14	0.645
Heart rate (bpm)	94 ± 21	95 ± 21	92 ± 21	0.456	93 ± 21	96 ± 21	0.520
CVP (mmHg)	10 (8–13)	10 (8–14)	10 (8–12)	0.678	10 (8–13)	10 (9–13)	0.683
Norepinephrine, *n* (%)	51 (53)	35 (55)	16 (50)	0.828	28 (52)	23 (55)	0.838
Norepinephrine (mcg/Kg/min)	0.02 (0.00–0.22)	0.02 (0.00–0.17)	0.02 (0.00–0.35)	0.676	0.01 (0.00–0.18)	0.07 (0.00–0.30)	0.391
Lactate (mmol/L)	1.7 (1.1–3.0)	1.5 (0.9–2.6)	2.1 (1.3–4.0)	*0.024*	1.3 (0.9–2.7)	2.1 (1.2–3.3)	*0.028*
Creatinine (mg/dL)	1.0 (0.7–1.4)	0.9 (0.7–1.3)	1.2 (0.8–1.7)	0.213	0.9 (0.7–1.2)	1.2 (0.7–1.7)	0.070
Renal failure *n* (%)	40 (42)	23 (37)	17 (53)	0.131	16 (30)	24 (57)	*0.012*
Total bilirubin (mg/dL)	0.7 (0.5–1.7)	0.6 (0.5–1.4)	1.1 (0.6–1.9)	*0.037*	0.6 (0.5–1.0)	1.1 (0.5–1.9)	0.096
Platelets ($x10^3/\mu L$)	168 (105–225)	182 (107–280)	136 (80–179)	*0.011*	183 (107–280)	136 (93–183)	*0.040*
Leukocytes (cells $x10^3/\mu L$)	12.0 (8.5–15.4)	11.2 (7.7–15.3)	12.5 (8.9–16.1)	0.455	11.2 (8.2–15.2)	12.4 (8.7–15.5)	0.624
Duration of mechanical ventilation (days)	4.5 (2.4–8.2)	4.3 (2.5–7.2)	5.6 (2.2–8.6)	0.756	3.6 (1.8–6.2)	7.2 (2.7–16.9)	*<0.001*
ICU length of stay (days)	6.4 (4.4–11.0)	7.1 (4.6–12.4)	6.0 (2.6–9.6)	0.140	6.0 (4.4–8.9)	8.3 (4.1–17.4)	0.109

n number of patients, *ARDS* acute respiratory distress syndrome, *FiO_2* inspired oxygen fraction, *PEEP* positive end-expiratory pressure, *PaO_2* arterial oxygen pressure, *$PaCO_2$* arterial carbon dioxide pressure, *MAP* mean arterial pressure, *CVP* central venous pressure, *ICU* intensive care unit

Statistically significant *p* values (<0.05) are shown in italics

the PaO_2/FiO_2 ratio at T1 ($r = 0.191$, $p = 0.07$), or with the change in the PaO_2/FiO_2 ratio between T0 and T1 ($r = 0.095$, $p = 0.36$). The changes in endocan concentrations between T0 and T1 were not significantly correlated with the changes in PaO_2/FiO_2 ratios between T0 and T1 ($r = 0.126$, $p = 0.23$).

In the subgroups of septic and non-septic patients ($n = 64$ and $n = 32$, respectively), there were no significant differences in endocan concentrations at T0 or T1 in patients with poor evolution or good evolution (Additional file 1: Table S3). In the subgroup of non-trauma patients ($n = 88$), endocan concentrations at T1 were higher in patients with a poor evolution than in those with a good evolution ($p = 0.03$), but not at T0 (Additional file 1: Table S3).

Discussion

Our results demonstrate that plasma endocan concentrations measured early in the course of ARDS can reflect disease severity and predict poor evolution, as assessed by death or prolonged dependence on mechanical ventilation.

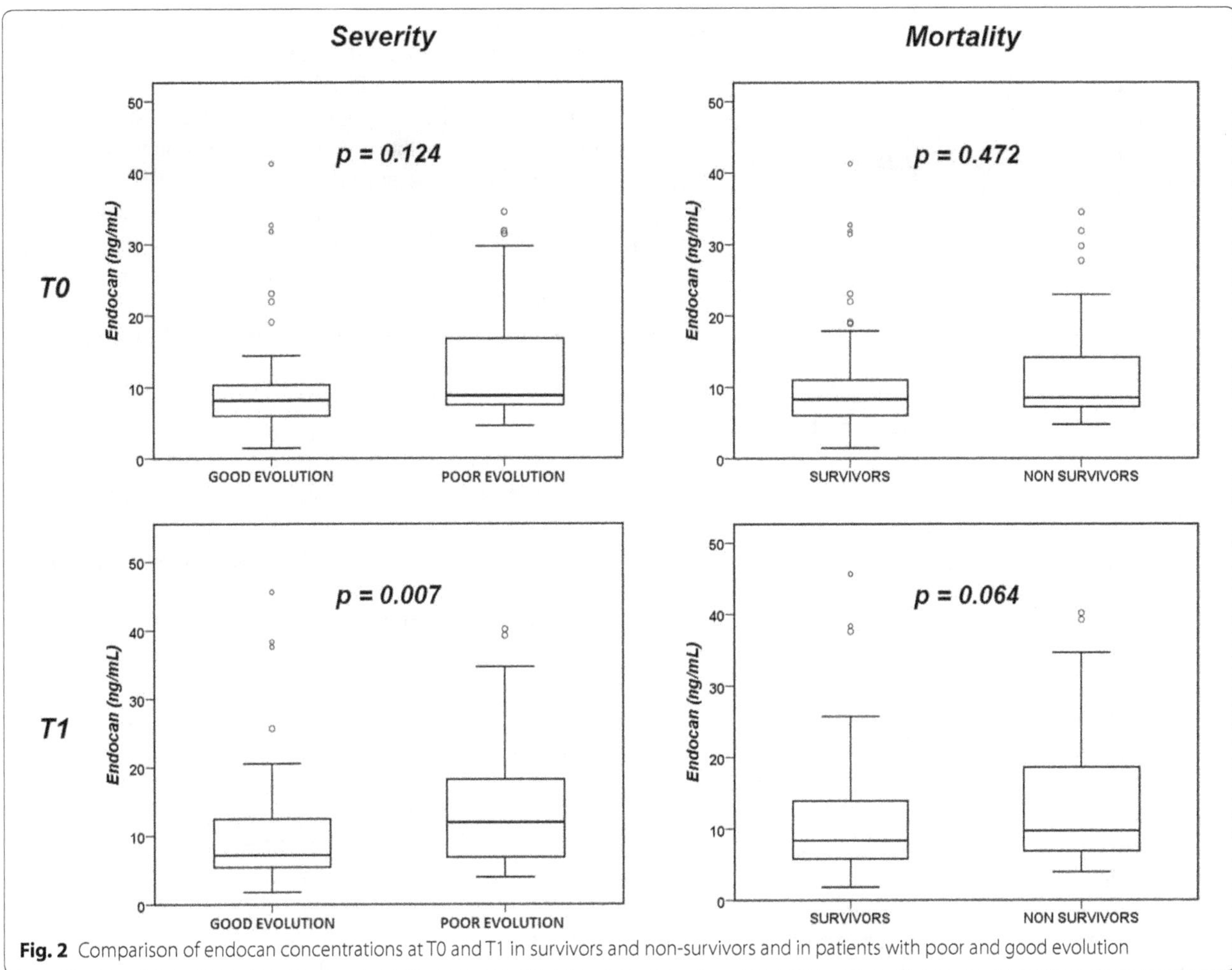

Fig. 2 Comparison of endocan concentrations at T0 and T1 in survivors and non-survivors and in patients with poor and good evolution

Data on endocan levels in patients with ARDS are limited. A retrospective study of 24 trauma patients reported that patients who developed ARDS had lower endocan levels on admission than matched patients without ARDS [22]. A prospective study in 20 septic ICU patients reported lower endocan concentrations at admission in patients who had developed respiratory failure by day 3 after admission than in those who had not; the endocan level at admission was correlated with the decrease in PaO_2/FiO_2 ratio on days 2 and 3 [11]. These studies only measured endocan concentrations on admission. In a more recent study in patients with sepsis, endocan concentrations were measured on admission and after 72 h or on development of new organ dysfunction; an increase in endocan concentrations was associated with development of ARDS [23]. Our results show that endocan concentrations are higher in patients with more severe ARDS who require prolonged mechanical ventilation. Similarly, in a small prospective cohort of 42 patients with ARDS (mainly due to sepsis), endocan concentrations (1 day after the diagnosis of ARDS) were higher in non-survivors than in survivors [19].

We measured endocan concentrations at two points during the early phase of ARDS, a period when prognostication is difficult. Several studies have shown that the PaO_2/FiO_2 ratio has only mild to moderate power to predict bad outcomes [3, 24, 25]. A score that combines PaO_2/FiO_2 ratios, cardiovascular dysfunction and age has been proposed, but data need to be collected for 3 days following diagnosis [26]. Others have suggested combining different clinical variables at the moment of ARDS diagnosis [25], but external validation is missing. Our data show that endocan concentrations have prognostic power already on the first day after ARDS diagnosis and that there was no correlation of endocan concentrations with PaO_2/FiO_2 ratios on admission or with changes in the ratio over the first 2 days after diagnosis.

Our data confirm previous findings of high endocan concentrations in septic patients. In an early study, Scherpereel and colleagues [17] showed that human in vitro endothelial cells secreted endocan after stimulation by

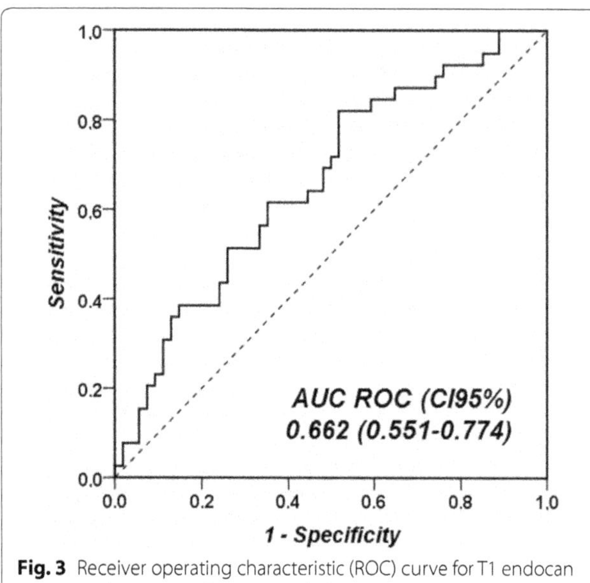

Fig. 3 Receiver operating characteristic (ROC) curve for T1 endocan concentrations to predict poor evolution

lipopolysaccharide and tumor necrosis factor-alpha. They also reported higher circulating endocan concentrations in septic patients than in healthy donors or patients with isolated systemic inflammatory response syndrome (SIRS) [17]. Mihajlovic and colleagues reported that higher initial endocan concentrations were related to later development of organ dysfunction and mortality in patients with sepsis [18]. However, although T0 endocan concentrations were higher in patients with sepsis than in those without, there were no differences in endocan concentrations at T0 and T1 in patients with poor or good evolution in the sepsis subgroup.

We observed higher endocan concentrations in patients with than in those without renal failure. In healthy human tissues, endocan is preferentially expressed in the lung endothelium, but also in the glomerular endothelial and tubular epithelial cells in the kidneys [9, 10]. A recent study showed that in patients who had received a kidney transplant, endocan concentrations were directly correlated with more advanced stages of chronic kidney disease [27]. In pathological conditions, renal expression of endocan may potentially be increased or renal excretion reduced, but there are no data in this field. Based on currently available data, renal function should be taken into consideration when interpreting endocan concentrations.

In addition to its potential role in the pathogenesis of ARDS and other inflammatory conditions, endocan may also be involved in the pathogenesis of other conditions. Recent data suggest that endocan may have a role in chronic cardiovascular disease [12], hypertension or diabetes, but endocan levels were similar in patients with and without these comorbid conditions in our database. One human study has suggested that endocan is also expressed in highly proliferative tissues, such as the neo-vasculature or the lymph nodes [10]. It has been shown that in some neoplasms, endocan is preferentially expressed in the tumor endothelium and its expression is regulated by tumor-derived factors [28]. Exposure of mice to high concentrations of endocan can also induce the development of tumors [29]. This observation may explain why elevated plasma concentrations have been found in patients with different types of cancer and are associated with the probability of survival [30–32]. The prevalence of active cancer in our population was low

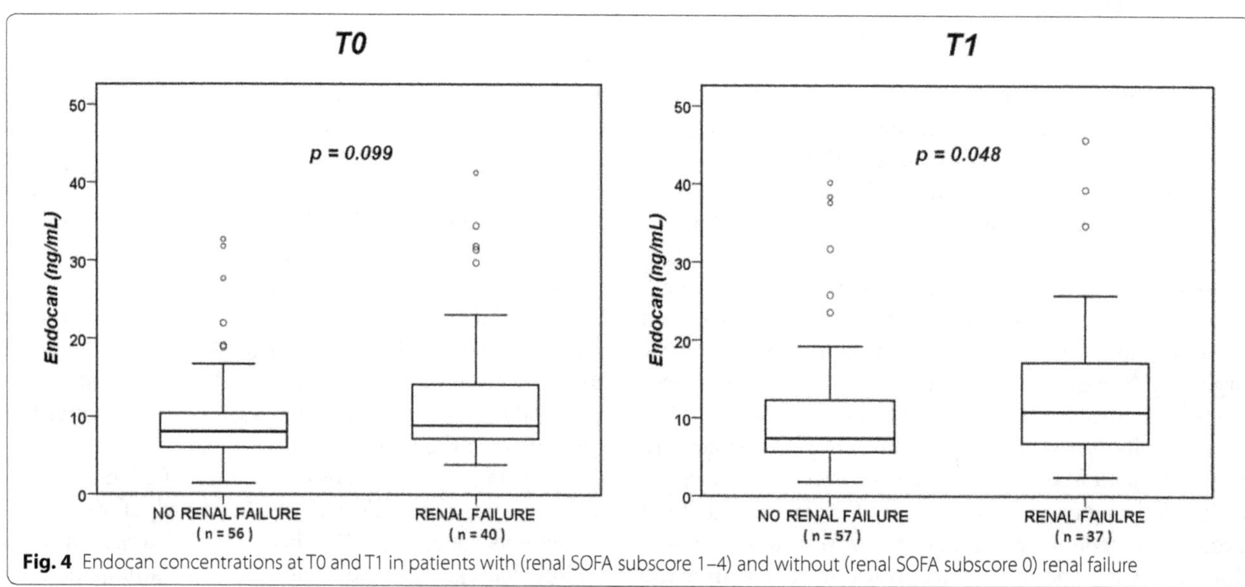

Fig. 4 Endocan concentrations at T0 and T1 in patients with (renal SOFA subscore 1–4) and without (renal SOFA subscore 0) renal failure

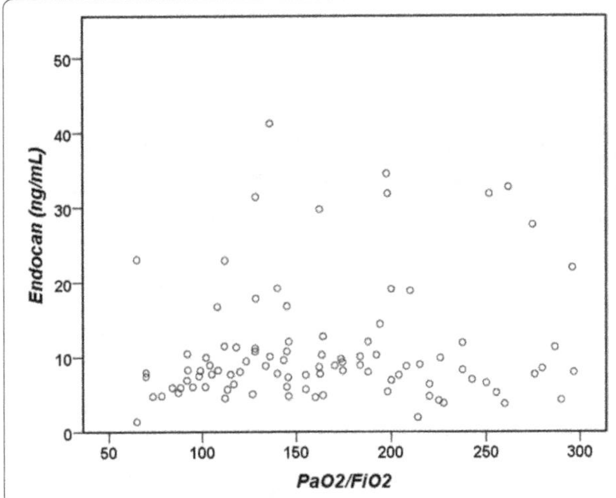

Fig. 5 Correlation of endocan concentrations with PaO_2/FiO_2 ratio at T0 ($r = 0.137, p = 0.18$)

and endocan concentrations were no different in these patients compared to those without cancer (data not shown); nevertheless, this factor may be relevant in oncologic ICUs.

Our study has several limitations. First, ARDS is a heterogeneous syndrome including various pathogenic mechanisms that may or may not be related to the endocan pathway. Second, we did not measure endocan concentrations after 24 h and therefore have no information on concentrations at later time points, but we were focusing on endocan as an early biomarker, because patient outcomes are highly influenced by subsequent clinical evolution. Third, including a control group of non-ARDS patients may have provided interesting information regarding the role of endocan as a diagnostic biomarker, but our aim was to determine whether endocan could be used as an early biomarker of severity in patients already diagnosed with ARDS. Finally, our study may have lacked power to detect some differences in the early stages of ARDS and in the analyzed subgroups, as suggested by the tendency for endocan concentrations to be higher in patients with worse outcomes even at the time of ARDS diagnosis.

Conclusion

In patients with ARDS, plasma endocan concentrations 24 h after diagnosis may be useful to predict poor evolution.

Abbreviations

APACHE: acute physiology and chronic health evaluation; ARDS: acute respiratory distress syndrome; AUC: area under the curve; CI: confidence interval; CVP: central venous pressure; EDTA: ethylenediaminetetraacetic acid; ELISA: enzyme-linked immunosorbent assay; ESM-1: endothelial cell-specific molecule 1; FiO_2: inspired oxygen fraction; ICU: intensive care unit; MAP: mean arterial pressure; PaO_2: arterial oxygen pressure; $PaCO_2$: arterial carbon dioxide pressure; PEEP: positive end-expiratory pressure; ROC: receiver operating characteristic; SIRS: systemic inflammatory response syndrome; SOFA: sequential organ failure assessment.

Authors' contributions

DO, LR, DDB, JC and JLV conceived and designed the study; DO, LR and FA performed all the endocan measurements; DO, LR, MI, FA and MM screened and collected data from the population; DO wrote the first draft of the manuscript. LR, MI, FA, MM, DDB, JC and JLV revised the text for intellectual content. All authors read and approved the final manuscript.

Competing interests

The authors declare that they have no competing interests.

Funding

No external funding.

References

1. Bellani G, Laffey JG, Pham T, Fan E, Brochard L, Esteban A, et al. Epidemiology, patterns of care, and mortality for patients with acute respiratory distress syndrome in intensive care units in 50 countries. JAMA. 2016;315:788–800.
2. Maca J, Jor O, Holub M, Sklienka P, Bursa F, Burda M, et al. Past and present ARDS mortality rates: a systematic review. Respir Care. 2017;62:113–22.
3. Ranieri VM, Rubenfeld GD, Thompson BT, Ferguson ND, Caldwell E, Fan E, et al. Acute respiratory distress syndrome: the Berlin definition. JAMA. 2012;307:2526–33.
4. Orfanos SE, Mavrommati I, Korovesi I, Roussos C. Pulmonary endothelium in acute lung injury: from basic science to the critically ill. Intensive Care Med. 2004;30:1702–14.
5. Orfanos SE, Armaganidis A, Glynos C, Psevdi E, Kaltsas P, Sarafidou P, et al. Pulmonary capillary endothelium-bound angiotensin-converting enzyme activity in acute lung injury. Circulation. 2000;102:2011–8.
6. Orbegozo Cortes D, Rahmania L, Irazabal M, Santacruz C, Fontana V, De Backer D, et al. Microvascular reactivity is altered early in patients with acute respiratory distress syndrome. Respir Res. 2016;17:59.
7. Bull TM, Clark B, McFann K, Moss M. Pulmonary vascular dysfunction is associated with poor outcomes in patients with acute lung injury. Am J Respir Crit Care Med. 2010;182:1123–8.
8. Moussa MD, Santonocito C, Fagnoul D, Donadello K, Pradier O, Gaussem P, et al. Evaluation of endothelial damage in sepsis-related ARDS using circulating endothelial cells. Intensive Care Med. 2015;41:231–8.
9. Lassalle P, Molet S, Janin A, Heyden JV, Tavernier J, Fiers W, et al. ESM-1 is a novel human endothelial cell-specific molecule expressed in lung and regulated by cytokines. J Biol Chem. 1996;271:20458–64.
10. Zhang SM, Zuo L, Zhou Q, Gui SY, Shi R, Wu Q, et al. Expression and distribution of endocan in human tissues. Biotech Histochem. 2012;87:172–8.
11. Palud A, Parmentier-Decrucq E, Pastre J, De Freitas CN, Lassalle P, Mathieu D. Evaluation of endothelial biomarkers as predictors of organ failures in septic shock patients. Cytokine. 2015;73:213–8.
12. Balta S, Mikhailidis DP, Demirkol S, Ozturk C, Celik T, Iyisoy A. Endocan: a novel inflammatory indicator in cardiovascular disease? Atherosclerosis. 2015;243:339–43.
13. Cross LJ, Matthay MA. Biomarkers in acute lung injury: insights into the pathogenesis of acute lung injury. Crit Care Clin. 2011;27:355–77.
14. Thille AW, Esteban A, Fernandez-Segoviano P, Rodriguez JM, Aramburu JA, Vargas-Errazuriz P, et al. Chronology of histological lesions in acute respiratory distress syndrome with diffuse alveolar damage: a prospective cohort study of clinical autopsies. Lancet Respir Med. 2013;1:395–401.
15. Cox LA, van Eijk LT, Ramakers BP, Dorresteijn MJ, Gerretsen J, Kox M, et al. Inflammation-induced increases in plasma endocan levels are associated with endothelial dysfunction in humans in vivo. Shock. 2015;43:322–6.
16. Lee W, Ku SK, Kim SW, Bae JS. Endocan elicits severe vascular inflammatory responses in vitro and in vivo. J Cell Physiol. 2014;229:620–30.

17. Scherpereel A, Depontieu F, Grigoriu B, Cavestri B, Tsicopoulos A, Gentina T, et al. Endocan, a new endothelial marker in human sepsis. Crit Care Med. 2006;34:532–7.
18. Mihajlovic DM, Lendak DF, Brkic SV, Draskovic BG, Mitic GP, Novakov Mikic AS, et al. Endocan is useful biomarker of survival and severity in sepsis. Microvasc Res. 2014;93:92–7.
19. Tang L, Zhao Y, Wang D, Deng W, Li C, Li Q, et al. Endocan levels in peripheral blood predict outcomes of acute respiratory distress syndrome. Mediators Inflamm. 2014;2014:625180.
20. Knaus WA, Draper EA, Wagner DP, Zimmerman JE. APACHE II: a severity of disease classification system. Crit Care Med. 1985;13:818–29.
21. Vincent JL, Moreno R, Takala J, Willatts S, De Mendonca A, Bruining H, et al. The SOFA (Sepsis-related Organ Failure Assessment) score to describe organ dysfunction/failure. On behalf of the Working Group on Sepsis-Related Problems of the European Society of Intensive Care Medicine. Intensive Care Med. 1996;22:707–10.
22. Mikkelsen ME, Shah CV, Scherpereel A, Lanken PN, Lassalle P, Bellamy SL, et al. Lower serum endocan levels are associated with the development of acute lung injury after major trauma. J Crit Care. 2012;27:522–7.
23. Ioakeimidou A, Pagalou E, Kontogiorgi M, Antoniadou E, Kaziani K, Psaroulis K et al. Increase of circulating endocan over sepsis follow-up is associated with progression into organ dysfunction. Eur J Clin Microbiol Infect Dis. 2017. https://doi.org/10.1007/s10096-017-2988-6.
24. Hernu R, Wallet F, Thiolliere F, Martin O, Richard JC, Schmitt Z, et al. An attempt to validate the modification of the American–European consensus definition of acute lung injury/acute respiratory distress syndrome by the Berlin definition in a university hospital. Intensive Care Med. 2013;39:2161–70.
25. Villar J, Perez-Mendez L, Basaldua S, Blanco J, Aguilar G, Toral D, et al. A risk tertiles model for predicting mortality in patients with acute respiratory distress syndrome: age, plateau pressure, and P(aO(2))/F(IO(2)) at ARDS onset can predict mortality. Respir Care. 2011;56:420–8.
26. Gajic O, Afessa B, Thompson BT, Frutos-Vivar F, Malinchoc M, Rubenfeld GD, et al. Prediction of death and prolonged mechanical ventilation in acute lung injury. Crit Care. 2007;11:R53.
27. Su YH, Shu KH, Hu CP, Cheng CH, Wu MJ, Yu TM, et al. Serum endocan correlated with stage of chronic kidney disease and deterioration in renal transplant recipients. Transplant Proc. 2014;46:323–7.
28. Abid MR, Yi X, Yano K, Shih SC, Aird WC. Vascular endocan is preferentially expressed in tumor endothelium. Microvasc Res. 2006;72:136–45.
29. Scherpereel A, Gentina T, Grigoriu B, Senechal S, Janin A, Tsicopoulos A, et al. Overexpression of endocan induces tumor formation. Cancer Res. 2003;63:6084–9.
30. Hatfield KJ, Lassalle P, Leiva RA, Lindas R, Wendelboe O, Bruserud O. Serum levels of endothelium-derived endocan are increased in patients with untreated acute myeloid leukemia. Hematology. 2011;16:351–6.
31. Ozaki K, Toshikuni N, George J, Minato T, Matsue Y, Arisawa T, et al. Serum endocan as a novel prognostic biomarker in patients with hepatocellular carcinoma. J Cancer. 2014;5:221–30.
32. Grigoriu BD, Depontieu F, Scherpereel A, Gourcerol D, Devos P, Ouatas T, et al. Endocan expression and relationship with survival in human non-small cell lung cancer. Clin Cancer Res. 2006;12:4575–82.

13

Internal jugular vein variability predicts fluid responsiveness in cardiac surgical patients with mechanical ventilation

Guo-guang Ma[†], Guang-wei Hao[†], Xiao-mei Yang, Du-ming Zhu, Lan Liu, Hua Liu, Guo-wei Tu[*] and Zhe Luo[*]

Abstract

Background: To evaluate the efficacy of using internal jugular vein variability (IJVV) as an index of fluid responsiveness in mechanically ventilated patients after cardiac surgery.

Methods: Seventy patients were assessed after cardiac surgery. Hemodynamic data coupled with ultrasound evaluation of IJVV and inferior vena cava variability (IVCV) were collected and calculated at baseline, after a passive leg raising (PLR) test and after a 500-ml fluid challenge. Patients were divided into volume responders (increase in stroke volume $\geq$ 15%) and non-responders (increase in stroke volume < 15%). We compared the differences in measured variables between responders and non-responders and tested the ability of the indices to predict fluid responsiveness.

Results: Thirty-five (50%) patients were fluid responders. Responders presented higher IJVV, IVCV and stroke volume variation (SVV) compared with non-responders at baseline ($P < 0.05$). The relationship between IJVV and SVV was moderately correlated ($r = 0.51$, $P < 0.01$). The areas under the receiver operating characteristic (ROC) curves for predicting fluid responsiveness were 0.88 (CI 0.78–0.94) for IJVV compared with 0.83 (CI 0.72–0.91), 0.97 (CI 0.89–0.99), 0.91 (CI 0.82–0.97) for IVCV, SVV, and the increase in stroke volume in response to a PLR test, respectively.

Conclusions: Ultrasound-derived IJVV is an accurate, easily acquired noninvasive parameter of fluid responsiveness in mechanically ventilated postoperative cardiac surgery patients, with a performance similar to that of IVCV.

Keywords: Internal jugular veins, Inferior vena cava, Stroke volume variation, Fluid responsiveness, Cardiac surgery

Background

Fluid management is one of the most important treatments for stabilizing hemodynamics in patients after cardiac surgery. Hypovolemia may lead to inadequate organ perfusion, whereas fluid overload may lead to postoperative complications such as congestive heart failure or pulmonary edema [1–3]. In addition, patients who underwent cardiac surgery have a certain degree of myocardial stunning [4], and hence, caution should be taken regarding fluid management in patients with a limited cardiac reserve.

It is imperative to predict the patient's fluid responsiveness before volume expansion [5]. Several parameters have been introduced in clinical practice to predict fluid responsiveness and to guide therapy [2]. Based on the influence of cycling intra-thoracic pressure on arterial pulse pressure or stroke volume, dynamic indicators such as arterial pulse pressure variation (PPV) or stroke volume variation (SVV) have been widely used as reliable predictors of fluid responsiveness [6–8]. However, these dynamic parameters have several limitations and can only be used under strict conditions.

Recently, noninvasive and point-of-care ultrasound seems to meet the criteria of an ideal bedside tool for fluid status assessment. Several studies have confirmed

*Correspondence: tu.guowei@zs-hospital.sh.cn; luo.zhe@zs-hospital.sh.cn
[†]Guo-guang Ma and Guang-wei Hao have contributed equally to this work
Department of Critical Care Medicine, Zhongshan Hospital, Fudan University, No. 180 Fenglin Road, Shanghai 200032, Xuhui District, People's Republic of China

that respiratory variations of the superior and inferior vena cava diameters (collapsibility index [CI] and distensibility index [DI]) accurately reflect volume responsiveness in mechanically ventilated patients [9, 10]. Unfortunately, measurements of the inferior vena cava (IVC) and superior vena cava (SVC) may fail to predict fluid responsiveness following cardiac surgery due to methodological problems such as poor subcostal caval image quality caused by mediastinal air, surgical drains, dressings, abdominal distension or morbid obesity [11–13]; a more accurate measurement would require transoesophageal echocardiography (TEE). It is well known that pressure and volume changes within the intra-thoracic systemic venous compartment can transmit to the extrathoracic veins, for example, the intra-abdominal IVC or extrathoracic internal jugular vein (IJV) [14–16]. The IJV is, technically, much more easily accessible for sonographic visualization than the IVC, and measurement of the IJV does not require TEE. Internal jugular vein variability (IJVV) has been studied in several studies [17–19], but its reliability has not been well confirmed in patients after cardiac surgery. The aim of this study was to evaluate the reliability of IJVV, as visualized by ultrasound, to predict fluid responsiveness in mechanically ventilated patients after cardiac surgery.

Methods

This study was approved by the Ethical Committee of Zhongshan Hospital affiliated to Fudan University (No. B2016077), and informed consent was obtained from all study participants. This trial has been registered at clinicaltrials.gov as NCT02852889.

Patient selection

Patients who underwent cardiac surgery between August and December 2016 in the Cardiac Surgery Intensive Care Unit (CSICU) of the Zhongshan Hospital of Fudan University were screened for inclusion by research personnel. All patients routinely underwent a TEE during the operation and a postoperative (after admission to ICU and prior to study enrollment) comprehensive transthoracic echocardiography (TTE). The TEE was used to monitor the hemodynamics and confirm the postoperative effect of surgery. TTE was used to identify different causes of hypotension in postoperative period such as obstructive shock, hypovolemia and reduced ventricular systolic function. The patients were included when they presented with circulatory instability and required a rapid fluid challenge based on the clinical judgment of the attending physician. The physician's decision was principally based on the presence of clinical signs of acute circulatory failure (low blood pressure or urine output, tachycardia, or mottling) and/or clinical signs of organ hypoperfusion (renal dysfunction or hyperlactatemia). The exclusion criteria included age < 18 years; evidence of cardiac arrhythmia (e.g., atrial fibrillation); evidence of jugular vein thrombosis; bilaterally inserted venous catheters (jugular or subclavian vein); echocardiographic examination that showed the existence of severe tricuspid or mitral regurgitation or right heart dysfunction (right ventricular fractional area change < 40% examined by TEE; tricuspid annular plane systolic excursion < 16 mm examined by TTE); a history of radiotherapy or surgery of the neck region or back (making it impossible to put the patient in a supine position with the head elevated to 30°); a contraindication to the passive leg raising (PLR) test; and the inability to obtain interpretable ultrasound images due to a difficult acoustic window.

All enrolled patients were sedated via propofol and morphine infusion, and with absence of inspiratory efforts according to the ventilator waveform and monitoring parameters. No muscular blocking agents were used in this study. All patients were ventilated in the intermittent positive pressure ventilation (IPPV) mode in the supine position with the head elevated to 30°. The ventilatory parameters were adjusted to the following criteria: tidal volume (Vt): 8 ml/kg predicted body weight (PBW), Pplat < 30 cmH_2O, positive end-expiratory pressure (PEEP): 5 cmH_2O, respiratory rate: 12–16 breaths per minute, $PaCO_2 \leq 45$ mmHg and oxygen saturation (SaO_2) > 96%. The following baseline data were recorded for each patient: age (years), weight (kg), height (cm), diagnosis, type of cardiac surgery, acute physiology and chronic health evaluation (APACHE) II score, European system for cardiac operative risk evaluation (EuroSCORE), vasoactive drug infusion rates and preoperative echocardiographic parameters [left ventricular ejection fraction (LVEF), presence of left ventricular hypertrophy, right ventricular end-diastolic diameter, and tricuspid regurgitation grade].

Measurements

We analyzed a series of measured hemodynamic variables from an indwelling radial arterial catheter and central venous catheter in each patient. These data included heart rate (HR) (beats/minute), mean arterial pressure (MAP) (mmHg), central venous pressure (CVP) (mmHg), stroke volume (SV) (ml), PLR-induced increase in stroke volume (PLR-ΔSV) (ml), and stroke volume variation (SVV) using the FloTrac/Vigileo (Edwards Lifesciences, Irvine, CA, USA) continuous hemodynamic monitoring system. The pressure transducers were consistently adjusted to the level of the patient's right atrium.

Intensivists with a certification of ultrasound evaluation performed all of the ultrasound examinations. An associate critical care professor supervised the entire course of examinations. The intensivists performing the ultrasound examinations were blinded to the hemodynamic data. (These were collected by another investigator.) Sonographic measurements of the IJV and IVC diameters were taken using a Philips CX50 ultrasound device (Philips Healthcare, Hamburg, Germany) equipped with a linear transducer (L12-3 Broadband Linear Array Transducer) and a transthoracic phased array transducer (S5-1 Phased Array Transducer), respectively.

Patients admitted at the ICU after cardiac surgery had a conventional right IJV catheter. To avoid any risk of infection at the puncture site, sonographic measurements were taken on the left IJV. The IJV was visualized by placing the ultrasound transducer perpendicular to the skin in the transverse plane on the patient's neck at the level of the cricoid cartilage in order to avoid interference from the probe-to-vein angle. The vein was identified by compression as well as by color Doppler imaging. To avoid any influence of external compression on the IJV diameter during the examination, sufficient ultrasound gel was used to prevent direct skin contact with the transducer [20], and thus, the least amount of pressure was applied (Fig. 1a).

An M-mode scan was recorded over a whole respiratory cycle (Fig. 1b, c), and then, the image was frozen. The maximum antero-posterior diameter of the IJV was measured at the end of inspiration [diamax (cm)], and the minimum diameter was measured at the end of expiration [diamin (cm)]. The IJV variability (IJVV) was calculated using the formula: IJVV (%) = (diamax − diamin)/[(diamax + diamin)/2] × 100. Using similar methods, the IVC was visualized longitudinally in the subxyphoid long-axis view, and its M-mode cursor was used to measure the IVC variability (IVCV) approximately 3 cm from the right atrium.

Study design

Ultrasound examinations and the collection of hemodynamic data were performed at baseline (*T*0, in a supine position with the head elevated to 30° for baseline measurements), 1 min after a PLR test (*T*1, the bed was automatically moved to a position with the head elevated to 0° and the legs up to 45°) and after a 500-mL Gelofusine challenge (T2, the bed was returned to the initial position, and fluid was infused over 30 min). PLR was performed in order to compare the predictive value of different parameters in predicting fluid responsiveness. Vasoactive drug infusion rates and ventilation settings were kept constant during the study procedures. Patients were classified as "volume responders" if there was an increase in SV ≥ 15% after the fluid challenge, and the remaining patients were classified as "volume non-responders" [21, 22].

Statistical analysis

The number of the enrolled patients was referred to similar studies evaluating the prediction ability of IJVV [17–19]. All continuous variables except the doses of norepinephrine and dobutamine were normally distributed (Kolmogorov–Smirnov test). The results are expressed as the mean ± SD (standard deviation) or median (25–75% inter-quartile range, IQR) as appropriate. After checking the homogeneity of variance for each parameter, the difference between values was compared using the independent sample *t* test, and the comparisons of hemodynamic variables between the different study times were assessed using paired Student *t* tests. Comparisons between responders and non-responders were assessed using two-sample Student's *t* tests. *P* values < 0.05 were considered statistically significant. Correlations were assessed by Pearson coefficient. Receiver operating characteristic (ROC) curves were constructed to establish the sensitivity and specificity of dynamic and static indicators in predicting fluid responsiveness. The areas under the ROC curves (AUCs) were compared using DeLong and colleagues' test. The optimal cutoff of each variable was estimated by maximizing the Youden index. A difference between two AUCs was considered statistically significant, when the *P* value of DeLong and colleagues' test

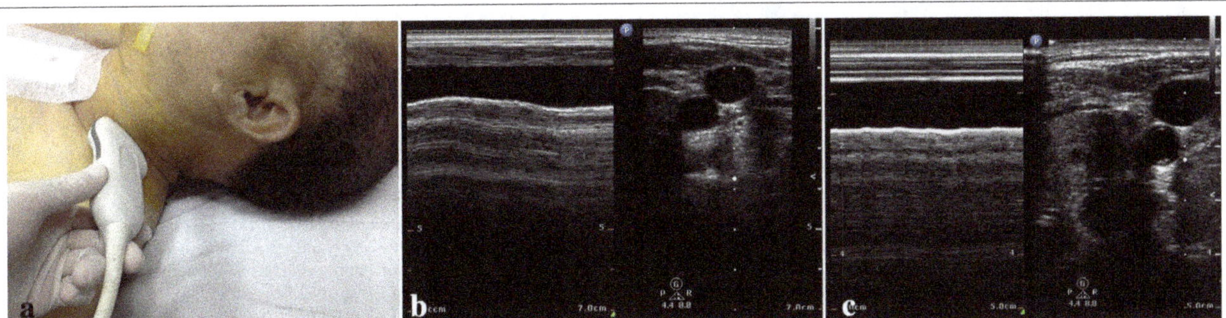

Fig. 1 Ultrasound probe position for IJV detection at the cricoid cartilage level (**a**). The patient is in the supine position at 30°. M-mode assessment of the antero-posterior diameter of the IJV in a responsive patient (**b**, a high variability of IJV diameter is seen) and in a non-responsive patient (**c**, lack of variation of the IJV diameter is seen) while on mechanical ventilation

was < 0.05. Statistical analyses were performed with the MedCalc 8.1.0.0 (Mariakerke, Belgium) and SPSS software (19.0).

Results

A total of seventy-five postoperative cardiac surgery patients were enrolled during a period of 5 months. Five patients were excluded because visualization of the IVC via ultrasound was technically difficult. Seventy patients (44 males and 26 females) were included in the final analysis. The reasons for hemodynamic instability were related to the hypovolemia (35 patients), cardiac dysfunction (27 patients) and vasoplegic shock (8 patients). The mean age of the patients was 61 ± 10 years, and the APACHE II scores were 9 ± 5. All patients were sedated and were in sinus rhythm. The patients' mean LVEF (Simpson's method) before surgery was 50%. Baseline patient characteristics and clinical data are shown in Table 1. Hemodynamic and ultrasound data in responders and non-responders at all study times [baseline (*T0*), during PLR (*T1*), and after fluid challenge (*T2*)] are reported in Table 2. Fluid challenge significantly increased SV by more than 15% in 35 (50%) patients (responders, from 39.87 ± 13.67 to 58.72 ± 22.16 ml, $P < 0.05$). The remaining 35 (50%) patients did not exhibit a significant change in SV (non-responders, from 49.86 ± 17.71 to 54.81 ± 16.53 ml). The results of PLR and fluid challenge in this study are shown in Additional file 1.

Table 1 Baseline characteristics of the patients ($n = 70$)

Characteristic	
Age (years)	61 ± 10
Male sex, *n* (%)	44 (62.86)
Body mass index (kg/m^2)	22 ± 3
Left ventricular ejection fraction (%)	50
Cardiac surgery category, *n* (%)	
Valve	37 (52.86)
CABG	12 (17.14)
CABG + valve	7 (10.00)
Aortic surgery	9 (12.86)
Others	5 (7.14)
Postoperative day, *n* (%)	
d0	62 (88.57%)
d1	8 (11.43%)
APACHE II scores	9 ± 5
EuroSCORE	4 ± 2
Tidal volume (mL)	520 ± 28
PEEP (cm H_2O)	5
PaO_2/FiO_2 (mmHg)	123 ± 57
Lactate (mmol/L)	3.23 ± 3.39
Patients receiving norepinephrine, *n* (%)	45 (64.29)
Patients receiving dobutamine, *n* (%)	9 (12.86)
Dose of norepinephrine (μg kg^{-1} min^{-1})	0.24 (0.15–0.35)
Dose of dobutamine (μg kg^{-1} min^{-1})	0.33 (0.28–0.43)

Values are expressed as mean ± SD, median (25–75% inter-quartile range) or number and frequency in %

CABG coronary artery bypass grafting, *APACHE II* acute physiology and chronic health evaluation, *EuroSCORE* European system for cardiac operative risk evaluation, *PEEP* positive end-expiratory pressure, PaO_2 arterial partial pressure of oxygen, FiO_2 inspiratory fraction of oxygen

Table 2 Hemodynamic parameters measured in responders and non-responders

	T0	*T1*	*T2*
HR (beats min^{-1})			
Responders	91 ± 20	89 ± 18	87 ± 14
Non-responders	88 ± 17	88 ± 17	87 ± 16
SBP (mmHg)			
Responders	87 ± 19	95 ± 29	119 ± 26^c
Non-responders	111 ± 17^a	116 ± 19^a	112 ± 23
DBP (mmHg)			
Responders	46 ± 8	53 ± 7^b	58 ± 8^c
Non-responders	55 ± 11^a	58 ± 9^a	54 ± 8^a
MAP (mmHg)			
Responders	58 ± 10	67 ± 9^b	73 ± 11^c
Non-responders	71 ± 10^a	75 ± 10^a	70 ± 9
CVP (mmHg)			
Responders	11 ± 4	11 ± 3	12 ± 3
Non-responders	12 ± 4	14 ± 4^{a,b}	13 ± 4
CO (L/min)			
Responders	3.60 ± 1.54	4.68 ± 1.79^b	5.11 ± 2.15^c
Non-responders	4.17 ± 0.93	4.50 ± 1.17	4.69 ± 1.44
SV (ml)			
Responders	39.87 ± 13.67	52.99 ± 16.22^b	58.72 ± 22.16^c
Non-responders	49.86 ± 17.71^a	53.52 ± 18.14	54.81 ± 16.53
SVV (%)			
Responders	14.94 ± 1.85	10.34 ± 5.26^b	8.71 ± 4.59^c
Non-responders	9.49 ± 2.67^a	7.74 ± 4.83^a	7.03 ± 2.67^c
IJVV (%)			
Responders	23.04 ± 16.76	9.88 ± 13.76^b	7.96 ± 8.72^c
Non-responders	9.90 ± 5.63^a	6.38 ± 2.37^b	5.73 ± 2.02^c
IVCV (%)			
Responders	15.97 ± 4.08	8.98 ± 4.52^b	8.08 ± 7.70^c
Non-responders	8.78 ± 5.42^a	8.14 ± 4.94	6.41 ± 2.76^c

Values are expressed as mean ± SD

HR heart rate, BP, *SBP* systolic blood pressure, *DBP* diastolic blood pressure, *MAP* mean arterial pressure, *CVP* central venous pressure, *CO* cardiac output, *SV* stroke volume, *SVV* stroke volume variation, *IJVV* internal jugular venous variability, *IVCV* inferior vena cava variability

T0 baseline, *T1* after passive leg raising test, *T2* after fluid expansion

[a] $P < 0.05$ non-responders versus responders

[b] $P < 0.05$ T1 versus T0

[c] $P < 0.05$ T2 versus T0

Basal HR was not different between the responders and non-responders either at T1 or T2 (T1 89 ± 18 vs. 88 ± 17 beats min^{-1}, T2 87 ± 14 vs. 87 ± 16 beats min^{-1}), although HR tended to decrease after the PLR test or fluid challenge in responders. Responders displayed an increase in SBP, DBP and MAP from T0 to T2 (87 ± 19 vs. 119 ± 26 mmHg, $P < 0.05$; 46 ± 8 vs. 58 ± 8 mmHg, $P < 0.05$; and 58 ± 10 vs. 73 ± 11 mmHg, $P < 0.05$, respectively), and the same changes are also observed from T0 to T1 in DBP and MAP but not in SBP. No significant change in arterial pressure or HR was observed in non-responders. Non-responders generally displayed a higher CVP than responders after PLR (T1 14 ± 4 vs. 11 ± 3 mmHg, $P < 0.05$, Table 2). Although CVP tended to increase after the PLR test or fluid challenge in non-responders, we found a significant increase in CVP only after PLR (12 ± 4 vs. 14 ± 4 mmHg, $P < 0.05$); a difference was not observed after volume expansion (12 ± 4 vs. 13 ± 4 mmHg). In responders, a significant change in CVP was not observed after the PLR test nor the fluid challenge (11 ± 4 vs. 11 ± 3 mmHg; 11 ± 4 vs. 12 ± 3 mmHg).

In volume responders, IJVV, IVCV and SVV were significantly higher compared with non-responders at baseline. All of these values significantly decreased after the PLR test or fluid administration in responders. However, we found that both responders and non-responders exhibited a significant reduction in IJVV from baseline to the PLR test time or post-volume expansion, and similar findings were also presented for IVCV after fluid challenge (Table 2). We determined that the relationship between IJVV and SVV was moderately correlated (Fig. 2a, $r = 0.51$, $P < 0.01$). IVCV and SVV were significantly correlated (Fig. 2b, $r = 0.75$, $P < 0.01$).

The AUCs established for SVV and PLR-ΔSV were comparable (0.97 vs. 0.91, $P = 0.61$). The AUC of SVV was significantly greater than that of IVCV (0.97 vs. 0.83, $P < 0.01$) and IJVV (0.97 vs. 0.88, $P = 0.03$) (Fig. 3a). The AUCs for static indicators (CVP, IVC diameter and IJV diameter) were significantly lower than that of dynamic indicators (Fig. 3b). An SVV value > 12% was able to identify volume responders with a sensitivity of 91.43%, a specificity of 94.29% and an AUC of 0.97 (CI 0.89–0.99). The PLR-ΔSV > 12.84% for the prediction of fluid responsiveness was associated with a sensitivity of 100%, a specificity of 82.86% and an AUC of 0.91 (CI 0.82–0.97). IJVV > 12.99% predicted fluid responsiveness with a sensitivity of 91.43%, a specificity of 82.86% and an AUC of 0.88 (CI 0.78–0.94). IVCV showed an AUC of 0.83 (CI 0.72–0.91) with a cutoff value of 13.39% (sensitivity 85.71% and specificity 85.71%) (Table 3). A significant difference between IJVV and IVCV was not observed (0.88 vs. 0.83, $P = 0.43$).

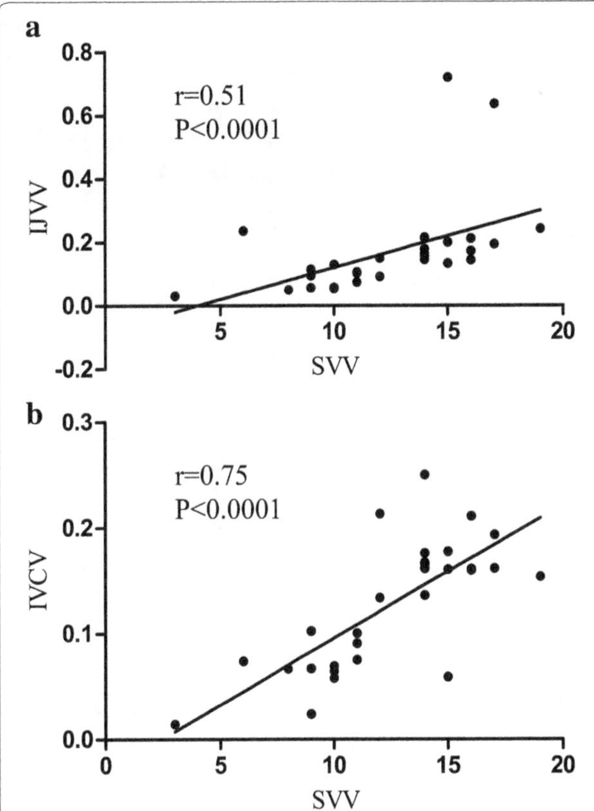

Fig. 2 Pearson correlation analysis. (**a**, association between IJVV and SVV; **b**, association between IVCV and SVV)

The intra-observer variability and inter-observer variability of IJVV measurement were further investigated in 30 patients. The results showed good concordance between estimation of IJVV by the two investigators, with a mean bias of − 0.01 and limits of agreement between − 0.1 and 0.08. The reliability of the measurements was also analyzed with intraclass correlation coefficients (ICCs) assessing intra-observer and inter-observer correlation (Additional file 2).

Discussion

The objective of this study was to evaluate whether ultrasound assessment of IJV respiratory diameter changes can serve as a simple indicator of fluid responsiveness in mechanically ventilated patients after cardiac surgery. Our data showed that IJVV was comparable to IVCV in predicting fluid responsiveness. There was a positive correlation between SVV and ventilator-induced IJVV. It was also found that the predictive value of PLR-ΔSV and SVV was superior to that of IVCV and IJVV.

Correcting hypovolemia is of paramount importance during the postoperative critical care of cardiac surgical patients. However, its correction should be carefully

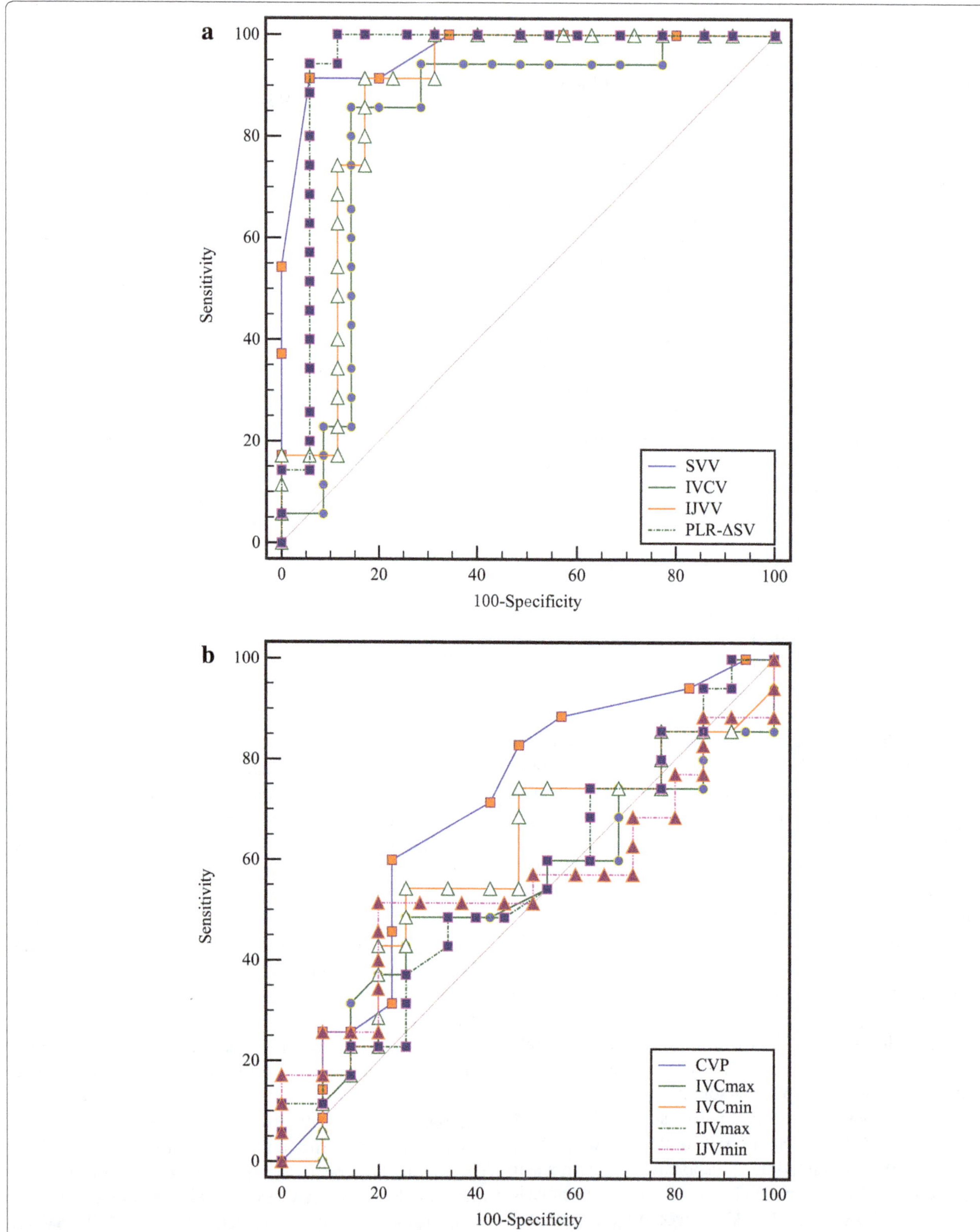

Fig. 3 Comparison of the areas under the ROC curves for the indicators used for predicting fluid responsiveness (**a**, dynamic indicators; and **b**, static indicators)

Table 3 Diagnostic ability of the different indices of fluid responsiveness

	AUC (95% CI)	Optimal cutoff (%)	Sensitivity (%)	Specificity (%)	Youden index	Positive predictive value	Negative predictive value	Positive likelihood ratio	Negative likelihood ratio
Dynamic indicators									
SVV	0.97 (0.89–0.99)	12.00	91.43	94.29	0.86	0.94	0.92	16.00	0.09
PLR-ΔSV	0.91 (0.82–0.97)	12.84	100.00	82.86	0.83	0.85	1.00	5.83	0.00
IJVV	0.88 (0.78–0.94)	12.99	91.43	82.86	0.74	0.84	0.91	5.33	0.10
IVCV	0.83 (0.72–0.91)	13.39	85.71	85.71	0.71	0.86	0.86	6.00	0.17
Static indicators									
CVP	0.70 (0.57–0.80)	11.00	60.00	77.14	0.37	0.72	0.66	2.63	0.52
IVCmax	0.53 (0.40–0.65)	1.57	48.57	74.29	0.23	0.65	0.59	1.89	0.69
IVCmin	0.58 (0.46–0.70)	1.40	54.29	74.29	0.29	0.68	0.62	2.11	0.62
IJVmax	0.55 (0.43–0.67)	0.86	48.57	65.71	0.14	0.59	0.56	1.42	0.78
IJVmin	0.55 (0.43–0.67)	0.64	51.43	80.00	0.31	0.72	0.62	2.57	0.61

AUC area under the receiver operating characteristic curve, *CI* confidence interval, *SVV* respiratory variation of stroke volume, *PLR-ΔSV* the increase in stroke volume in response to a passive leg raising test, *IJVV* internal jugular venous variability, *IVCV* inferior vena cava variability, *CVP* central venous pressure, *IVCmax* the maximum inferior vena cava diameter, *IVCmin* the minimum inferior vena cava diameter, *IJVmax* the maximum internal jugular venous diameter, *IJVmin* the minimum internal jugular venous diameter

guided to avoid unnecessary volume expansion [23]. Therefore, many investigators have explored reliable techniques with the goal of predicting fluid responsiveness in critically ill patients. Static parameters, such as CVP, are poor predictors of fluid responsiveness as previously reported and as shown in our study [23–25]. Based on the hemodynamic consequences of the heart–lung interactions, the use of dynamic indices of preload that result from respiratory variations is well-accepted bedside parameters of fluid responsiveness [7]. It was worth mentioning that tidal volume should be large enough to promote adequate preload variations. Fluid responsiveness cannot be reliably predicted if the tidal volume is < 8 ml/kg PBW [26]. Therefore, a Vt 8 mL/kg PBW was set in the present study. As higher PEEP may have adverse effects such as overinflation and hemodynamic deterioration, a PEEP of 5 cm H_2O was set initially after cardiac surgery according to our routine practice.

Mechanical ventilation-induced cyclic variations in vena cava diameter have been shown to be accurate predictors of fluid responsiveness. In our study, we have shown that the IVCV was a good predictor of fluid responsiveness for mechanically ventilated patients following cardiac surgery. IVCV threshold values of 13.39% have been reported in the literature to be able to discriminate between responders and non-responders with a sensitivity of 85.71% and a specificity of 85.71%. Based on the associations of intra-thoracic venous pressure and volume with extrathoracic venous pressure, we hypothesized that fluid responsiveness may also be reflected by changes in IJV pressure as assessed by IJVV. Measuring IJV diameter change is easily achieved with ultrasound with minimal training, as this approach is frequently used for ultrasound-guided central vein catheterization. We demonstrated the reliability of IJVV with a value of 12.99% in detecting fluid responsiveness, having a sensitivity of 91.43% and a specificity of 82.86% in mechanically ventilated cardiac surgical patients.

Several studies have investigated the ability of respiratory variations in IJV diameter to evaluate hypovolemia or a hemodynamic response to a fluid challenge. Guarracino et al. have reported that IJV distensibility [(diamax − diamin)/diamin × 100] accurately predicts volume responsiveness in mechanically ventilated septic patients [19]. A cutoff value of 18% IJV distensibility resulted in 80% sensitivity and 85% specificity for predicting a fluid response, which was defined as an increase in cardiac index ≥ 15%. However, this study did not include patients with cardiac disease who have different hemodynamic characteristics. Moreover, the authors did not compare the predictive values of IVCV and IJVV. Thudium et al. showed that ultrasound evaluation of IJV extensibility can change in response to preload-altering orthostatic maneuvers and pulse pressure variation alterations [17]. However, this study was conducted at the cardiac surgery intensive care unit, and all of the patients were included after elective cardiac surgery; the reporters did not perform the standard fluid challenge, and the subgroup analysis showed that different surgery categories had different results. Broilo et al. verified the hypothesis that respiratory variations of the IVC and IJV were correlated [18]. These two indicators showed a significant agreement in evaluating fluid responsiveness. However, they did not identify changes in cardiac output following a fluid challenge, and they did not evaluate changes in the vein diameters before and after a fluid challenge.

There were other studies demonstrating its utility, using measurements of the IJV to detect early hemorrhage in healthy volunteers that were donating blood [27, 28]. To our knowledge, this was the first study to evaluate the value of IJVV in predicting fluid responsiveness based on a standard fluid challenge in mechanically ventilated cardiac surgical patients.

Our study has several limitations. First, all subjects were on mechanical ventilation and absence of spontaneous breathing under sedation. Whether the conclusions can be extrapolated to patients with spontaneous breathing remains uncertain. Second, an uncalibrated system for hemodynamic monitoring was used in this study. Although the validation of FloTrac/vigileo system in measuring cardiac output has been assessed by numerous studies, the reliability of uncalibrated devices is still under debate [29–31]. Compared with pulmonary artery catheter (PAC) or transpulmonary thermodilution devices, FloTrac/vigileo system can be directly connected to the arterial catheter and has the advantage of auto-calibration. It theoretically meets the needs for rapidly assessing hemodynamic changes. Moreover, the dynamic indicator of SVV that could continuously displayed by the FloTrac/Vigileo system has also been shown to be able to predict fluid responsiveness in cardiac surgical patients [32–34]. Third, we did not enroll patients with right heart failure, as severe right heart failure or high CVP could influence IJV pressure and diameter and may decrease the relative variability even in the presence of preload responsiveness. Fourth, technical errors were possible, because even a slight pressure could have caused a great change in the cross-sectional image and diameter of the IJV during the acquisition of the measurements. We have made further efforts on the reproducibility and agreement of IJVV in 30 patients. The results showed good concordance between estimation of IJVV by the two investigators. Fifth, the initial semirecumbent position of the patient was 30° head of the bed (HOB) elevated instead of 45° (standard baseline position of PLR), because this was the recommended position for supine ventilated patient in the ICU. It was believed that this was more consistent with clinical scenario. Furthermore, taking sonographic measurements of the IVC diameters seems more easily in the position with HOB 30° than HOB 45°. The predict value of IJVV in other positions (such as the horizontal position) remains to be assessed.

Conclusions

Ultrasound evaluation of IJVV is a simple, easy and readily accessible bedside measurement that predicts volume responsiveness in mechanically ventilated cardiac surgical patients. The respiratory variations of the IJV and IVC showed comparable value in the prediction of fluid responsiveness.

Abbreviations

HR: Heart rate; MAP: Mean arterial pressure; CVP: Central venous pressure; SV: Stroke volume; SVV: Stroke volume variation; IJV: Internal jugular venous; IJVV: Internal jugular venous variability; IVC: Inferior vena cava; IVCV: Inferior vena cava variability; PLR: Passive leg raising; PLR-ΔSV: The increase in stroke volume in response to a passive leg raising test; CSICU: Cardiac surgery intensive care unit; PEEP: Positive end-expiratory pressure; PBW: Predicted body weight; IPPV: Intermittent positive pressure ventilation; LVEF: Left ventricular ejection fraction; ROC: Receiver operating characteristic.

Authors' contributions

G-gM, G-wH, G-wT performed the literature search, extracted date and drafted the manuscript. X-mY, LL and HL reviewed studies for inclusion and extracted data. G-wT, D-mZ and ZL performed the analysis and helped draft the manuscript. G-wT and ZL conceived the idea, participated in manuscript writing and revision. All authors read and approved the final manuscript.

Acknowledgements

None.

Competing interests

The authors declare that they have no competing interests.

Funding

This article was supported by grants from the National Natural Science Foundation of China (81500067), Natural Science Foundation of Shanghai (16ZR1405600), Health and Family Planning Commission of Shanghai (20154Y011) and the research funds of Zhong Shan Hospital (2017ZSYXQN23 and 2016ZSQN23).

References

1. Lee J, de Louw E, Niemi M, Nelson R, Mark RG, Celi LA, et al. Association between fluid balance and survival in critically ill patients. J Intern Med. 2015;277:468–77.
2. Carsetti A, Cecconi M, Rhodes A. Fluid bolus therapy: monitoring and predicting fluid responsiveness. Curr Opin Crit Care. 2015;21:388–94.
3. Kalus JS, Caron MF, White CM, Mather JF, Gallagher R, Boden WE, et al. Impact of fluid balance on incidence of atrial fibrillation after cardiothoracic surgery. Am J Cardiol. 2004;94:1423–5.
4. Mentzer RM Jr. Myocardial protection in heart surgery. J Cardiovasc Pharmacol Ther. 2011;16:290–7.
5. Donati A, Carsetti A, Damiani E, Adrario E, Romano R, Pelaia P. Fluid responsiveness in critically ill patients. Indian J Crit Care Med. 2015;19:375–6.
6. Suzuki S, Woinarski NC, Lipcsey M, Candal CL, Schneider AG, Glassford NJ, et al. Pulse pressure variation-guided fluid therapy after cardiac surgery: a pilot before-and-after trial. J Crit Care. 2014;29:992–6.
7. Marik PE, Cavallazzi R, Vasu T, Hirani A. Dynamic changes in arterial waveform derived variables and fluid responsiveness in mechanically ventilated patients: a systematic review of the literature. Crit Care Med. 2009;37:2642–7.
8. Michard F, Boussat S, Chemla D, Anguel N, Mercat A, Lecarpentier Y, et al. Relation between respiratory changes in arterial pulse pressure and fluid responsiveness in septic patients with acute circulatory failure. Am J Respir Crit Care Med. 2000;162:134–8.
9. Vieillard-Baron A, Chergui K, Rabiller A, Peyrouset O, Page B, Beauchet A, et al. Superior vena caval collapsibility as a gauge of volume status in ventilated septic patients. Intensive Care Med. 2004;30:1734–9.
10. Barbier C, Loubieres Y, Schmit C, Hayon J, Ricome JL, Jardin F, et al. Respiratory changes in inferior vena cava diameter are helpful in predicting

fluid responsiveness in ventilated septic patients. Intensive Care Med. 2004;30:1740–6.
11. Tavazzi G, Price S, Fletcher N. Bedside ultrasonographic measurement of the inferior vena cava. J Cardiothorac Vasc Anesth. 2015;29:e54–5.
12. Sobczyk D, Nycz K, Andruszkiewicz P. Bedside ultrasonographic measurement of the inferior vena cava fails to predict fluid responsiveness in the first 6 hours after cardiac surgery: a prospective case series observational study. J Cardiothorac Vasc Anesth. 2015;29:663–9.
13. Nagdev AD, Merchant RC, Tirado-Gonzalez A, Sisson CA, Murphy MC. Emergency department bedside ultrasonographic measurement of the caval index for noninvasive determination of low central venous pressure. Ann Emerg Med. 2010;55:290–5.
14. Chua Chiaco JM, Parikh NI, Fergusson DJ. The jugular venous pressure revisited. Cleve Clin J Med. 2013;80:638–44.
15. Conn RD, O'Keefe JH. Simplified evaluation of the jugular venous pressure: significance of inspiratory collapse of jugular veins. Mo Med. 2012;109:150–2.
16. Constant J. Using internal jugular pulsations as a manometer for right atrial pressure measurements. Cardiology. 2000;93:26–30.
17. Thudium M, Klaschik S, Ellerkmann RK, Putensen C, Hilbert T. Is internal jugular vein extensibility associated with indices of fluid responsiveness in ventilated patients? Acta Anaesthesiol Scand. 2016;60:723–33.
18. Broilo F, Meregalli A, Friedman G. Right internal jugular vein distensibility appears to be a surrogate marker for inferior vena cava vein distensibility for evaluating fluid responsiveness. Rev Bras Ter Intensiva. 2015;27:205–11.
19. Guarracino F, Ferro B, Forfori F, Bertini P, Magliacano L, Pinsky MR. Jugular vein distensibility predicts fluid responsiveness in septic patients. Crit Care. 2014;18:647.
20. Prekker ME, Scott NL, Hart D, Sprenkle MD, Leatherman JW. Point-of-care ultrasound to estimate central venous pressure: a comparison of three techniques. Crit Care Med. 2013;41:833–41.
21. Cecconi M, Parsons AK, Rhodes A. What is a fluid challenge? Curr Opin Crit Care. 2011;17:290–5.
22. Vincent JL, Weil MH. Fluid challenge revisited. Crit Care Med. 2006;34:1333–7.
23. Preisman S, Kogan S, Berkenstadt H, Perel A. Predicting fluid responsiveness in patients undergoing cardiac surgery: functional haemodynamic parameters including the Respiratory Systolic Variation Test and static preload indicators. Br J Anaesth. 2005;95:746–55.
24. Marik PE, Baram M, Vahid B. Does central venous pressure predict fluid responsiveness? A systematic review of the literature and the tale of seven mares. Chest. 2008;134:172–8.
25. Osman D, Ridel C, Ray P, Monnet X, Anguel N, Richard C, et al. Cardiac filling pressures are not appropriate to predict hemodynamic response to volume challenge. Crit Care Med. 2007;35:64–8.
26. De Backer D, Heenen S, Piagnerelli M, Koch M, Vincent JL. Pulse pressure variations to predict fluid responsiveness: influence of tidal volume. Intensive Care Med. 2005;31:517–23.
27. Unluer EE, Kara PH. Ultrasonography of jugular vein as a marker of hypovolemia in healthy volunteers. Am J Emerg Med. 2013;31:173–7.
28. Akilli NB, Cander B, Dundar ZD, Koylu R. A new parameter for the diagnosis of hemorrhagic shock: jugular index. J Crit Care. 2012;27(530):e13–8.
29. Marque S, Gros A, Chimot L, Gacouin A, Lavoue S, Camus C, et al. Cardiac output monitoring in septic shock: evaluation of the third-generation Flotrac-Vigileo. J Clin Monit Comput. 2013;27:273–9.
30. Monnet X, Anguel N, Jozwiak M, Richard C, Teboul JL. Third-generation FloTrac/Vigileo does not reliably track changes in cardiac output induced by norepinephrine in critically ill patients. Br J Anaesth. 2012;108:615–22.
31. De Backer D, Marx G, Tan A, Junker C, Van Nuffelen M, Huter L, et al. Arterial pressure-based cardiac output monitoring: a multicenter validation of the third-generation software in septic patients. Intensive Care Med. 2011;37:233–40.
32. Krige A, Bland M, Fanshawe T. Fluid responsiveness prediction using Vigileo FloTrac measured cardiac output changes during passive leg raise test. J Intensive Care. 2016;4:63.
33. Kim SY, Song Y, Shim JK, Kwak YL. Effect of pulse pressure on the predictability of stroke volume variation for fluid responsiveness in patients with coronary disease. J Crit Care. 2013;28(318):e1–7.
34. Cannesson M, Musard H, Desebbe O, Boucau C, Simon R, Henaine R, et al. The ability of stroke volume variations obtained with Vigileo/FloTrac system to monitor fluid responsiveness in mechanically ventilated patients. Anesth Analg. 2009;108:513–7.

14

Patient–ventilator asynchrony during conventional mechanical ventilation in children

Guillaume Mortamet[1,2,3], Alexandrine Larouche[1,3], Laurence Ducharme-Crevier[1,3], Olivier Fléchelles[4], Gabrielle Constantin[1,3], Sandrine Essouri[3,5], Amélie-Ann Pellerin-Leblanc[6], Jennifer Beck[7,8,9], Christer Sinderby[7,9,10], Philippe Jouvet[1,3] and Guillaume Emeriaud[1,3*]

Abstract

Background: We aimed (1) to describe the characteristics of patient–ventilator asynchrony in a population of critically ill children, (2) to describe the risk factors associated with patient–ventilator asynchrony, and (3) to evaluate the association between patient–ventilator asynchrony and ventilator-free days at day 28.

Methods: In this single-center prospective study, consecutive children admitted to the PICU and mechanically ventilated for at least 24 h were included. Patient–ventilator asynchrony was analyzed by comparing the ventilator pressure curve and the electrical activity of the diaphragm (Edi) signal with (1) a manual analysis and (2) using a standardized fully automated method.

Results: Fifty-two patients (median age 6 months) were included in the analysis. Eighteen patients had a very low ventilatory drive (i.e., peak Edi < 2 μV on average), which prevented the calculation of patient–ventilator asynchrony. Children spent 27% (interquartile 22–39%) of the time in conflict with the ventilator. Cycling-off errors and trigger delays contributed to most of this asynchronous time. The automatic algorithm provided a NeuroSync index of 45%, confirming the high prevalence of asynchrony. No association between the severity of asynchrony and ventilator-free days at day 28 or any other clinical secondary outcomes was observed, but the proportion of children with good synchrony was very low.

Conclusion: Patient–ventilator interaction is poor in children supported by conventional ventilation, with a high frequency of depressed ventilatory drive and a large proportion of time spent in asynchrony. The clinical benefit of strategies to improve patient–ventilator interactions should be evaluated in pediatric critical care.

Keywords: Diaphragm function, Mechanical ventilation, Patient–ventilator asynchrony, Patient–ventilator interaction, Pediatric intensive care unit, Pediatrics

Background

Mechanical ventilation is commonly used in pediatric intensive care units (PICUs) [1]. Maintaining the patient's own spontaneous breathing effort during ventilation is key. Assisted (or patient-triggered) ventilation may improve ventilation perfusion matching and forestall the development of ventilator-induced diaphragmatic dysfunction [2]. As the patient contributes in the ventilation, good interaction between the patient and the ventilator is essential.

Children have higher respiratory rates, smaller tidal volumes, and weaker inspiratory efforts when compared with adults, and patient–ventilator synchrony is difficult to achieve in pediatric patients [3]. These can lead to a mismatch between the patient and the ventilator, defined as a patient–ventilator asynchrony (PVA). PVA

*Correspondence: guillaume.emeriaud@umontreal.ca
[1] Pediatric Intensive Care Unit, CHU Sainte-Justine, 3175 Côte Sainte-Catherine, Montreal, QC, Canada
Full list of author information is available at the end of the article

includes the inspiratory and expiratory timing errors (delays between patient demand and ventilator response), efforts undetected by the ventilator, assist delivered in the absence of patient demand, and double triggering (two rapidly successive assists following a single effort).

In critically ill adults, asynchronies occur frequently and are associated with prolonged ventilator support, sleep disorders, poor lung aeration, longer stay in the intensive care unit and mortality [4–9]. Pediatric data in this field are lacking. PVA seems frequent in PICU [10–13], but little is known about the risk factors of PVA and the association with patient outcome.

In the present study, we aimed to describe the characteristics of PVA in critically ill children, to identify risk factors associated with PVA, and to evaluate the association between PVA and patient outcome.

Methods

This prospective observational study was conducted in the PICU of CHU Sainte-Justine, a university-affiliated pediatric hospital, from August 2010 to October 2012. The study protocol was approved by the ethics committee of CHU Sainte-Justine. Written informed consent was obtained from the parents or legal tutor.

Patients

Consecutive children aged between 7 days and 18 years admitted to the PICU and mechanically ventilated for at least 24 h were eligible. The screening was performed daily by a research assistant. Eligible patients reached inclusion criteria when the presence of spontaneous breathing was evidenced by clinical respiratory efforts or by a respiratory rate sustainably higher than the set ventilator rate. Patients were excluded if they had one of the following criteria: chronic respiratory insufficiency with prior ventilatory support longer than 1 month, tracheostomy, neuromuscular disease, contraindications to nasogastric tube exchange (i.e., local trauma, recent local surgery, or severe coagulation disorder), suspected bilateral diaphragm paralysis, immediate postcardiac surgery period, expected death in the next 24 h, or a limitation of life support treatment.

No modification of the ventilator settings was done for the study. The attending physicians set the ventilator mode and settings according to the local practices. Patients were ventilated with the Evita XL (Dräger, Lubeck, Germany) or the Servo-I ventilator (Maquet, Solna, Sweden). Sedation and analgesia were decided by the treating team and usually involved a combination of benzodiazepines and opioids. There was no local written protocol regarding the ventilator management or the sedation during the study. The ventilation support was reassessed every 1 or 2 h by respiratory therapists according to local practice. At the time of the study, neurally adjusted ventilatory assist (NAVA) was not routinely used in clinical practice in our unit.

Protocol

PVA was recorded at two different times during the PICU stay. We obtained a first 30-min recording in acute phase, i.e., as soon as possible after inclusion in the study, and an esophageal catheter was installed to record the electrical activity of diaphragm (Edi). The second (pre-extubation) recording was performed during 15 min in the 4 h preceding extubation, if the Edi catheter was still in place.

Data recording

PVA was analyzed by comparing the ventilator pressure curve and the Edi signal. Edi was recorded using a specific nasogastric catheter (Edi catheter, Maquet, Solna, Sweden) connected to a dedicated Servo-I ventilator (Maquet, Solna, Sweden). This ventilator was used only to continuously process and record the Edi signal, the patient being ventilated with his own ventilator as before the study. The catheter was positioned according to the recommendations of the manufacturer as previously described [12, 14].

Demographic data and patient's characteristics, including age, gender, weight, time of measurements, admission diagnostic and comorbidities, Pediatric Index of Mortality (PIM) II and Pediatric Logistic Organ Dysfunction (PELOD) scores, were collected. The sedation score was calculated for the 4-h period preceding the first recording, as suggested by Randolph et al. [15], using a score for which one point was given for the amount of each drug that would be equivalent to 1 h of sedation in a nontolerant subject. The Comfort B scale was used to determine the level of comfort (comfort is better when score is lower).

Clinical outcomes

The primary outcome was the number of ventilator-free days at day 28 (since intubation). Patients who died were considered having zero ventilation-free day. The secondary clinical outcomes were first extubation success (no need for invasive ventilation support within 48 h of extubation), duration of mechanical ventilation, and length of PICU stay.

PVA manual analysis

As previously described [12, 16, 17], for each recording, Edi and ventilator pressure curves were analyzed in a breath-by-breath manner over a continuous 5-min period exempt of artifacts linked to agitation or patient care. Timings of the beginning and the end of inspiration and expiration phases on the Edi and the ventilatory pressure signals were semiautomatically identified: Main timings were automatically identified, and a visual inspection was performed breath by breath, permitting to validate and/or adjust the timing cursors if necessary. All analyses were performed by two independent investigators. By comparing the ventilator and Edi timings, PVA was identified, including wasted efforts (clear effort observed on Edi with no ventilator assist), auto-triggered breath (ventilator assist delivered in the absence of Edi increase), double triggering (two rapidly successive assists following a single effort), and inspiratory trigger and cycling-off errors. As the response of the ventilator for triggering or cycling off could be frequently either retarded or premature [12], we reported both types of asynchrony.

The main PVA variable of interest was the percentage of time spent in asynchrony, calculated from the total duration spent in each type of PVA (wasted efforts, auto-triggering, double triggering, trigger and cycling off errors) divided by the duration of the recording. A priori, we defined severe PVA when the percentage of time spent in asynchrony was superior to the 75th percentile of the entire cohort, i.e., the quarter of patients with the worst synchrony.

In order to facilitate the comparison with other studies [18], we also calculated the asynchrony index (AI), defined as the number of asynchronous events (i.e., the sum of wasted efforts, ineffective triggering, double triggering, and cycles with important trigger and cycling-off errors) divided by the total respiratory rate (i.e., the sum of ventilator cycles and wasted efforts), and expressed as a percentage. Important trigger and cycling-off errors were considered when the error (i.e., premature or delayed response) exceeded 33% of inspiratory and expiratory times, respectively. An AI > 10% was considered as a high incidence of asynchrony [5, 18].

PVA automatic analysis

Asynchrony was also analyzed using a standardized automated method over the same period, to prevent interobserver variability and to avoid observer subjectivity [19]. Inspiratory and expiratory timings were fully automatically detected on ventilator pressure and Edi signals based on predetermined thresholds (0.5 μV for Edi amplitude). Asynchrony was quantified using the NeuroSync index, a global index considering both inspiratory and cycling-off errors. A higher NeuroSync index reflects worse asynchrony, and synchrony can be considered as poor when NeuroSync index exceeds 20% [20, 21].

Sample size calculation

Based on studies conducted in adults, we expected a difference in ventilator-free days of 6 days. With a group distribution of 3/1 and a type-1 error risk of 0.05, the inclusion of 56 patients was necessary to achieve a power of 80%. We planned to enroll a sample of 60 patients to take into account the attrition risk.

Statistical analysis

Data are expressed as median values (with interquartiles, IQR) for continuous variables, and number and/or frequency (%) for categorical data. Differences in categorical variables were tested using Chi-square or Fisher's exact test. Differences in continuous variables were assessed by the nonparametric Mann–Whitney test, the paired *t* test, or the Wilcoxon test.

Patients with peak inspiratory Edi < 2 μV were a posteriori excluded from PVA analysis (both manual and automated) because the reality of the spontaneous activity in those patients appeared questionable, and the identification of PVA is complex. intraclass correlation coefficient (ICC, two-way random model) was calculated to assess interobserver reproducibility for manual PVA analysis and to compare the results from the manual and the automatic methods. After confirmation of an excellent interobserver agreement (ICC > 0.75), the averages of the two observer's results were calculated and used in further analysis.

The association of potential risk factors with severe PVA was studied by univariate logistic regression analysis. Noncollinear factors associated with a univariate association with $p < 0.05$ were included in a multivariate logistic regression. The relationship between PVA and clinical outcomes was described using univariate analysis.

All p values are two-tailed and considered significant if $p < 0.05$. Statistical analyses were performed using SPSS 24.0 (SPSS, Inc, Chicago, IL).

Results

Study population

During the study period, 2090 patients were admitted to the PICU. Among the 406 eligible patients, 60 patients reached inclusion criteria and were enrolled (Fig. 1). Exploitable signals were finally available in 52 patients, who were included in the analysis. Median age of eligible patients who were not included was 8 (1–48) months old, which is similar to analyzed patients ($p = 0.96$). Twenty-two of these patients also had a second recording in the pre-extubation period. The patient characteristics are presented in Table 1. They were studied 4 (IQR: 1–10) days after PICU admission.

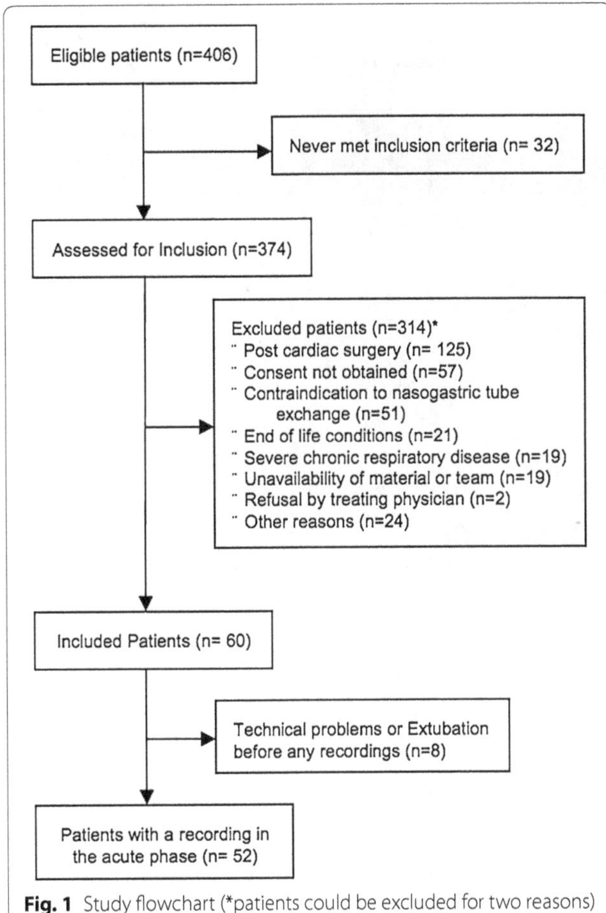

Fig. 1 Study flowchart (*patients could be excluded for two reasons)

Eighteen patients had a very low ventilatory drive (peak Edi < 2 μV on average), which prevented the calculation of PVA. As detailed in Table 1, these patients tended to be older, were affected less frequently by a respiratory disease, and had a lower $PaCO_2$ and a lower comfort score as compared to patients with higher drive.

Magnitude of PVA

A total of 9806 breaths were analyzed with the manual method, with a median of 168 (IQR: 123–258) breaths analyzed per recording. The interrater agreement for PVA manual analysis was excellent, with ICC > 0.85 for all PVA parameters. The total proportion of time spent in PVA was 27% (IQR: 22–39) of the time. As illustrated in Fig. 2, cycling-off errors and trigger delays contributed to most of this asynchronous time 12% (IQR: 8–15) and 11% (IQR: 8–16), respectively. Auto-triggered cycles, wasted efforts, and double triggering were also highly prevalent, with two (IQR: 0–3), two (IQR: 1–10), and one (IQR: 0–5) events per minute, respectively.

The median AI was 25% (IQR: 18–35), and 33 (97%) patients had an AI greater than 10%.

Characteristics of patients with severe asynchrony

Nine patients were considered as severely asynchronous, with a proportion of time spent in asynchrony > 75th percentile, i.e., > 39% of time (Table 2). Patients with severe asynchrony were younger (p = 0.007), had more frequently a narrower and noncuffed ETT (p = 0.001 and p = 0.019, respectively), and were less frequently ventilated in pressure-support ventilation (PSV, p = 0.034). All but one of these patients were admitted for a respiratory failure as a first reason, and five of them had bronchiolitis. In the multivariate logistic regression model in which age, presence of a cuffed ETT, and PSV mode were tested, none of these variables were independently associated with severe PVA (all p > 0.17).

The patients with severe asynchrony were enrolled earlier in the PICU course (2 days (1–5) vs 8 (2–11), p = 0.054), which must be considered while looking at the relationship between PVA and length of stay or ventilation duration.

Evolution of PVA

As illustrated in Fig. 3, when comparing the recordings from acute phase and pre-extubation phase, the level of PVA tended to decrease over time (p = 0.01), and both period data were correlated ($R^2 = 0.41$). Peak Edi increased between the two phases (p = 0.01).

Automatic analysis of PVA

The automatic algorithm provided a NeuroSync index of 45% (32–70%), confirming the high prevalence of asynchrony. As shown in Fig. 4, a good correlation was observed between NeuroSync index and the percentage of time spent in asynchrony derived from the manual analysis, with an ICC of 0.88.

Outcome

We did not observe any association between the level of asynchrony and neither ventilator-free days at day 28, nor the secondary outcomes (Table 2). This holds true with the manual classification as severe PVA or not (Table 2), as well as with the automated NeuroSync index (correlation with ventilation duration: $R^2 = 0.12$; p = 0.58). None of the patient characteristics were associated with the duration of mechanical ventilation.

Discussion

The incidence of PVA is very high during pediatric conventional ventilation. As a whole, children spend about one-third of the time in conflict with their ventilator. We described an a priori defined group with severe PVA, but marked PVA was present even in the other children, and the proportion of children which could be considered as "well synchronized" is low. Besides, an unexpected form

Table 1 Characteristics of population (n = 52)

	Total $n = 52$	Peak Edi < 2 μV $n = 18$	Peak Edi > 2 μV $n = 34$
Age (months)	10 (2–42)	21 (1–135)	6 (2–29)
Weight (kg)	6.5 (4.3–17.4)	11 (4.8–38.4)	5.3 (4.0–12.0)
Male, n (%)	31 (60%)	11 (61%)	20 (59%)
Days between admission and inclusion	4 (1–10)	3 (1–7)	4 (1–10)
Days between MV initiation and inclusion	3 (1–7)	2 (1–6)	4 (2–7)
Main reasons for PICU admission, *n* (%)			
Respiratory failure	31 (60%)	5 (28%)	26 (76%)*
Including bronchiolitis	11 (21%)	1 (6%)	10 (29%)
Hemodynamic failure	3 (6%)	2 (11%)	1 (3%)
Neurologic disorder	9 (17%)	6 (33%)	3 (9%)
Metabolic disorder	2 (4%)	0 (0%)	2 (6%)
Trauma	2 (4%)	2 (11%)	0 (0%)
Postoperative admission	5 (10%)	3 (17%)	2 (6%)
Chronic condition, *n* (%)			
Respiratory disease	8 (15%)	2 (11%)	6 (18%)
Cardiac disease	9 (17%)	3 (17%)	6 (18%)
Neurological disease	11 (21%)	4 (22%)	7 (21%)
Immuno-oncologic disease	3 (6%)	0 (0%)	3 (9%)
Clinical status			
PIM-2 score	1.7 (0.8–4.3)	2.3 (0.9–4.5)	1.6 (0.8–4.4)
PELOD score	2 (1–1)	1 (1–11)	1 (1–11)
Set respiratory rate, min^{-1}	25 (20–35)	23 (14–38)	31 (25–42)*
Measured respiratory rate, min^{-1}	29 (20–36)	20 (15–29)	34 (28–40)*
pH	7.40 (7.35–7.42)	7.40 (7.36–7.43)	7.39 (7.34–7.43)
$PaCO_2$, mmHg	46 (42–53)	42 (38–47)	48 (45–57)*
HCO_3^-, mmHg	28 (24–32)	27 (23–30)	30 (25–33)
PEEP, cmH_2O	5 (5–6)	5 (5–5)	5 (5–6)
FiO_2	0.35 (0.29–0.41)	0.30 (0.24–0.35)	0.35 (0.30–0.50)
Comfort score	13 (10–15)	11 (8–13)	15 (12–16)*
Score sedation	11 (6–21)	10 (1–14)	15 (6–25)
Edi analysis			
Peak inspiratory Edi, μV	3.6 (1.2–7.6)	1.1 (0.6–1.3)	6.6 (3.8–11.5)
Tonic expiratory Edi, μV	0.7 (0.4–1.9)	0.4 (0.3–0.5)	1.1 (0.7–2.5)

Data are expressed as median (interquartile range) or *n* (%)

Edi electrical activity of the diaphragm, *MV* mechanical ventilation, *PICU* pediatric intensive care unit, *PEEP* positive end-expiratory pressure

*Significant difference between the two groups (p < 0.05)

of bad interaction was observed, with the high prevalence of low ventilatory drive.

The magnitude of PVA that we observed is in agreement with that previously described [10–12]. In a recent study conducted in a PICU, Blokpoel et al. [10] showed that PVA occurred in 33% of breaths. These authors identified PVA using the analysis of ventilator waveforms, a method which has a low sensitivity [6]. We used the Edi signal which clearly facilitates the detection of PVA, in particular the calculation of timing errors for triggering or cycling off [3, 12, 13, 17, 22, 23]. We were therefore able to show that most of the time spent in asynchrony results from delayed or premature reactions of the ventilator. These timing errors are important, especially when the normal inspiratory time is frequently around 400 ms in this population. We hypothesize that this delay in ventilator response is the consequence of small tidal volumes and short inspiratory and expiratory times in children as compared to adults. Although considered as the classical method [12, 17, 24], the breath-by-breath manual analysis of PVA could be criticized because of its dependency on an investigator, as well as being highly time

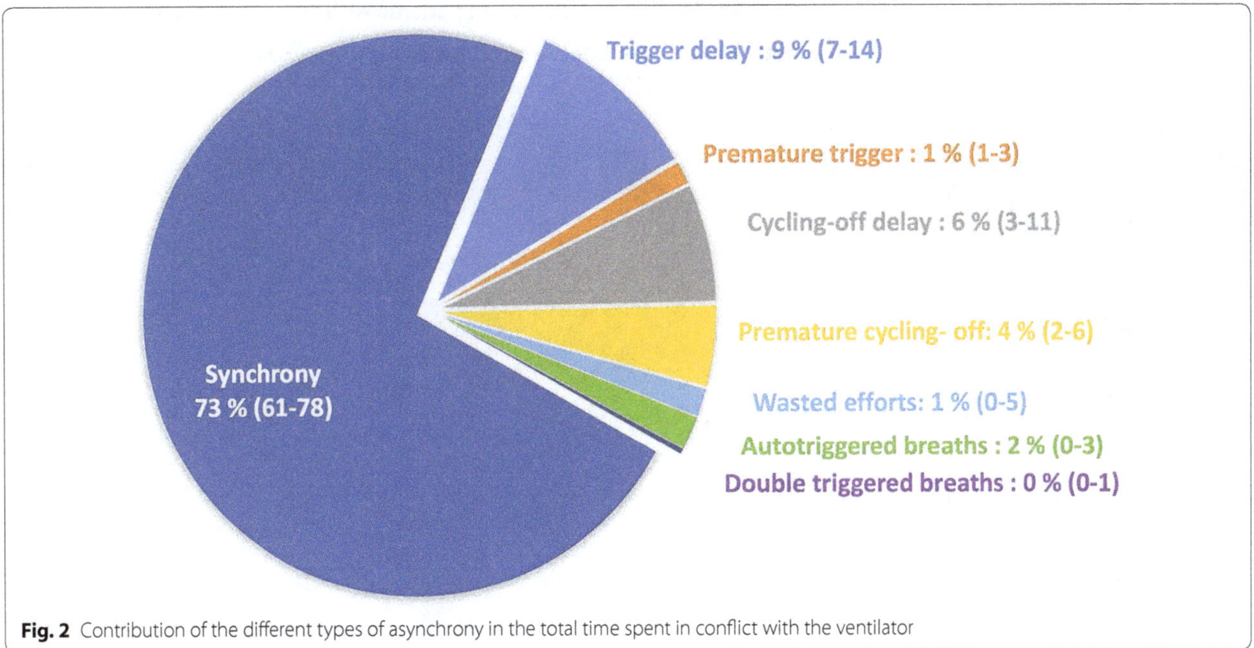

Fig. 2 Contribution of the different types of asynchrony in the total time spent in conflict with the ventilator

consuming. However, our findings were supported by the good agreement between the two independent investigators, and by the concordance also observed between the automatically calculated NeuroSync index and the manually calculated PVA.

To date, no definition of severe PVA in children had been standardized. Some authors use the specific index described in adults by Thille et al. [5, 25] and others the percentage of asynchronous breaths [3, 10, 12]. In the present study, we primarily assessed the magnitude of PVA according to the time spent in asynchrony, because it illustrates well the burden of asynchrony while taking into account different types of patient–ventilator conflict [17]. As expressed using the AI, our results confirm the severity of PVA, a huge proportion of the patients having an AI > 10%. A recent meta-analysis reported that the mean reported AI varied from 13 to 37% in adults, and from 38 to 74% in children during conventional ventilation, while a significant decrease in AI was observed with NAVA [18]. Consistent with the other PVA indices, only two patients in our series had a NeuroSync index < 20%, which corresponds to an adequate synchrony [20, 21]. The nonsevere group can therefore not be assumed as "well synchronized." In agreement with Blokpoel et al. [10], who observed that only 20% children had an acceptable level of PVA, our study highlights that PVA is a major problem in PICU and concerns more than three-quarters of the children, as opposed to one-quarter of adult patients.

Younger age, smaller tracheal tubes, and absence of a cuff on the tracheal tube were associated with severe PVA, and PSV mode was more frequent in patients with less severe PVA. The smaller size and the absence of cuff may suggest that increased leaks could have played a role, as suggested by Blokpoel et al. [10]. The magnitude of the leaks was not different between the two groups, but the precision of this measure is not perfect [26]. None of the patients ventilated in PSV was classified as severe PVA. We may hypothesize that the patients ventilated in PSV have a stronger ventilatory drive, leading to a better detection of the breathing efforts by the ventilator [5]. However, a confounding factor may also explain this association, PSV being mostly used in our unit in older and less sedated patients.

Overall, we did not observe any association between severe asynchrony and adverse outcomes during the PICU course, in contrast to studies in adults [4, 5, 7]. Similarly, Blokpoel et al. did not observe prolonged ventilation in patients with higher levels of asynchrony. While this may be the consequence of the limited power of these two pediatric studies, several explanations could be hypothesized to explain this difference with adult studies. In adults, adverse outcome was observed in severe PVA groups, while the remaining patients were appropriately synchronized [4, 5, 7]. In contrast, the number of children with good patient–ventilator interaction is quite low. In our study, patients with severe PVA frequently had diseases usually associated with good outcome (e.g.,

Table 2 Characteristics of patients depending on the level of asynchrony (in patients with Edi > 2 μV, *n* = 34)

	% time spent in asynchrony < 39% (*n* = 25)	% time spent in asynchrony > 39% (*n* = 9)	p value
Age (m)	14 (2–40)	2 (1–3)	0.007
Weight (kg)	7.0 (4.5–17.3)	4.3 (3.6–5.4)	0.049
Male, *n* (%)	14 (56%)	6 (67%)	0.70
Days between admission and inclusion	8 (2–11)	2 (1–5)	0.054
Main reasons for PICU admission, *n* (%)			0.56
Respiratory failure	18 (72%)	8 (89%)	0.40
Including bronchiolitis	5 (20%)	5 (56%)	0.08
Hemodynamic failure	1 (4%)	0 (0%)	1
Neurologic disorder	3 (12%)	0 (0%)	0.55
Metabolic disorder	1 (4%)	1 (11%)	0.46
Trauma	0 (0%)	0 (0%)	1
Post-surgery	2 (8%)	0 (0%)	1
Chronic condition, *n* (%)			
Respiratory disease	5 (20%)	1 (11%)	1
Cardiac disease	6 (24%)	0 (0%)	0.16
Neurological disease	6 (24%)	1 (11%)	0.64
Immuno-oncologic disease	3 (12%)	0 (0%)	0.55
Clinical status			
PIM-2 score	2.5 (0.9–4.4)	0.9 (0.5–7.0)	0.40
PELOD score	1 (1–11)	11 (1–12)	0.38
pH	7.40 (7.33–7.42)	7.37 (7.33–7.42)	0.63
HCO_3^-, mmHg	30.0 (25.1–32.9)	28.8 (24.9–32.0)	0.84
$PaCO_2$, mmHg	48.0 (44.4–53.4)	48.9 (45.8–57.5)	0.57
Hb, g/dL	10.2 (7.3–10.7)	10.4 (7.9–12.3)	0.33
Lactate, mmol/L	1.5 (0.8–2.1)	1.5 (1.2–1.9)	1
Comfort score	15 (13–16)	15 (11–17)	0.95
Sedation score	11 (6–23)	21 (11–39)	0.15
ETT size	4.0 (3.5–4.5)	3.5 (3.5–3.5)	0.013
Cuffed ETT	17 (68%)	2 (22%)	0.019
Ventilatory settings			
Set RR	25 (20–35)	30 (28–38)	0.13
Measured RR	34 (28–40)	35 (29–40)	0.92
Mode PSV	10 (40%)	0 (0%)	0.034
Mode ACV-P	4 (16%)	3 (33%)	0.35
Mode IACV-P	7 (28%)	3 (33%)	1
Mode ACV-V	0 (0%)	0 (0%)	1
Mode IACV-V	1 (4%)	2 (22%)	0.16
Mode PRVC	3 (12%)	1 (11%)	1
PEEP, cmH_2O	5 (5–5)	6 (5–7)	0.06
FiO_2	0.35 (0.26–0.44)	0.35 (0.30–0.60)	0.45
Leaks (%)	7 (4–15)	2 (0–7)	0.17
Analysis			
Peak inspiratory Edi, μV	7.2 (3.8–15.3)	5.5 (3.4–7.2)	0.20
Tonic expiratory Edi, μV	0.9 (0.6–2.4)	2.0 (1.1–2.9)	0.058
Type of asynchrony			
Wasted Efforts, % of breath analyzed	4.5 (1.6–15.8)	30.6 (18.7–39.8)	0.002
Auto-triggering, % of breath analyzed	6.1 (1.3–9.9)	8.4 (0.9–23.3)	0.36
Double triggering, % of breath analyzed	2.1 (0.0–3.2)	0.0 (0.0–0.8)	0.08
Trigger error, ms	136 (104–176)	284 (190–302)	0.008

Table 2 continued

	% time spent in asynchrony < 39% (*n* = 25)	% time spent in asynchrony > 39% (*n* = 9)	p value
Cycling-off error, ms	64 (40–131)	255 (184–297)	0.018
Time spent in asynchrony			
Total time spent in asynchrony, %	24 (17–28)	47 (43–50)	< 0.001
Wasted Effort, %	0.6 (0.2–3.5)	5.3 (2.8–13.6)	0.03
Auto-triggering, %	1.6 (0.3–2.4)	2.3 (0.3–4.7)	0.40
Double triggering, %	0.1 (0.0–0.4)	0.0 (0.0–0.1)	0.053
Trigger error			
Delay, %	7.6 (7.6–11.2)	15.5 (12.2–19.1)	0.001
Premature, %	0.8 (0.5–2.1)	2.3 (1.4–2.9)	0.058
Cycle-off error			
Delay, %	3.8 (1.8–6.3)	15.0 (10.2–17.5)	< 0.001
Premature, %	4.1 (2.2–5.9)	3.2 (2.0–6.7)	0.98
NeuroSync index, %	38 (31–47)	81 (69–83)	< 0.001
Outcome			
Death in PICU	1 (4.0%)	1 (11.1%)	1
Days in PICU	14 (5–22)	7 (4–14)	0.17
Days in PICU after inclusion	6 (4–12.5)	5 (3–6)	0.66
Days on MV	9 (4–15)	4 (3–12)	0.23
Days on MV after inclusion	2.5 (1–6.5)	3 (1–4)	0.9
NIV post extubation	4 (16.0%)	1 (11.1%)	1
Reintubation	5 (20.0%)	1 (11.1%)	1

Edi electrical activity of the diaphragm, *PICU* pediatric intensive care unit, *RR* respiratory rate, *PSV* pressure-support ventilation, *ACV-P* pressure-regulated assist control ventilation, *IACV-P* pressure-regulated intermittent assist control ventilation, *ACV-V* volume-regulated assist control ventilation, *IACV-V* volume-regulated intermittent assist control ventilation, *PRVC* pressure-regulated volume control ventilation, *PEEP* positive end-expiratory pressure, *ETT* endo-tracheal tube, *MV* mechanical ventilation, *NIV* noninvasive ventilation

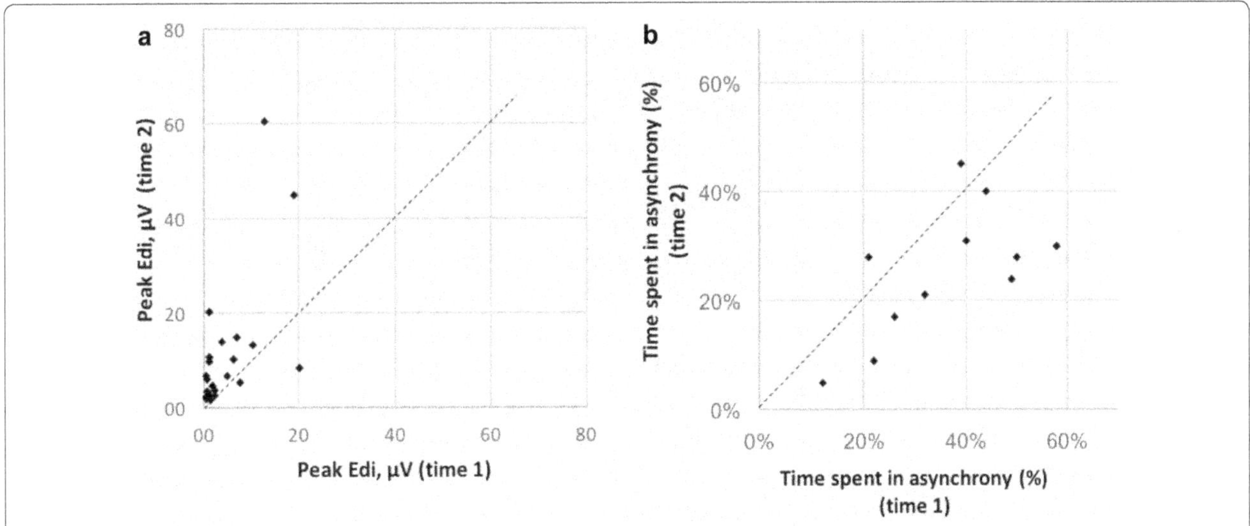

Fig. 3 Evolution of inspiratory Edi (panel a) and of the time spent in asynchrony (panel b) from inclusion time (time 1) to pre-extubation period (time 2)

bronchiolitis). It is also important to note that the patients with more severe PVA were recorded earlier in the PICU course. This baseline discrepancy makes it difficult to assess the relationship between PVA and ventilation duration.

The question remains whether those children would have a better outcome providing the PVA was improved. Only a controlled interventional trial, for example using a specific mode like NAVA, could confirm the independent role of PVA on outcome. Such evidence remains limited

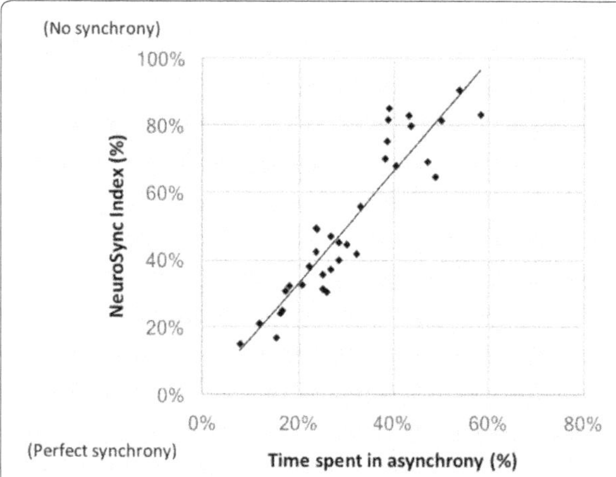

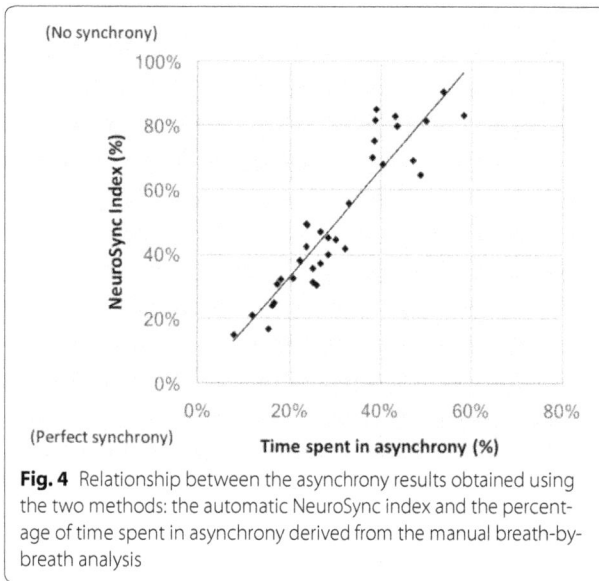

Fig. 4 Relationship between the asynchrony results obtained using the two methods: the automatic NeuroSync index and the percentage of time spent in asynchrony derived from the manual breath-by-breath analysis

in PICU. In a crossover trial conducted in 12 children, De la Oliva et al. [13] observed that the improvement in PVA with NAVA was associated with an improvement in comfort score. This has been supported by another study by Piastra et al. [27]. This finding is interesting when sedation is sometimes needed in cases of severe asynchrony. In the present study, we were not able to confirm that a better synchrony leads to a better comfort for the patient, as similar comfort score was observed in both groups. However, the patient with sever asynchrony tended to require more sedatives, as illustrated by higher sedation score (21 (11–39) vs 11 (6–23), although this difference did not reach significance ($p = 0.15$). An improved synchrony might have the potential to reduce sedation needs and its associated side effects. In a large randomized controlled trial, Kallio et al. [28] observed an interesting trend for shorter ventilation and ICU length of stay using NAVA ($p = 0.03$ and $p = 0.07$, respectively).

Finally, some authors hypothesize that improved PVA could also have deleterious effects that counterbalance the benefits [29]. It is, however, difficult to retain this hypothesis here while very few patients had good synchrony.

Interestingly, the peak Edi in the present study was relatively low (IQR 1.2–7.6) as compared to values observed in extubated children, which usually are between 5 and 30 mcV, depending on the lung condition [30, 31]. Many patients had low respiratory drive after several days of intubation, while they were deemed to be actively breathing. We consider this finding as a new form of poor patient–ventilator interaction, although not an asynchrony. This low respiratory activity has previously been reported [14, 32]. It could be the consequence of overassistance, oversedation, their combination, or more rarely of an abnormal output by the central respiratory center or by bilateral phrenic nerve palsy [33, 34]. In this study group, many patients were admitted for nonrespiratory reasons. Even low level of ventilator support can be sufficient in such conditions to suppress the patient breaths [35]. We previously reported that the ventilatory drive increased in these patients after the extubation, so the central or peripheral neurological explanation seems unlikely [31]. Oversedation may have contributed, as suggested by higher degree of comfort observed in these patients. As described by Vaschetto et al., the combination of overassistance and sedation has a synergistic impact on the drive suppression. More attention should be paid to this frequent complication, especially since such respiratory behavior has clearly been linked to diaphragm dysfunction [30, 36, 37].

Several limitations of our study need to be discussed. We included in the analysis fewer patients than expected. It is possible that our study was underpowered in particular to conduct subgroup analysis or to truly assess the impact on patient outcome. This is a single-center study, and the results may have been influenced by the local practice, especially regarding ventilator settings. NAVA was not used in routine practice during the study period in our PICU. NAVA can improve patient–ventilator interactions [12, 18, 38], and the results of our study would probably be different in population treated with this mode. Many patients were not included, which could limit the external validity of our findings. Certain medical conditions, as chronic respiratory insufficiency with prior ventilatory support, tracheostomy or neuromuscular disease, were a priori excluded, preventing us to generalize our findings to these patients. Two ventilators (Evita XL and Servo-I) were used during the study. Similar studies are necessary to confirm our findings with other ventilators. Due to the study design and the need to observe active breathing for considering patient inclusion, patients were not recorded at the same time after admission. Although the degree of PVA did not seem to change so much over the PICU course, this difference in inclusion timing made it difficult to interpret the relationship between asynchrony and outcome.

Conclusion

Patient–ventilator interaction is poor in critically ill children supported by conventional ventilation. The study did not permit to ascertain if these poor interactions have important clinical consequence. But the magnitude of PVA and the prevalence of low ventilatory drive warrant further studies to assess whether strategies to optimize patient–ventilator interactions can improve the outcome of PICU patients.

Abbreviations

Edi: electrical activity of the diaphragm; ETT: endotracheal tube; NAVA: neurally adjusted ventilatory assist; PICU: pediatric intensive care unit; PSV: pressure support ventilation; PVA: patient–ventilator asynchrony.

Authors' contributions

AL, GE, OF, SE, and PJ designed the study. GM, AL, GC, AAPL, OF, JB, CS, and GE performed the analysis and carried out the chart review and data collection. GM, JB, CS, PJ, and GE wrote the manuscript, which was reviewed, edited, and approved by all authors. As the corresponding author, GE has full access to all the data in the study and has final responsibility for the decision to submit for publication. All authors read and approved the final manuscript.

Author details

[1] Pediatric Intensive Care Unit, CHU Sainte-Justine, 3175 Côte Sainte-Catherine, Montreal, QC, Canada. [2] INSERM U 955, Equipe 13, Créteil, France. [3] CHU Sainte-Justine Research Center, Université de Montréal, Montreal, Canada. [4] Pediatric Intensive Care Unit, CHU Fort-de-France, Fort-de-France, France. [5] Department of Pediatrics, CHU Sainte-Justine, Montreal, QC, Canada. [6] Queen's University, Kingston, Canada. [7] Keenan Research Centre for Biomedical Science, Li Ka Shing Knowledge Institute, St. Michael's Hospital, Toronto, ON, Canada. [8] Department of Pediatrics, University of Toronto, Toronto, Canada. [9] Institute for Biomedical Engineering and Science Technology (iBEST), Ryerson University and St-Michael's Hospital, Toronto, Canada. [10] Department of Medicine, University of Toronto, Toronto, Canada.

Acknowledgements

The authors are indebted to the patients and their families for their willingness to participate in our study. We thank Mariana Dumitrascu, Laurence Bertout, and Noémie Loron for their help in the screening and enrollment process, Lucy Clayton for the study management support, the respiratory therapists for their logistic help, the PICU fellows, attending healthcare providers, and PICU nurses for their collaboration, and Norman Comtois for his invaluable support regarding signal recording and analysis. This work was performed in CHU Sainte-Justine, Pediatric Intensive Care Unit, Montreal, Quebec, Canada.

Competing interests

GM, LDC, OF, GC, SE, and AAPL have no conflict of interest to declare. GE's research program is supported by a scholarship award by the Fonds de Recherche du Québec – Santé. He is currently leading a feasibility study in neonatal ventilation, which is financially supported by Maquet Critical Care. PJ is supported by a scholarship award by the Fonds de Recherche du Québec – Santé, Ministry of Health and Sainte-Justine Hospital. He was a consultant for Sage Therapeutic inc. and was invited to a congress by Medunik Inc and Covidien. JB and CS have made inventions related to neural control of mechanical ventilation that are patented. The patents are assigned to the academic institution(s) where inventions were made. The license for these patents belongs to Maquet Critical Care. Future commercial uses of this technology may provide financial benefit to JB and CS through royalties. JB and CS each own 50% of Neurovent Research Inc (NVR). NVR is a research and development company that builds the equipment and catheters for research studies. NVR has a consulting agreement with Maquet Critical Care. Neurovent research Inc. provided a recording device. Maquet Critical Care provided the ventilator and catheters for the study. This company was not involved in the result analysis and reporting.

Funding

The study was supported by a Young Investigator Award of the Respiratory Health Network of the Fonds de la Recherche du Québec–Santé and by an operating grant for applied clinical research of CHU Sainte-Justine and Sainte-Justine Research Center.

References

1. Payen V, Jouvet P, Lacroix J, Ducruet T, Gauvin F. Risk factors associated with increased length of mechanical ventilation in children. Pediatr Crit Care Med. 2012;13(2):152–7.
2. Petrof BJ, Hussain SN. Ventilator-induced diaphragmatic dysfunction: what have we learned? Curr Opin Crit Care. 2016;22(1):67–72.
3. Beck J, Reilly M, Grasselli G, Mirabella L, Slutsky AS, Dunn MS, et al. Patient–ventilator interaction during neurally adjusted ventilatory assist in low birth weight infants. Pediatr Res. 2009;65(6):663–8.
4. de Wit M, Miller KB, Green DA, Ostman HE, Gennings C, Epstein SK. Ineffective triggering predicts increased duration of mechanical ventilation. Crit Care Med. 2009;37(10):2740–5.
5. Thille AW, Rodriguez P, Cabello B, Lellouche F, Brochard L. Patient–ventilator asynchrony during assisted mechanical ventilation. Intensive Care Med. 2006;32(10):1515–22.
6. Colombo D, Cammarota G, Alemani M, Carenzo L, Barra FL, Vaschetto R, et al. Efficacy of ventilator waveforms observation in detecting patient–ventilator asynchrony. Crit Care Med. 2011;39(11):2452–7.
7. Blanch L, Villagra A, Sales B, Montanya J, Lucangelo U, Lujan M, et al. Asynchronies during mechanical ventilation are associated with mortality. Intensive Care Med. 2015;41(4):633–41.
8. Bosma K, Ferreyra G, Ambrogio C, Pasero D, Mirabella L, Braghiroli A, et al. Patient–ventilator interaction and sleep in mechanically ventilated patients: pressure support versus proportional assist ventilation. Crit Care Med. 2007;35(4):1048–54.
9. Kacmarek RM, Villar J, Blanch L. Cycle asynchrony: always a concern during pressure ventilation! Minerva Anestesiol. 2016;82(7):728–30.
10. Blokpoel RG, Burgerhof JG, Markhorst DG, Kneyber MC. Patient–ventilator asynchrony during assisted ventilation in children. Pediatr Crit Care Med. 2016;17(5):e204–11.
11. Vignaux L, Grazioli S, Piquilloud L, Bochaton N, Karam O, Jaecklin T, et al. Optimizing patient–ventilator synchrony during invasive ventilator assist in children and infants remains a difficult task*. Pediatr Crit Care Med. 2013;14(7):e316–25.
12. Bordessoule A, Emeriaud G, Morneau S, Jouvet P, Beck J. Neurally adjusted ventilatory assist improves patient–ventilator interaction in infants as compared with conventional ventilation. Pediatr Res. 2012;72(2):194–202.
13. de la Oliva P, Schuffelmann C, Gomez-Zamora A, Villar J, Kacmarek RM. Asynchrony, neural drive, ventilatory variability and COMFORT: NAVA versus pressure support in pediatric patients. A non-randomized cross-over trial. Intensive Care Med. 2012;38(5):838–46.
14. Ducharme-Crevier L, Du Pont-Thibodeau G, Emeriaud G. Interest of monitoring diaphragmatic electrical activity in the pediatric intensive care unit. Crit Care Res Pract. 2013;2013:384210.
15. Randolph AG, Wypij D, Venkataraman ST, Hanson JH, Gedeit RG, Meert KL, et al. Effect of mechanical ventilator weaning protocols on respiratory outcomes in infants and children: a randomized controlled trial. JAMA. 2002;288(20):2561–8.
16. Larouche A, Massicotte E, Constantin G, Ducharme-Crevier L, Essouri S, Sinderby C, et al. Tonic diaphragmatic activity in critically ill children with and without ventilatory support. Pediatr Pulmonol. 2015;50:1304–12.
17. Ducharme-Crevier L, Beck J, Essouri S, Jouvet P, Emeriaud G. Neurally adjusted ventilatory assist (NAVA) allows patient–ventilator synchrony during pediatric noninvasive ventilation: a crossover physiological study. Crit Care (London, England). 2015;19:44.
18. Sehgal IS, Dhooria S, Aggarwal AN, Behera D, Agarwal R. Asynchrony index in pressure support ventilation (PSV) versus neurally adjusted ventilator assist (NAVA) during non-invasive ventilation (NIV) for respiratory failure: systematic review and meta-analysis. Intensive Care Med. 2016;42(11):1813–5.
19. Sinderby C, Liu S, Colombo D, Camarotta G, Slutsky AS, Navalesi P, et al. An automated and standardized neural index to quantify patient–ventilator interaction. Crit Care (London, England). 2013;17(5):R239.
20. Doorduin J, Sinderby CA, Beck J, van der Hoeven JG, Heunks LM. Assisted ventilation in patients with acute respiratory distress syndrome: lung-distending pressure and patient–ventilator interaction. Anesthesiology. 2015;123(1):181–90.
21. Doorduin J, Sinderby CA, Beck J, van der Hoeven JG, Heunks LM. Automated patient–ventilator interaction analysis during neurally adjusted non-invasive ventilation and pressure support ventilation in chronic obstructive pulmonary disease. Crit Care (London, England). 2014;18(5):550.
22. Beck J, Tucci M, Emeriaud G, Lacroix J, Sinderby C. Prolonged neural expiratory time induced by mechanical ventilation in infants. Pediatr Res. 2004;55(5):747–54.
23. Vignaux L, Grazioli S, Piquilloud L, Bochaton N, Karam O, Levy-Jamet Y,

et al. Patient–ventilator asynchrony during noninvasive pressure support ventilation and neurally adjusted ventilatory assist in infants and children. Pediatr Crit Care Med. 2013;14(8):e357–64.

24. Piquilloud L, Vignaux L, Bialais E, Roeseler J, Sottiaux T, Laterre PF, et al. Neurally adjusted ventilatory assist improves patient–ventilator interaction. Intensive Care Med. 2011;37(2):263–71.
25. Azoulay E, Kouatchet A, Jaber S, Lambert J, Meziani F, Schmidt M, et al. Noninvasive mechanical ventilation in patients having declined tracheal intubation. Intensive Care Med. 2013;39(2):292–301.
26. Kim P, Salazar A, Ross PA, Newth CJ, Khemani RG. Comparison of tidal volumes at the endotracheal tube and at the ventilator. Pediatr Crit Care Med. 2015;16(9):e324–31.
27. Piastra M, De Luca D, Costa R, Pizza A, De Sanctis R, Marzano L, et al. Neurally adjusted ventilatory assist vs pressure support ventilation in infants recovering from severe acute respiratory distress syndrome: nested study. J Crit Care. 2014;29(2):312e1-5.
28. Kallio M, Peltoniemi O, Anttila E, Pokka T, Kontiokari T. Neurally adjusted ventilatory assist (NAVA) in pediatric intensive care—a randomized controlled trial. Pediatr Pulmonol. 2015;50(1):55–62.
29. Richard JC, Lyazidi A, Akoumianaki E, Mortaza S, Cordioli RL, Lefebvre JC, et al. Potentially harmful effects of inspiratory synchronization during pressure preset ventilation. Intensive Care Med. 2013;39(11):2003–10.
30. Beck J, Emeriaud G, Liu Y, Sinderby C. Neurally adjusted ventilatory assist (NAVA) in children: a systematic review. Minerva Anestesiol. 2016;82:874–83.
31. Emeriaud G, Larouche A, Ducharme-Crevier L, Massicotte E, Flechelles O, Pellerin-Leblanc AA, et al. Evolution of inspiratory diaphragm activity in children over the course of the PICU stay. Intensive Care Med. 2014;40(11):1718–26.
32. Alander M, Peltoniemi O, Pokka T, Kontiokari T. Comparison of pressure-, flow-, and NAVA-triggering in pediatric and neonatal ventilatory care. Pediatr Pulmonol. 2012;47(1):76–83.
33. Szczapa T, Beck J, Migdal M, Gadzinowski J. Monitoring diaphragm electrical activity and the detection of congenital central hypoventilation syndrome in a newborn. J Perinatol. 2013;33(11):905–7.
34. Liet JM, Dejode JM, Joram N, Gaillard Le Roux B, Pereon Y. Bedside diagnosis of bilateral diaphragmatic paralysis. Intensive Care Med. 2013;39(2):335.
35. Khemani RG, Smith LS, Zimmerman JJ, Erickson S. Pediatric acute respiratory distress syndrome: definition, incidence, and epidemiology: proceedings from the Pediatric Acute Lung Injury Consensus Conference. Pediatr Crit Care Med. 2015;16(5 Suppl 1):S23–40.
36. Levine S, Nguyen T, Taylor N, Friscia ME, Budak MT, Rothenberg P, et al. Rapid disuse atrophy of diaphragm fibers in mechanically ventilated humans. N Engl J Med. 2008;358(13):1327–35.
37. Jaber S, Petrof BJ, Jung B, Chanques G, Berthet JP, Rabuel C, et al. Rapidly progressive diaphragmatic weakness and injury during mechanical ventilation in humans. Am J Respir Crit Care Med. 2011;183(3):364–71.
38. Demoule A, Clavel M, Rolland-Debord C, Perbet S, Terzi N, Kouatchet A, et al. Neurally adjusted ventilatory assist as an alternative to pressure support ventilation in adults: a French multicentre randomized trial. Intensive Care Med. 2016;42(11):1723–32.

15

End-inspiratory pause prolongation in acute respiratory distress syndrome patients: effects on gas exchange and mechanics

Hernan Aguirre-Bermeo[1], Indalecio Morán[1], Maurizio Bottiroli[2], Stefano Italiano[1], Francisco José Parrilla[1], Eugenia Plazolles[1], Ferran Roche-Campo[3] and Jordi Mancebo[1*]

Abstract

Background: End-inspiratory pause (EIP) prolongation decreases dead space-to-tidal volume ratio (Vd/Vt) and $PaCO_2$. We do not know the physiological benefits of this approach to improve respiratory system mechanics in acute respiratory distress syndrome (ARDS) patients when mild hypercapnia is of no concern.

Methods: The investigation was conducted in an intensive care unit of a university hospital, and 13 ARDS patients were included. The study was designed in three phases. First phase, baseline measurements were taken. Second phase, the EIP was prolonged until one of the following was achieved: (1) EIP of 0.7 s; (2) intrinsic positive end-expiratory pressure $\geq$1 cmH_2O; or (3) inspiratory–expiratory ratio 1:1. Third phase, the Vt was decreased (30 mL every 30 min) until $PaCO_2$ equal to baseline was reached. FiO_2, PEEP, airflow and respiratory rate were kept constant.

Results: EIP was prolonged from 0.12 $\pm$ 0.04 to 0.7 s in all patients. This decreased the Vd/Vt and $PaCO_2$ (0.70 $\pm$ 0.07 to 0.64 $\pm$ 0.08, $p < 0.001$ and 54 $\pm$ 9 to 50 $\pm$ 8 mmHg, $p = 0.001$, respectively). In the third phase, the decrease in Vt (from 6.3 $\pm$ 0.8 to 5.6 $\pm$ 0.8 mL/Kg PBW, $p < 0.001$) allowed to decrease plateau pressure and driving pressure (24 $\pm$ 3 to 22 $\pm$ 3 cmH_2O, $p < 0.001$ and 13.4 $\pm$ 3.6 to 10.9 $\pm$ 3.1 cmH_2O, $p < 0.001$, respectively) and increased respiratory system compliance from 29 $\pm$ 9 to 32 $\pm$ 11 mL/cmH_2O ($p = 0.001$). PaO_2 did not significantly change.

Conclusions: Prolonging EIP allowed a significant decrease in Vt without changes in $PaCO_2$ in passively ventilated ARDS patients. This produced a significant decrease in plateau pressure and driving pressure and significantly increased respiratory system compliance, which suggests less overdistension and less dynamic strain.

Keywords: End-inspiratory pause, Dead space, Tidal volume, Acute respiratory distress syndrome, Mechanical ventilation

Background

Mechanical ventilation in patients with acute respiratory distress syndrome (ARDS) must combine both low tidal volumes (Vt) and adequate positive end-expiratory pressure (PEEP) [1, 2]. However, in patients with ARDS, respiratory acidosis and high airway plateau pressures (P_{plat}) may limit management of ventilatory adjustments. In particular, the functional consequences of hypercapnia and respiratory acidosis may differ considerably depending on a patient's condition, and they may involve almost any physiological function [3–6].

Optimization of mechanical ventilation parameters is associated with a reduction in dead space and is a useful strategy to reduce hypercapnia in ARDS patients [7]. Many other strategies have also been developed to decrease hypercapnia at the bedside, such as increases in respiratory rate [8], use of active humidifiers [9] and the tracheal gas insufflation [10] or aspiration of dead space [11]. At bedside, the dead space could be calculated using the Enghoff modification of the Bohr equation. The use of this equation implies the use of $PaCO_2$ as surrogate for

*Correspondence: jmancebo@santpau.cat
[1] Servei de Medicina Intensiva, Hospital de la Santa Creu i Sant Pau, Universidad Autònoma de Barcelona (UAB), Sant Quintí, 89, 08041 Barcelona, Spain
Full list of author information is available at the end of the article

alveolar carbon dioxide. Therefore, this equation measures a global index of efficiency of gas exchange because it takes also shunt effect into account [12].

Some authors have also shown that prolonging the end-inspiratory pause (EIP) is a feasible maneuver to achieve similar targets [13, 14]. In experimental models [15] and in ARDS patients [14, 16–18], EIP prolongation has proven effective at enhancing CO_2 elimination and decreasing partial pressure of carbon dioxide in arterial blood ($PaCO_2$) and also physiological dead space (Vd_{phys}). Prolonging EIP extends the time available for an enhanced diffusion between inhaled Vt and resident alveolar gas, thus facilitating the transfer of CO_2 from alveoli toward the airways [17, 18].

Although several of the physiological studies described above have reported that EIP prolongation improves gas exchange, none have investigated the potential physiological benefits of this approach in terms of Vt reduction or improved respiratory system mechanics when hypercapnia is of no concern. To address this gap, the objective of our study was to ascertain whether EIP prolongation decreases $PaCO_2$ and whether this effect can be used to decrease Vt while keeping $PaCO_2$ constant. We hypothesized that this approach may have beneficial effects on respiratory system mechanics in ARDS patients.

Methods

The study was performed in the Intensive Care Unit at Hospital de la Santa Creu i Sant Pau, Barcelona (Spain). The institutional ethics committee approved the study (Reference: 10/089), and the patients' relatives gave signed informed consent.

Patients

Fourteen patients who met the criteria for ARDS [19] were included in the study. Exclusion criteria were: age <18 years, pregnancy, hemodynamic or respiratory instability, and variation of more than 0.5 °C in body temperature in the last 12 h before the study was planned [20]. One patient was excluded during the study period (see Results).

All patients were under sedation and analgesia with intravenous perfusion of midazolam and opiates. Neuromuscular blockade was used in all patients to prevent triggering of the ventilator. Careful endotracheal suctioning was performed before the protocol was started. Heated humidifiers (Fisher & Paykel; MR 290 chamber and MR 850 ALU electric heater; Panmure, New Zealand) were used for airway humidification in all patients. These humidifiers were placed in the inspiratory limb of the circuit in accordance with the manufacturer's recommendations. The respiratory rate, FiO_2, inspiratory flow (square pattern) and PEEP were kept constant throughout the study.

Protocol

All patients were in steady state in the 60-min preceding data recording, and all of them were in a semirecumbent position. The study was performed in three consecutive 30-min phases. Measurements in the first phase (baseline phase) were taken under the mechanical ventilation parameters set by the patient's attending physician. In the second phase (EIP prolongation phase), the EIP was prolonged until one of the following parameters was reached: (1) EIP of 0.7 s; (2) intrinsic positive end-expiratory pressure (PEEPi) $\geq$1 cmH_2O; or (3) inspiratory–expiratory ratio (I/E) of 1:1. We chose the EIP prolongation time (0.7 s) based on findings from a previous study by Devaquet et al. [18] in which a 20 % prolongation of the inspiratory time induced a significant decrease in $PaCO_2$ and dead space. In the third phase (Vt reduction phase), the Vt was diminished in steps of 30 mL every 30 min until $PaCO_2$ reached baseline levels.

The following data were collected at inclusion: demographic variables (age, sex, height), simplified acute physiology score II, ARDS etiology and days of mechanical ventilation.

During the last minute of each phase, we collected the following respiratory variables: peak airway pressure, Pplat, mean airway pressure, PEEPi, PEEP, driving airway pressure (ΔPaw), Vt, dead space-to-Vt ratio (Vd/Vt), static compliance of the respiratory system (Crs) and airway resistance. At the same time, we recorded the following gas exchange variables: pH, partial pressure of arterial oxygen (PaO_2), $PaCO_2$ and end-tidal carbon dioxide concentration in the mixed expired gas ($EtCO_2$). PEEPi was measured with a prolonged end-expiratory pause of 4 s, performed using the ventilator expiratory hold button. $EtCO_2$ was measured continuously with a CO_2 mainstream sensor (General Electric Capnostat, Milwaukee, WI, USA). The mean value of the last 10 recorded $EtCO_2$ values in each phase of the study was used for analysis.

Ventilatory settings and airway pressures were recorded directly from the ventilator monitoring system. Plateau pressure was measured during an end-inspiratory pause. Dead space was calculated using the Enghoff modification of the Bohr equation [21]: $Vd/Vt = (PaCO_2 - PeCO_2)/PaCO_2$, being $PeCO_2$ the partial pressure of carbon dioxide in mixed expired gas. Expired gas was measured by collecting gas for 3 min with a Douglas bag (P-341–60; Warren E. Collins Inc., Boston, MA, USA) attached directly to the expiratory port of the ventilator. An automated analyzer (ABL 520; Radiometer A/S, Copenhagen, Denmark) was used to measure expired and arterial gases. Dead space data were expressed as physiological dead space (Vd_{phys} in mL), defined as the sum of instrumental, anatomic and alveolar dead space [22]. Driving pressure (cmH_2O) was calculated as Pplat-PEEP. Crs (mL/cmH_2O) was calculated as Vt/[Pplat-(PEEP + PEEPi)], and airway resistance (cmH_2O/L/s) was calculated as (peak airway pressure − plateau pressure)/Flow. Predicted body weight (PBW) was calculated as follows: 50 + 0.91(height in cm-152.4) for men and 45.5 + 0.91(height in cm-152.4) for women [8]. Arterial to end-tidal CO_2 gradient (P(a-et) CO_2) was calculated in each study phase. We used Puritan Bennett™ 840 (Covidien, Galway, Ireland) and Dräger Evita XL (Dräger Medical, Lübeck, Germany) ventilators. All the ventilators used have a compressible volume compensation system.

Statistical analysis

Data are expressed as mean ± standard deviation. The results were analyzed using one-way analysis of variance for repeated measures (ANOVA) with the Greenhouse–Geisser correction. We performed the Kolmogorov–Smirnov test to confirm normal data distribution. Since the distribution of the data was normal, we used the Student's *t* test and the Pearson linear correlation to compare data and correlations between phases and variables, respectively. A two-tailed *p* value less than 0.05 was considered statistically significant. The SPSS® Statistics (version 20.0, Chicago, IL, USA) statistical software was used for statistical analysis.

Results

One of the 14 patients enrolled in the study was excluded from the analysis due to fever, tachypnea and unstable $EtCO_2$ during the second phase of the study. The study was performed 5 ± 4 days after starting mechanical ventilation. Table 1 shows demographic data at admission, ARDS etiology and baseline characteristics at study day.

Baseline EIP was 0.12 ± 0.04 s, and it was increased to 0.7 ± 0 s in all patients ($p < 0.001$). This EIP change was performed maintaining PEEPi <1 cmH_2O (0.2 ± 0.2 to 0.5 ± 0.4 cmH_2O, $p = 0.06$) and without the I/E inverse ratio ventilation (1:4.7 ± 0:1.3 to 1:1.7 ± 0:0.4, $p = <0.001$). EIP prolongation decreased Vd_{phys} and $PaCO_2$ significantly with respect to basal conditions (267 ± 71 to 244 ± 65 mL and 54 ± 9 to 50 ± 8 mmHg, respectively; $p < 0.001$ for both comparisons). The decrease in $PaCO_2$ levels due to EIP prolongation was correlated with the drop in Vd_{phys} ($r = 0.871$; $p < 0.001$). Individual changes in $PaCO_2$ and in Vd_{phys} are shown in Figs. 1 and 2, respectively.

Between the first and second phase, significant decreases were observed in both the Vd/Vt ratio (0.70 ± 0.07 to 0.64 ± 0.08; $p < 0.001$) and $EtCO_2$ (41 ± 6 to 39 ± 6 mmHg; $p = 0.006$). Basal Vd_{phys} and P(a-et) CO_2 had a close correlation ($r = 0.75$; $p = 0.003$). The change in Vd_{phys} and the change in P(a-et)CO_2 between the first and second phase also showed a close correlation ($r = 0.68$; $p = 0.001$).

In the third phase (EIP prolongation and Vt reduction), the Vt was significantly reduced as compared to previous phases (6.3 ± 0.8 to 5.6 ± 0.8 mL/Kg PBW; $p < 0.001$). In the third phase, as per protocol design, the $PaCO_2$ and pH values were statistically identical to those at baseline (54 ± 9 vs. 54 ± 10 mmHg; $p = 0.90$ and 7.31 ± 0.07 vs. 7.31 ± 0.08; $p = 0.90$, respectively).

The Vd_{phys} decreased progressively and significantly during all phases of the study (267 ± 71 to 244 ± 65 to 216 ± 58 mL; $p < 0.001$). The Vd_{phys} and Vt at baseline were strongly correlated ($r = 0.946$; $p < 0.001$). Additionally, the Vt reduction was tightly correlated with the decrease in Vd_{phys} ($r = 0.894$; $p < 0.001$). Respiratory system mechanics, gas exchange, hemodynamics, and temperature data throughout the study are also given in Table 2.

Discussion

The main finding of our study was that the end-inspiratory pause prolongation allowed to decrease tidal volume while maintaining similar $PaCO_2$ levels. Indeed, the decrease in tidal volume led to a significant decrease in Pplat and ΔPaw, and it also improved the respiratory system compliance.

Several studies have shown that prolongation of EIP enhances CO_2 elimination and decreases dead space and $PaCO_2$ levels [14–18]. Diffusion of CO_2 is time dependent, and EIP prolongation increases the time available for alveolar gas exchange [14, 23, 24]. Devaquet et al. [18] extended inspiratory time from 0.7 ± 0.2 to 1.4 ± 0.3 s by increasing the inspiratory pause time from 0 to 20 % of the total breathing cycle. They observed that this modification significantly decreased both Vd/Vt (around 10 %) and $PaCO_2$ (around 11 %). Despite these beneficial effects of prolonged EIP and the direct relationship between inspiratory time and enhanced CO_2 elimination [16, 18], EIP prolongation may lead to potentially adverse effects such as PEEPi production and inversion of the I/E ratio together with increases in mean airway pressure. These effects might also provoke hyperinflation, thus altering cardiac performance [25, 26]. Nevertheless, Devaquet and colleagues [18] showed that EIP could be prolonged without significantly increasing PEEPi (I/E ratio 1:1.5). Not surprisingly, and in spite of a significant increase in EIP, we did not induce any significant increase in PEEPi since the expiratory time was long enough to avoid air trapping at the end of a passive expiration (average expiratory time 1.7 ± 0.3 s). Actually (see Table 2), the average product of three time constants (the time needed to

Table 1 Demographic data at admission and baseline characteristics of patients on the study day

Admission							Study day					
Patient	**Age (years)**	**Gender**	**SAPS II**	**PBW (kg)**	**Measured weight (kg)**	**ARDS etiology**	**Days of MV before study**	**PaO2/FiO2 (mmHg)**	**FiO2a**	**PEEP (cmH_2O)[a]**	**Flow (L/min)[a]**	**RR (bpm)[a]**
1	75	M	59	67.7	58.5	Pneumonia	8	112	0.7	10	70	22
2	52	M	42	68.7	78	Aspiration	13	185	0.65	12	57	20
3	46	F	30	52.4	61	Multiple Trauma	7	118	0.7	12	60	25
4	62	F	69	47.9	55	Pneumonia	5	131	0.6	10	60	25
5	56	F	23	52.4	61.5	Pneumonia	3	100	0.8	12	60	22
6	66	M	40	63.2	72.5	Pneumonia	1	184	0.5	10	60	20
7	57	M	62	69.6	83	Pneumonia	1	147	0.5	8	60	17
8	36	M	24	61.4	90	Pneumonia	4	242	0.5	14	75	23
9	55	M	49	66.8	72	Pneumonia	2	219	0.6	14	70	21
10	51	F	60	43.3	64	Sepsis	12	269	0.4	8	50	21
11	74	F	61	47.9	62.5	Sepsis	1	266	0.5	10	60	21
12	43	M	61	59.6	80.5	Sepsis	3	194	0.7	10	60	22
13	63	M	30	83.1	106	Pneumonia	6	283	0.35	8	60	30
Mean ± SD	57 ± 11		47 ± 16	60.3 ± 11.2	72.6 ± 14.6		5 ± 4	188 ± 64	0.58 ± 0.13	11 ± 2	61 ± 7	22 ± 3

ARDS acute respiratory distress syndrome, *FiO_2* fraction of inspired oxygen, *MV* mechanical ventilation, *PaO_2/FiO_2* partial pressure of arterial oxygen over fraction of inspired oxygen, *PBW* predicted body weight, *PEEP* positive end-expiratory pressure, *RR* respiratory rate, *SAPS II* simplified acute physiology score II

[a] These settings were kept constant throughout the study

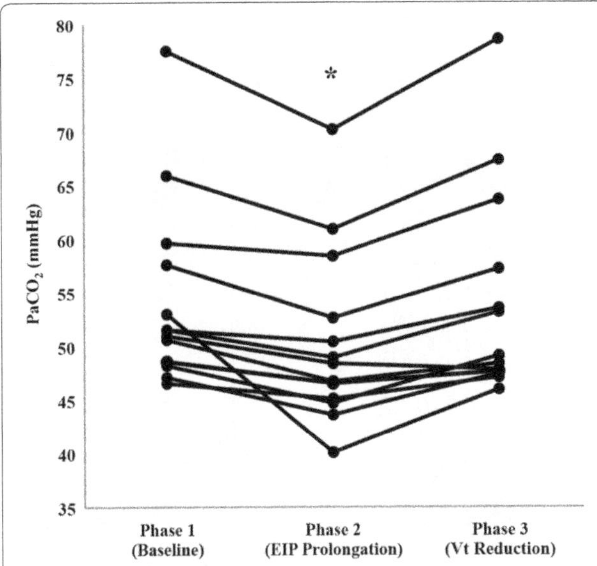

Fig. 1 Individual values for $PaCO_2$ during the study. The *asterisk* denotes statistically significant differences ($p < 0.001$) during prolongation of end-inspiratory pause. *EIP* end-inspiratory pause, *$PaCO_2$* partial pressure of carbon dioxide in arterial blood, *Vt* tidal volume

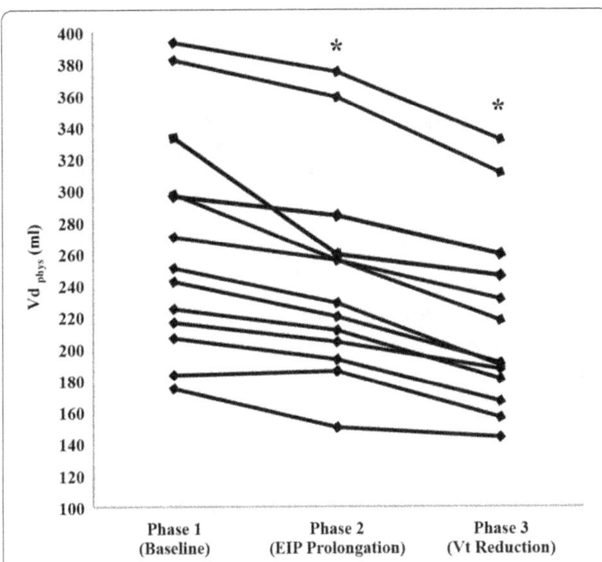

Fig. 2 Individual values for Vd_{phys} during the study. The *asterisks* denote a significant, progressive decrease in Vd_{phys} ($p < 0.001$) during prolongation of end-inspiratory pause (EIP) and during Vt reduction. *EIP* end-inspiratory pause, *Vd_{phys}* physiological dead space, *Vt* tidal volume

passively exhale 96 % of inhaled tidal volume) was in our patients about 1.1 s. ($0.373 \times 3 = 1.1$ s), well below to the average expiratory time.

Prolongation of EIP in our patients caused a significant decrease in dead space and $PaCO_2$ levels that was similar to previously reported [14–18]. When comparing phase 1 (baseline) and phase 2 (isolated EIP prolongation), we found that the decrease in the Vd/Vt correlated well with the drop in $PaCO_2$ ($r = 0.810$; $p < 0.001$). These changes observed in our patients may be explained by the increase on the time available for distribution and diffusion of inspired tidal gas within resident alveolar gas during EIP prolongation [14]. Indeed, total PEEP levels, airflow, respiratory rate, tidal volume and respiratory mechanics were totally unchanged in this phase of our study [14, 27, 28].

Comparing the second (isolated EIP prolongation) and third (EIP prolongation and Vt reduction) phases, our data showed that the Vd/Vt ratio remained unchanged. However, the Vd_{phys}, expressed in mL, decreased significantly between phases 2 and 3. This is explained by the significant reduction in Vt (that also provoked a decrease in Vd_{phys}) during the third phase as compared to the previous phases, and thus Vd/Vt ratio did not change. The fact that the reduction in Vt in the third phase was accompanied by a significant decrease in Vd_{phys} and ΔPaw (with a significant increase in compliance) suggests that some degree of overdistension might be present at baseline.

As previously described, low tidal volume ventilation in ARDS may induce hypercapnia and, secondarily, induce pulmonary artery hypertension that may impair right ventricular function [29] and eventually cause acute cor pulmonale [30]. To reduce hypercapnia in ARDS ventilated patients, active heated humidifiers are often used. These devices significantly decrease dead space, $PaCO_2$ and ventilator mechanical load [9] without increasing airflow resistance [31]. Although active humidification is recommended over heat and moisture exchangers in ARDS patients [32], two studies focussing on the effects of EIP prolongation on gas exchange [16, 17] did not describe the type of humidification used in their patients. A third study used passive or active humidification (10 and 5 patients, respectively) [18]. However, the effects on $PaCO_2$ in all these studies [16–18] were consistently the same, thus suggesting that humidification type per se does not influence the effects of EIP on $PaCO_2$.

Another technique used to decrease hypercapnia is to increase the respiratory rate. However, in ARDS patients, several studies have shown that a high respiratory rate led to gas trapping and induced PEEPi [33, 34]. In addition, experimental models suggested that higher respiratory rates may contribute to the development of ventilator-induced lung injury [35, 36]. Vieillard-Baron et al. [25] compared two respiratory rate strategies, 30 versus 15 breaths/min. They found that the high respiratory rate did not reduce $PaCO_2$ levels but produced dynamic hyperinflation and reduced the cardiac index. In our patients, EIP prolongation was achieved with a relatively

Table 2 Respiratory system mechanics, gas exchange and hemodynamic data during the study

	Phase 1 (baseline)	Phase 2 (EIP prolongation)	Phase 3 (Vt reduction)	Overall p value	Intergroup differences
EIP (s)	0.12 ± 0.04	0.7 ± 0	0.7 ± 0	<0.001	a, b
Ppeak (cmH_2O)	38 ± 6	38 ± 6	35 ± 5	<0.001	b, c
Pmean (cmH_2O)	15 ± 3	18 ± 2	17 ± 2	<0.001	a, b, c
Pplat (cmH_2O)	24 ± 3	24 ± 3	22 ± 3	<0.001	b, c
PEEPi (cmH_2O)	0.2 ± 0.2	0.5 ± 0.4	0.5 ± 0.4	0.06	
Vt (mL)	378 ± 73	378 ± 73	336 ± 61	<0.001	b, c
Vt (PBW; mL/Kg)	6.3 ± 0.8	6.3 ± 0.8	5.6 ± 0.8	<0.001	b, c
Vd_{phys} (mL)	267 ± 71	244 ± 65	216 ± 58	<0.001	a, b, c
Vd/Vt	0.70 ± 0.07	0.64 ± 0.08	0.64 ± 0.08	<0.001	a, b
Crs (mL/cmH_2O)	29 ± 9	29 ± 9	32 ± 11	0.001	b, c
Δ Paw (cmH_2O)	13.6 ± 3.6	13.4 ± 3.6	10.9 ± 3.1	<0.001	a, b, c
R_{aw} ($cmH_2O/L/s$)	14 ± 5	13 ± 5	13 ± 4	0.28	
pH	7.31 ± 0.07	7.34 ± 0.09	7.31 ± 0.08	<0.001	a, c
PaO_2 (mmHg)	102 ± 23	98 ± 23	105 ± 29	0.35	
$PaCO_2$ (mmHg)	54 ± 9	50 ± 8	54 ± 10	<0.001	a, c
$EtCO_2$ (mmHg)	41 ± 6	39 ± 6	43 ± 7	0.002	a, c
$P(a\text{-}et)CO_2$ (mmHg)	13 ± 6	12 ± 8	12 ± 9	0.27	
MAP (mmHg)	80 ± 12	76 ± 9	77 ± 12	0.08	
HR (beats/min)	87 ± 19	83 ± 20	86 ± 21	0.14	
Temperature (°C)	36.7 ± 0.9	36.7 ± 0.9	36.6 ± 0.8	0.61	

Data are presented as number (%) or mean ± SD

Intergroup differences ($p < 0.05$): a, phase 1 versus phase 2; b, phase 1 versus phase 3; c, phase 2 versus phase 3

Crs static compliance of the respiratory system, *EIP* end-inspiratory pause, *$EtCO_2$* end-tidal carbon dioxide concentration in the expired air, *FiO_2* fraction of inspired oxygen, *HR* heart rate, *MAP* mean arterial pressure, *PaO_2* partial pressure of oxygen in arterial blood, *$PaCO_2$* partial pressure of carbon dioxide in arterial blood, *PBW* predicted body weight, *PEEPi* intrinsic positive end-expiratory pressure, *Pmean* mean airway pressure, *Ppeak* peak airway pressure, *Pplat* plateau airway pressure, $P(a\text{-}et)CO_2$ arterial to end-tidal CO_2 gradient, *Raw* airway resistance, *Vd_{phys}* physiological dead space, *Vd/Vt* dead space-to-Vt ratio, *Vt* tidal volume, *ΔPaw* driving airway pressure

high inspiratory flow rate (1 L/s), thus avoiding inverse I/E ratio. This was a safe strategy to decrease $PaCO_2$ levels, while keeping respiratory rate constant (22 breaths/min) and not generating PEEPi.

In our study, the reduction in Vt to maintain isocapnia was modest. Should major reductions in Vt were required, then the use of invasive extracorporeal carbon dioxide removal devices had to be considered in order to avoid acute hypercapnia [37].

Studies analyzing the EIP prolongation did not describe changes in PaO_2 [14, 18], except one study by Mercat et al. [16]. This latter study found a slight, but not statistically significant, increase in PaO_2 levels during EIP prolongation. This finding was not confirmed in our study. We speculate that the length of time that patients are maintained with EIP prolongation and the mean airway pressure achieved during extended EIP may have contributed to this finding. Indeed, in Mercat's study [16], EIP prolongation was continued for 1 h with a mean airway pressure of 21 cmH_2O and an I/E ratio 1.1. In contrast, in Devaquet's study [18] and in our own study, EIP prolongation was shorter (30 min in both), mean airway pressure was lower (15 and 17 cmH_2O, respectively), and the I/E ratios achieved were 1:1.5 in Devaquet's study and 1:1.7 in ours.

The main novelty of our study is that prolonging EIP allowed to reduce Vt by 11 % (from 6.3 ± 0.8 to 5.6 ± 0.8 mL/kg of PBW; $p < 0.001$), maintaining $PaCO_2$ levels equal to baseline. These sequential ventilatory changes were accompanied by a reduction in Vd_{phys}. Also, when $PaCO_2$ returned to baseline due to a reduction in Vt, we found a significant decrease in Pplat and an increase in Crs. In addition, these changes in ventilatory mechanics were accompanied by a significant decrease in ΔPaw. All those findings could be explained by a degree of baseline overinflation even though our initial Vt was low [38]. We further support our contention by the tight correlation between Vt and Vd_{phys} at the onset of the study and the tight correlation between the decrease in Vt and Vd_{phys} at the end of the study. Our patients were basally ventilated with parameters similar to those used in previous studies [16–18] in terms of Vt and PEEP, and

Vd/Vt was also similar. Moreover, in our patients, Crs was lower (29 mL/cmH_2O) than in Mercat and Devaquet studies (37 and 50 mL/cmH_2O, respectively). Our findings thus suggest that if $PaCO_2$ is clinically tolerable, EIP prolongation in ARDS provides physiological benefits including a small and consistent decrease in Vt which may help decrease dynamic strain [39].

In our study, a slight but not statistically significant decrease in mean arterial pressure was observed. Such trend could have been the result of complex interactions of $PaCO_2$ and mean airway pressure in cardiovascular system.

We think that EIP prolongation is a feasible maneuver to optimize the consequences of mechanical ventilation in ARDS patients. Physicians may consider using an EIP prolongation in the early phase of ARDS when patients often require sedation and neuromuscular blocking agents. In our study, we have effectively implemented this strategy by using active humidification, relatively high inspiratory flow rates and close monitoring of PEEPi. This bundle decreases $PaCO_2$, which in turn will allow to further decrease Vt and the consequent lung strain when isocapnic conditions are met.

One of the limitations of our study is the relatively small number of patients, the majority with pneumonia, and the fact that the study is short term. Studies with patients with different ARDS etiologies and larger numbers are warranted to confirm our data. Also, we did not measure other parameters such as inflammatory mediators or lung volumes. The calculation of dead space using the Enghoff modification of Bohr equation in patients with large shunt fractions (>20–30 %) could underestimate dead space fraction [12]. In our study, we did not measure intrapulmonary shunt. However, according to the gas exchange values that we obtained, shunt fractions above 30 % are unlikely. Additionally, the EIP prolongation increases the mechanical inflation time and it could extend into neural expiration. Asynchronies may thus develop and cause an inadequate patient–ventilator interaction when the patients are not paralyzed [39–41]. Our results could be dependent on our routine management of mechanical ventilation in ARDS patients, but our findings have been consistent in all patients and we consider they could be extrapolated to other ARDS patients. Finally, the absolute decrease in tidal volume, although statistically significant, is moderate.

Conclusions

In conclusion, our data indicate that EIP prolongation is a simple and feasible strategy to decrease dead space and $PaCO_2$ levels. In addition, when $PaCO_2$ levels are of no clinical concern, EIP prolongation allows us to further decrease tidal volume. This, in turn, decreases plateau airway pressure, driving airway pressure and improves respiratory system compliance, suggesting less overdistension and less risk of dynamic strain and lung injury. Therefore, the use of this simple ventilator maneuver during mechanical ventilation in sedated and paralyzed ARDS patients merits consideration.

Abbreviations

ARDS: acute respiratory distress syndrome; Crs: static compliance of the respiratory system; EIP: end-inspiratory pause; $EtCO_2$: end-tidal carbon dioxide concentration in the mixed expired gas; IE: inspiratory–expiratory ratio; $PaCO_2$: partial pressure of carbon dioxide in arterial blood; PaO_2: partial pressure of arterial oxygen; PBW: predicted body weight; $PeCO_2$: partial pressure of carbon dioxide in mixed expired gas; PEEP: positive end-expiratory pressure; PEEPi: intrinsic positive end-expiratory pressure; P_{plat}: plateau airway pressure; P(a-et) CO_2: arterial to end-tidal CO_2 gradient; Vd/Vt: dead space-to-Vt ratio; Vd_{phys}: physiological dead space; Vt: tidal volume; ΔPaw: driving airway pressure.

Authors' contributions

All authors participated in the study design, data collection and analysis, manuscript writing and final approval. All authors read and approved the final manuscript.

Author details

[1] Servei de Medicina Intensiva, Hospital de la Santa Creu i Sant Pau, Universidad Autònoma de Barcelona (UAB), Sant Quintí, 89, 08041 Barcelona, Spain. [2] Anestesia e Rianimazione 3, Ospedale Niguarda Ca' Granda, Milan, Italy. [3] Servei de Medicina Intensiva, Hospital Verge de la Cinta, Tortosa, Spain.

Competing interests

The authors declare that they have no competing interests.

References

1. Eichacker PQ, Gerstenberger EP, Banks SM, Cui X, Natanson C. Meta-analysis of acute lung injury and acute respiratory distress syndrome trials testing low tidal volumes. Am J Respir Crit Care Med. 2002;166:1510–4.
2. Briel M, Meade M, Mercat A, Brower RG, Talmor D, Walter SD, Slutsky AS, Pullenayegum E, Zhou Q, Cook D, Brochard L, Richard JC, Lamontagne F, Bhatnagar N, Stewart TE, Guyatt G. Higher vs lower positive end-expiratory pressure in patients with acute lung injury and acute respiratory distress syndrome: systematic review and meta-analysis. JAMA. 2010;303:865–73.
3. Feihl F, Perret C. Permissive hypercapnia. How permissive should we be? Am J Respir Crit Care Med. 1994;150:1722–37.
4. Laffey JG, Engelberts D, Kavanagh BP. Buffering hypercapnic acidosis worsens acute lung injury. Am J Respir Crit Care Med. 2000;161:141–6.
5. Feihl F, Eckert P, Brimioulle S, Jacobs O, Schaller MD, Melot C, Naeije R. Permissive hypercapnia impairs pulmonary gas exchange in the acute respiratory distress syndrome. Am J Respir Crit Care Med. 2000;162:209–15.
6. O'Croinin DF, Nichol AD, Hopkins N, Boylan J, O'Brien S, O'Connor C, Laffey JG, McLoughlin P. Sustained hypercapnic acidosis during pulmonary infection increases bacterial load and worsens lung injury. Crit Care Med. 2008;36:2128–35.
7. Richecoeur J, Lu Q, Vieira SR, Puybasset L, Kalfon P, Coriat P, Rouby JJ. Expiratory washout versus optimization of mechanical ventilation during permissive hypercapnia in patients with severe acute respiratory distress syndrome. Am J Respir Crit Care Med. 1999;160:77–85.
8. Network The Acute Respiratory Distress Syndrome. Ventilation with lower tidal volumes as compared with traditional tidal volumes for acute lung injury and the acute respiratory distress syndrome. N Engl J Med. 2000;342:1301–8.

9. Moran I, Bellapart J, Vari A, Mancebo J. Heat and moisture exchangers and heated humidifiers in acute lung injury/acute respiratory distress syndrome patients. Effects on respiratory mechanics and gas exchange. Intensive Care Med. 2006;32:524–31.
10. Ravenscraft SA, Burke WC, Nahum A, Adams AB, Nakos G, Marcy TW, Marini JJ. Tracheal gas insufflation augments CO2 clearance during mechanical ventilation. Am Rev Respir Dis. 1993;148:345–51.
11. De Robertis E, Servillo G, Tufano R, Jonson B. Aspiration of dead space allows isocapnic low tidal volume ventilation in acute lung injury. Relationships to gas exchange and mechanics. Intensive Care Med. 2001;27:1496–503.
12. Suarez-Sipmann F, Bohm SH, Tusman G. Volumetric capnography: the time has come. Curr Opin Crit Care. 2014;20:333–9.
13. Astrom E, Uttman L, Niklason L, Aboab J, Brochard L, Jonson B. Pattern of inspiratory gas delivery affects CO_2 elimination in health and after acute lung injury. Intensive Care Med. 2008;34:377–84.
14. Aboab J, Niklason L, Uttman L, Brochard L, Jonson B. Dead space and CO_2 elimination related to pattern of inspiratory gas delivery in ARDS patients. Crit Care. 2012;16:R39.
15. Uttman L, Jonson B. A prolonged postinspiratory pause enhances CO_2 elimination by reducing airway dead space. Clin Physiol Funct Imaging. 2003;23:252–6.
16. Mercat A, Diehl JL, Michard F, Anguel N, Teboul JL, Labrousse J, Richard C. Extending inspiratory time in acute respiratory distress syndrome. Crit Care Med. 2001;29:40–4.
17. Aboab J, Niklason L, Uttman L, Kouatchet A, Brochard L, Jonson B. CO_2 elimination at varying inspiratory pause in acute lung injury. Clin Physiol Funct Imaging. 2007;27:2–6.
18. Devaquet J, Jonson B, Niklason L, Si Larbi AG, Uttman L, Aboab J, Brochard L. Effects of inspiratory pause on CO_2 elimination and arterial PCO_2 in acute lung injury. J Appl Physiol. 2008;105:1944–9.
19. Ranieri VM, Rubenfeld GD, Thompson BT, Ferguson ND, Caldwell E, Fan E, Camporota L, Slutsky AS. Acute respiratory distress syndrome: the Berlin definition. JAMA. 2012;307:2526–33.
20. Bacher A. Effects of body temperature on blood gases. Intensive Care Med. 2005;31:24–7.
21. Fletcher R, Jonson B, Cumming G, Brew J. The concept of deadspace with special reference to the single breath test for carbon dioxide. Br J Anaesth. 1981;53:77–88.
22. Lucangelo U, Blanch L. Dead space. Intensive Care Med. 2004;30:576–9.
23. Knelson JH, Howatt WF, DeMuth GR. Effect of respiratory pattern on alveolar gas exchange. J Appl Physiol. 1970;29:328–31.
24. Shanholtz C, Brower R. Should inverse ratio ventilation be used in adult respiratory distress syndrome? Am J Respir Crit Care Med. 1994;149:1354–8.
25. Vieillard-Baron A, Prin S, Augarde R, Desfonds P, Page B, Beauchet A, Jardin F. Increasing respiratory rate to improve CO_2 clearance during mechanical ventilation is not a panacea in acute respiratory failure. Crit Care Med. 2002;30:1407–12.
26. Armstrong BW Jr, MacIntyre NR. Pressure-controlled, inverse ratio ventilation that avoids air trapping in the adult respiratory distress syndrome. Crit Care Med. 1995;23:279–85.
27. Blanch L, Fernandez R, Benito S, Mancebo J, Net A. Effect of PEEP on the arterial minus end-tidal carbon dioxide gradient. Chest. 1987;92:451–4.
28. Beydon L, Uttman L, Rawal R, Jonson B. Effects of positive end-expiratory pressure on dead space and its partitions in acute lung injury. Intensive Care Med. 2002;28:1239–45.
29. Carvalho CR, Barbas CS, Medeiros DM, Magaldi RB, Lorenzi Filho G, Kairalla RA, Deheinzelin D, Munhoz C, Kaufmann M, Ferreira M, Takagaki TY, Amato MB. Temporal hemodynamic effects of permissive hypercapnia associated with ideal PEEP in ARDS. Am J Respir Crit Care Med. 1997;156:1458–66.
30. Vieillard-Baron A, Schmitt JM, Augarde R, Fellahi JL, Prin S, Page B, Beauchet A, Jardin F. Acute cor pulmonale in acute respiratory distress syndrome submitted to protective ventilation: incidence, clinical implications, and prognosis. Crit Care Med. 2001;29:1551–5.
31. Moran I, Cabello B, Manero E, Mancebo J. Comparison of the effects of two humidifier systems on endotracheal tube resistance. Intensive Care Med. 2011;37:1773–9.
32. Restrepo RD, Walsh BK. Humidification during invasive and noninvasive mechanical ventilation: 2012. Respir Care. 2012;57:782–8.
33. Richard JC, Brochard L, Breton L, Aboab J, Vandelet P, Tamion F, Maggiore SM, Mercat A, Bonmarchand G. Influence of respiratory rate on gas trapping during low volume ventilation of patients with acute lung injury. Intensive Care Med. 2002;28:1078–83.
34. de Durante G, del Turco M, Rustichini L, Cosimini P, Giunta F, Hudson LD, Slutsky AS, Ranieri VM. ARDSNet lower tidal volume ventilatory strategy may generate intrinsic positive end-expiratory pressure in patients with acute respiratory distress syndrome. Am J Respir Crit Care Med. 2002;165:1271–4.
35. Hotchkiss JR Jr, Blanch L, Murias G, Adams AB, Olson DA, Wangensteen OD, Leo PH, Marini JJ. Effects of decreased respiratory frequency on ventilator-induced lung injury. Am J Respir Crit Care Med. 2000;161:463–8.
36. Conrad SA, Zhang S, Arnold TC, Scott LK, Carden DL. Protective effects of low respiratory frequency in experimental ventilator-associated lung injury. Crit Care Med. 2005;33:835–40.
37. Fanelli V, Ranieri MV, Mancebo J, Moerer O, Quintel M, Morley S, Moran I, Parrilla F, Costamagna A, Gaudiosi M, Combes A. Feasibility and safety of low-flow extracorporeal carbon dioxide removal to facilitate ultra-protective ventilation in patients with moderate acute respiratory distress sindrome. Crit Care. 2016;20:36.
38. Terragni PP, Rosboch G, Tealdi A, Corno E, Menaldo E, Davini O, Gandini G, Herrmann P, Mascia L, Quintel M, Slutsky AS, Gattinoni L, Ranieri VM. Tidal hyperinflation during low tidal volume ventilation in acute respiratory distress syndrome. Am J Respir Crit Care Med. 2007;175:160–6.
39. Mauri T, Yoshida T, Bellani G, Goligher EC, Carteaux G, Rittayamai N, Mojoli F, Chiumello D, Piquilloud L, Grasso S, Jubran A, Laghi F, Magder S, Pesenti A, Loring S, Gattinoni L, Talmor D, Blanch L, Amato M, Chen L, Brochard L, Mancebo J. Esophageal and transpulmonary pressure in the clinical setting: meaning, usefulness and perspectives. Intensive Care Med 2016. doi:10.1007/s00134-016-4400-x.
40. Georgopoulos D. Effects of mechanical ventilation on control of breathing. In: Tobin M, editor. Principles and practice of mechanical ventilation. New York: McGraw-Hill; 2013. p. 805–20.
41. Murias G, Lucangelo U, Blanch L. Patient-ventilator asynchrony. Curr Opin Crit Care. 2016;22:53–9.

16

Increase in intra-abdominal pressure during airway suctioning-induced cough after a successful spontaneous breathing trial is associated with extubation outcome

Yasuhiro Norisue[1,2,4*], Jun Kataoka[1], Yosuke Homma[1], Takaki Naito[2], Junpei Tsukuda[2], Kentaro Okamoto[2], Takeshi Kawaguchi[2], Lonny Ashworth[3], Shimada Yumiko[1], Yuiko Hoshina[1], Eiji Hiraoka[1] and Shigeki Fujitani[2]

Abstract

Background: A patient's ability to clear secretions and protect the airway with an effective cough is an important part of the pre-extubation evaluation. An increase in intra-abdominal pressure (IAP) is important in generating the flow rate necessary for a cough. This study investigated whether an increase from baseline in IAP during a coughing episode induced by routine pre-extubation airway suctioning is associated with extubation outcome after a successful spontaneous breathing trial (SBT).

Methods: Three hundred thirty-five (335) mechanically ventilated patients who passed an SBT were enrolled. Baseline IAP and peak IAP during successive suctioning-induced coughs were measured with a fluid column connected to a Foley catheter.

Results: Extubation was unsuccessful in 24 patients (7.2%). Unsuccessful extubation was 3.40 times as likely for patients with a delta IAP (ΔIAP) of ≤ 30 cm H_2O than for those with a ΔIAP > 30 cm H_2O, after adjusting for APACHE II score (95% CI, 1.39–8.26; $p = .007$).

Conclusion: ΔIAP during a coughing episode induced by routine pre-extubation airway suctioning is significantly associated with extubation outcome in patients with a successful SBT.

Keywords: Cough, Airway suctioning, Extubation, Intra-abdominal pressure, Mechanical ventilation

Background

Although cough strength for clearing secretions is important in successful extubation, it is not routinely objectively evaluated in daily practice after a successful spontaneous breathing trial (SBT). The inability to produce an adequate cough—because of muscle weakness or pain—increases the risks of atelectasis, oxygen desaturation, re-intubation, and, possibly, pneumonia [1–3].

Cough strength, as measured by voluntary and involuntary cough peak expiratory flow (CPEF), has been proposed as an independent predictor of successful extubation [4–10]. Previous studies reported that an involuntary CPEF of < 60 L/min was significantly associated with increased risk of extubation failure [5, 9, 10]. In addition to methods that focus on CPEF, clinicians desire a procedure that would allow evaluation of involuntary cough strength among patients who are unable or unwilling to produce maximal cough effort without special devices. Ideally, this procedure would not require disconnecting the patient from the ventilator circuit during routine pre-extubation airway suctioning, as this almost always induces cough.

*Correspondence: norisue.yasuhiro@gmail.com
[4] Department of Pulmonary and Critical Care Medicine, Tokyo Bay Urayasu Ichikawa Medical Center, 3-4-32 Todaijima, Urayasu, Chiba 2790001, Japan
Full list of author information is available at the end of the article

Physiologically, a cough begins with a deep inspiratory phase, followed by an expiratory phase of bursts of intercostal and abdominal muscle contractions [11]. This results in "the compressive phase" and an abrupt rise in intrapleural and intra-abdominal pressure (IAP) [12] with the relaxed diaphragm. IAP is then transmitted into intrapleural pressure [13], which abruptly increases airway pressure and cough. The increase in intra-abdominal pressure (ΔIAP) during an episode of continuous coughing is thus positively correlated with cough strength [13–16]. Use of a Foley catheter to measure bladder pressure during cough is straightforward and can be performed in most centers. We tested the hypothesis that low ΔIAP is associated with extubation failure after a successful SBT.

Methods

Study design

This is a single-center, prospective, cohort study. The study was approved by the Institutional Review Board at Tokyo Bay Urayasu Ichikawa Medical Center (TBUIMC). A waiver of informed consent was obtained because the study exposed patients to less than minimal risk.

Patients

The study was performed in the medical–surgical ICU during the period from April 2015 through November 2015. All mechanically ventilated patients 18 years or older who had been endotracheally intubated and had passed an SBT of longer than 30 min were eligible for inclusion. The SBT was conducted on pressure support ventilation with a pressure support of 5 cm H_2O, a positive end-expiratory pressure (PEEP) of ≤ 8 cm H_2O, and a fraction of inspiratory oxygen (FiO_2) of ≤ 0.50. Patients were excluded from the study if they had "comfort care" or "do not re-intubate" status or had been previously extubated during the same hospitalization. Patients were also excluded if they had documented or suspected upper airway obstruction, end-stage renal disease requiring hemodialysis, or no Foley catheter at the time of extubation. Successful completion of an SBT was determined using the standard Tokyo Bay Urayasu Ichikawa Medical Center (TBUIMC) Respiratory Care Weaning Protocols (no evidence of severe anxiety, dyspnea, or excessive accessory muscle use; a rapid shallow breathing index [RSBI] of ≤ 105 breaths/min/L; and adequate gas exchange, i.e., $SaO_2 \geq 90\%$ with $FiO_2 \leq 0.50$ and PEEP ≤ 8 cm H_2O).

Observations and measurements

A water-column technique was used to measure IAP [17], which was determined in the ICU by resident physicians using the following protocol, after all sedatives and analgesics were discontinued for at least 60 min: (1) the drainage tube of the patient's Foley bladder catheter was clamped; (2) sterile normal saline (20 ml) was instilled into the bladder via the aspiration port of the Foley catheter with a needleless connection system; (3) a fluid column consisting of two extension tubes (length 75 cm, inner diameter 3.1 mm; Terumo, Tokyo, Japan) was constructed, connected to the aspiration port of the Foley catheter, and then placed at the level of the mid-axillary line; (4) with the patient in supine position, fluid level in the absence of cough at end expiration was marked on the extension tube and recorded as the baseline bladder pressure; (5) airway suctioning was performed by advancing the closed-system suction catheter while the patient was connected to the ventilator, which is part of the standard pre-extubation procedure; and (6) the recorder observed changes in fluid level and marked the highest fluid level on the extension tube during successive coughs, which was recorded as the highest bladder pressure. The patient was extubated within 10 min after IAP measurement. Attending physicians and fellows responsible for clinical decisions, including extubation, were blinded to the results of the IAP and ΔIAP measurements.

Definitions of extubation success and failure

Successful extubation was defined as the absence of the need for re-intubation within 72 h after extubation. Extubation failure was defined as re-intubation within 72 h after extubation. Patients were followed until hospital discharge or death. The use of prophylactic or therapeutic noninvasive positive pressure ventilation without consequent re-intubation was not considered as extubation failure.

Sample size

Because at least 10 episodes of extubation failure were required in order to conduct multiple regression analysis adjusted for APACHE II score—the most important confounding factor for extubation outcomes—the estimated minimum sample size needed for the statistical analysis was 135 with a predicted extubation failure rate of 8%, as indicated by the past extubation failure rate in this ICU [18]. With a planned study duration of 9 months, the predicted number of patients to be recruited in the study was 400, assuming an average of approximately 45 extubations per month in our ICU.

Statistical analysis

The primary outcome of this study was extubation failure. Secondary outcomes included in-hospital mortality, ICU days, and length of hospital stay. A ΔIAP cutoff value for extubation failure was estimated with receiver operator characteristic (ROC) analysis. A multivariable-adjusted logistic regression model was used to calculate the odds ratio for extubation failure based on ΔIAP adjusted for APACHE II score. Mean baseline IAP, ΔIAP, and other variables were compared in relation to extubation success and failure. The Student *t* test was used to compare the means for variables. The Fisher exact test was used to compare grouped data such as sex, Confusion Assessment Method for the Intensive Care Unit (CAM-ICU), and mortality. For measures of association, 95% confidence intervals (CI) were computed, and statistical significance was defined as a two-tailed *p* value of less than .05. Using a multivariable-adjusted logistic regression model, we estimated the odds ratio (OR) for re-intubation adjusted for APACHE II score. We also conducted a secondary analysis to investigate the relationship between ΔIAP and extubation outcomes in patients who were mechanically ventilated for longer than 72 h. All statistical analyses, except for sample size estimation, were performed with the IBM Statistical Package for the Social Sciences version 22.0 (IBM, Corp, Armonk, NY, USA).

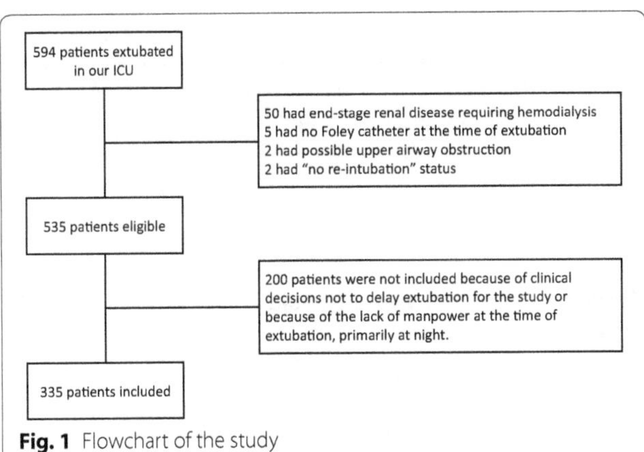

Fig. 1 Flowchart of the study

Results

Patients

A total of 335 patients were included in the analyses (Fig. 1), 24 (7.2%) of whom were re-intubated within 72 h after extubation. Tables 1 and 2 show patient baseline characteristics and indications for intubation, respectively. Univariate analysis showed that CAM-ICU, APACHE II score, Simplified Acute Physiology Score II score, intubation days, length of ICU stay, length of hospital stay, 28-day mortality, and in-hospital mortality were significantly higher, and P/F ratio was significantly lower, in the extubation failure group than in the extubation success group. Figures 2 and 3 show the distributions of baseline IAP and ΔIAP for the patients. The median (interquartile range) baseline IAP was 8 (4–11) cm H_2O, and the median (interquartile range) ΔIAP was 38 (23–55) cm H_2O (range, 0–120 cm H_2O).

Table 1 Baseline characteristics of patients in each group

Characteristics	Extubation success	Extubation failure	*p* value
Number of patients, *n*	311	24	
Male sex, *n* (%)	193 (62.1)	17 (70.8)	0.512
Age, median (IQR)	71 (62–79)	72 (64–78)	0.581
BMI, median (IQR)	22.7 (20.3–25.2)	21.05 (17.3–24.8)	0.115
GCS, median (IQR)	11 (10–11)	11 (10–11)	0.667
CAM-ICU, positive (%)	40 (12.9)	8 (33.3)	0.012
APACHE II score, median (IQR)	20 (17–24)	24 (22–28)	< 0.001
SAPS II score, median (IQR)	41 (32–51)	51 (46–59)	< 0.001
In–out balance, median ml (IQR)	2959 (1000–5322)	2676 (793–4500)	0.701
Intubation days, median (IQR)	2 (1–3)	4 (2–6)	0.001
P/F ratio, median (IQR)	300 (250–367)	275 (218–326)	0.036
TV, median L (IQR)	0.44 (0.36–0.55)	0.47 (0.40–0.66)	0.139
MV, median L (IQR)	6.90 (5.60–8.19)	7.90 (5.76–9.75)	0.087
RSBI, median breaths/min/L (IQR)	37.2 (26.4-48.9)	38.2(16.9-51.3)	0.691
Length of ICU stay, median (IQR)	4 (2–6)	12 (6–16)	< 0.001
Length of hospital stay, median (IQR)	20 (14–36)	48 (27–55)	< 0.001
28-Day mortality, *n* (%)	3 (1.0)	3 (12.5)	0.006
In-hospital mortality, *n* (%)	10 (3.2)	5 (20.8)	0.002
Baseline IAP, mm H_20, median (IQR)	7.9 (4.0–10.0)	8.0 (5.7–13.0)	0.19
ΔIAP, mm H_2O, median (IQR)	39.0 (24.0–57.0)	25.5 (19.8–38.3)	0.012

Table 2 Indications for intubation in each group

Indications for intubation	Extubation success (*n*)	Extubation failure (*n*)	*p* value
Emergent abdominal surgery	13	1	0.22
Emergent non-abdominal surgery	48	5	
Elective abdominal surgery	10	1	
Elective non-abdominal surgery	110	3	
Altered mental status	3	0	
Acute myocardial infarction	7	1	
Congestive heart failure	19	0	
Asthma	1	0	
Pneumonia	13	1	
Sepsis	22	3	
COPD	2	1	
Drug intoxication	5	0	
Hemorrhagic stroke	9	1	
Ischemic stroke	2	0	
Gastrointestinal bleeding	4	0	
Status epilepticus	6	1	
Others	37	6	

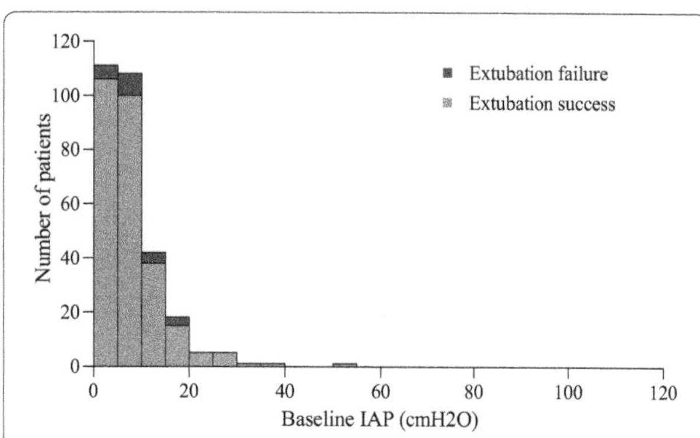

Fig. 2 Histogram showing the number of patients and baseline intra-abdominal pressure (IAP)

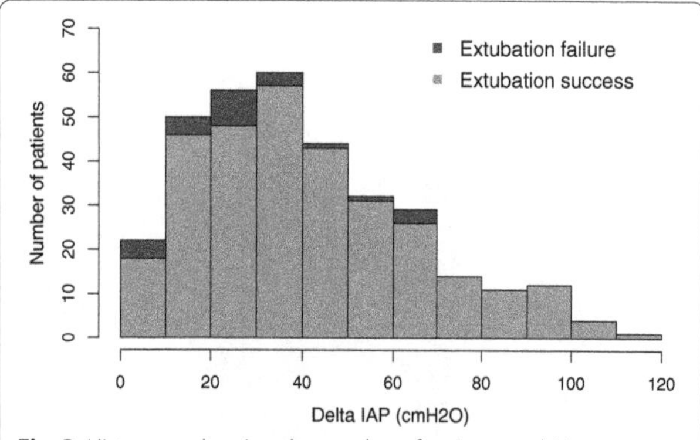

Fig. 3 Histogram showing the number of patients and Δintra-abdominal pressure (ΔIAP)

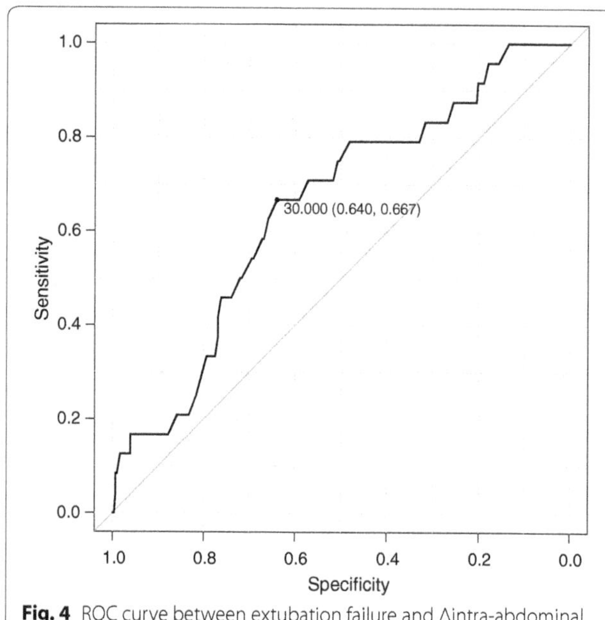

Fig. 4 ROC curve between extubation failure and Δintra-abdominal pressure (ΔIAP)

Table 3 Unadjusted and adjusted odds ratio of low ΔIAP for extubation failure

	OR	95% CI	*p* value
Unadjusted	3.56	1.47–8.55	0.005
Adjusted*	3.40	1.39–8.26	0.007

*Adjusted for APACHE II score

ΔIAP and outcome measures

ΔIAP was significantly higher in the extubation success group than in the extubation failure group ($p=0.012$; median, 39.00 vs 25.50 cm H_2O, respectively). Figure 4 shows the ROC curve between ΔIAP and extubation failure. The area under the ROC curve was 0.654 (95% CI 0.544–0.764), and the cutoff value was 30 cm H_2O (sensitivity, 64%; specificity, 67%). ΔIAP was classified as ≤ 30 cm H_2O (low ΔIAP group) or >30 cm H_2O (high ΔIAP group). Table 3 shows that low ΔIAP was significantly associated with extubation failure after adjusting for APACHE II score (adjusted OR, 3.40; 95% CI, 1.39–8.26, $p=.007$). The positive predictive value and negative predictive value of a ΔIAP value of ≤ 30 cm H_2O for extubation failure were 1.85 and 0.52, respectively.

ΔIAP and outcome measures in patients who were mechanically ventilated for longer than 72 h

A secondary analysis including only patients who were mechanically ventilated for longer than 72 h (124 patients with successful extubation and 17 patients with extubation failure) yielded an AUC of 0.708 (95% CI

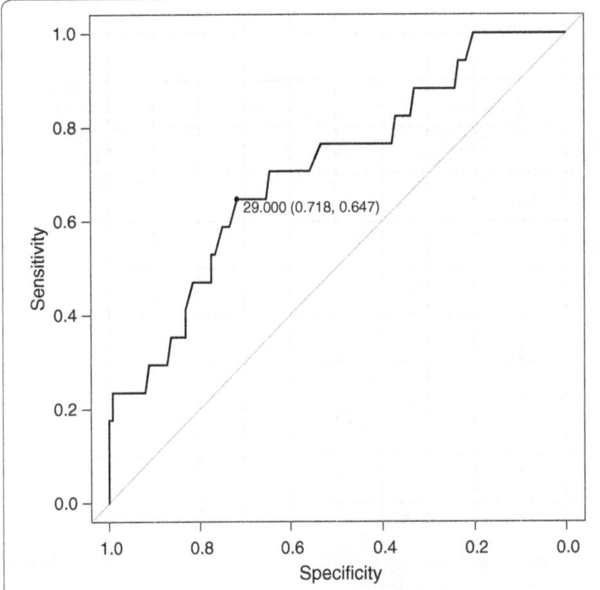

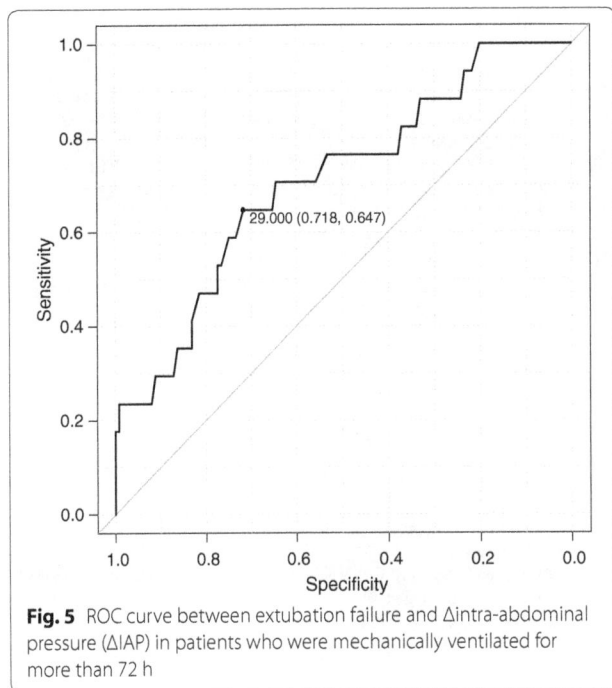

Fig. 5 ROC curve between extubation failure and Δintra-abdominal pressure (ΔIAP) in patients who were mechanically ventilated for more than 72 h

Table 4 Unadjusted and adjusted odds ratio of low ΔIAP for extubation failure in patients were mechanically ventilated for more than 72 h

	OR	95% CI	*p* value
Unadjusted	3.93	1.39–11.20	0.01
Adjusted*	3.79	1.32–10.75	0.01

*Adjusted for APACHE II score

0.571–0.845) with a cutoff value of 29 cm H_2O (Fig. 5). Multiple regression analysis (Table 4) showed that a low ΔIAP (≤29 cm H_2O) was significantly associated with extubation failure, after adjusting for APACHE II score (adjusted OR, 3.79; 95% CI, 1.32–10.75, $p=0.01$). The positive predictive value and negative predictive value of a ΔIAP value of ≤29 cm H_2O for extubation failure were 2.21 and 0.56, respectively.

Discussion

This study showed that diminished ΔIAP during coughing induced by routine pre-extubation suctioning was significantly associated with extubation failure. Expiratory muscle strength is important in producing a successful cough [19]. However, CPEF is the only widely accepted method of evaluating pre-extubation expiratory muscle strength during cough production. Smina et al. [5] reported that a CPEF ≤60 L/min yielded an AUC of 0.7 (sensitivity 69%; specificity 74%) in predicting extubation failure. Our ΔIAP data indicated similar predictive values, especially in patients mechanically ventilated for longer than 72 h. These findings suggest that ΔIAP is a potentially useful parameter for assessing expiratory muscle strength.

The cough reflex protects the airway by means of a continuous series of expiratory coughs with subsequent inspiratory efforts [20–22]. The continuous increase in IAP during such an episode provides sustained expiratory force [14]. The present results are consistent with these physiological characteristics of the cough reflex and support the hypothesis that an inability to increase IAP predicts extubation failure. Moreover, our secondary analysis of patients intubated for longer than 72 h yielded a better AUC in predicting extubation failure. The present results are attributable to the significant association between duration of mechanical ventilation and ICU-acquired weakness (ICUAW) [23]; thus, our method might be more relevant and useful for patients at high risk of ICUAW, including expiratory muscle weakness.

The proposed method of estimating cough strength has several practical strengths. Most mechanically ventilated patients already have a Foley catheter, and IAP measurement is feasible in most ICUs. Second, airway suctioning is part of the pre-extubation process; therefore, ΔIAP measurement can be included in routine pre-extubation evaluation. Finally, cough strength induced by airway suctioning does not depend on patient effort and is thus feasible for most mechanically ventilated patients, including those who are uncooperative because of dementia, delirium, or altered mental status.

Future studies should investigate how to apply ΔIAP to clinical decision making. For example, a patient who has passed an SBT but has a low ΔIAP may need appropriate preparation for possible re-intubation. Unlike the present patients with a low ΔIAP, none of those with a ΔIAP > 70 cm H_2O had extubation failure (Fig. 3). Thus, a ΔIAP > 70 cm H_2O may be potentially used to exclude the possibility of extubation failure in patients with a successful SBT and no airway obstruction.

This study has limitations that warrant mention. ΔIAP was measured with a fluid column rather than by connecting the Foley catheter to a digital pressure transducer. Because of resistance in the extension tube, the fluid level might not have reached the true maximum pressure level during a coughing episode. Moreover, the accuracy of visual IAP measurement has not been validated and may not be accurate. The present cutoff value might therefore be more accurately regarded as a cutoff value for the fluid column method than as the true ΔIAP cutoff value.

Conclusion

In conclusion, ΔIAP during a coughing episode induced by routine pre-extubation airway suctioning is significantly associated with extubation outcome in patients with a successful SBT.

Abbreviations

APACHE: Acute Physiology and Chronic Health Evaluation; CAM-ICU: Confusion Assessment Method for the Intensive Care Unit; CI: confidence interval; ESRD: end-stage renal disease; FiO2: fraction of inspired oxygen; GCS: Glasgow Coma Scale; IAP: intra-abdominal pressure; ICU: intensive care unit; OR: odds ratio; PEEP: positive end-expiratory pressure; PEF: peak expiratory flow; ROC: receiver operator characteristic; RSBI: rapid shallow breathing index; SBT: spontaneous breathing trial; SAPS: Simplified Acute Physiology Score; TBUIMC: Tokyo Bay Urayasu Ichikawa Medical Center.

Author contributions

YN is the guarantor of the content of the manuscript, including the data and analysis. YN had full access to all study data and takes responsibility for the integrity of the data and the accuracy of the data analysis. YN, TN, JT, KO, TK, EH, and SF substantially contributed to the study design, YH, YH, YS, LA, and JT contributed to data interpretation and drafting of the manuscript. YH, JK, and YH analyzed the data.

Author details

[1] Department of Emergency and Critical Care Medicine, Tokyo Bay Urayasu Ichikawa Medical Center, 3-4-32 Todaijima, Urayasu, Chiba 2790001, Japan. [2] Department of Emergency and Critical Care Medicine, St. Marianna University Hospital, 2-16-1 Sugao, Kawasaki, Kanagawa 2168511, Japan. [3] Department of Respiratory Care, Boise State University, 1910 W University Drive, Boise, ID 83725, USA. [4] Department of Pulmonary and Critical Care Medicine, Tokyo Bay Urayasu Ichikawa Medical Center, 3-4-32 Todaijima, Urayasu, Chiba 2790001, Japan.

Acknowledgements

We thank Professor Daniel Talmor for his valuable advice on this study and for reviewing the manuscript.

Competing interests

The authors declare that they have no competing interests.

References

1. Wang ZY, Bai Y. Cough-another important factor in extubation readiness in critically ill patients. Crit Care. 2012;16(6):461.
2. Jiang C, Esquinas A, Mina B. Evaluation of cough peak expiratory flow as a predictor of successful mechanical ventilation discontinuation: a narrative review of the literature. J Intensive Care. 2017;5:33.
3. Krinsley JS, Reddy PK, Iqbal A. What is the optimal rate of failed extubation? Crit Care. 2012;16(1):111.
4. Khamiees M, Raju P, DeGirolamo A, Amoateng-Adjepong Y, Manthous CA. Predictors of extubation outcome in patients who have successfully completed a spontaneous breathing trial. Chest. 2001;120(4):1262–70.
5. Smina M, Salam A, Khamiees M, Gada P, Amoateng-Adjepong Y, Manthous CA. Cough peak flows and extubation outcomes. Chest. 2003;124(1):262–8.
6. Duan J, Liu J, Xiao M, Yang X, Wu J, Zhou L. Voluntary is better than involuntary cough peak flow for predicting re-intubation after scheduled extubation in cooperative subjects. Respir Care. 2014;59(11):1643–51.
7. Bai L, Duan J. Use of cough peak flow measured by a ventilator to predict re-intubation when a spirometer is unavailable. Respir Care. 2017;62(5):566–71.
8. Beuret P, Roux C, Auclair A, Nourdine K, Kaaki M, Carton MJ. Interest of an objective evaluation of cough during weaning from mechanical ventilation. Intensive Care Med. 2009;35(6):1090–3.
9. Salam A, Tilluckdharry L, Amoateng-Adjepong Y, Manthous CA. Neurologic status, cough, secretions and extubation outcomes. Intensive Care Med. 2004;30(7):1334–9.
10. Su WL, Chen YH, Chen CW, Yang SH, Su CL, Perng WC, Wu CP, Chen JH. Involuntary cough strength and extubation outcomes for patients in an ICU. Chest. 2010;137(4):777–82.
11. Grelot L, Milano S. Diaphragmatic and abdominal muscle activity during coughing in the decerebrate cat. NeuroReport. 1991;2(4):165–8.
12. McCool FD. Global physiology and pathophysiology of cough: ACCP evidence-based clinical practice guidelines. Chest. 2006;129(1 Suppl):48S–53S.
13. Irwin RS, Rosen MJ, Braman SS. Cough. A comprehensive review. Arch Intern Med. 1977;137(9):1186–91.
14. Addington WR, Stephens RE, Phelipa MM, Widdicombe JG, Ockey RR. Intra-abdominal pressures during voluntary and reflex cough. Cough. 2008;4:2.
15. Luginbuehl H, Baeyens JP, Kuhn A, Christen R, Oberli B, Eichelberger P, Radlinger L. Pelvic floor muscle reflex activity during coughing—an exploratory and reliability study. Ann Phys Rehabil Med. 2016;59(5–6):302–7.
16. Stephens RE, Addington WR, Miller SP, Anderson JW. Videofluoroscopy of the diaphragm during voluntary and reflex cough in humans. Am J Phys Med Rehabil. 2003;82(5):384.
17. Malbrain ML, Cheatham ML, Kirkpatrick A, Sugrue M, Parr M, De Waele J, Balogh Z, Leppaniemi A, Olvera C, Ivatury R, et al. Results from the international conference of experts on intra-abdominal hypertension and abdominal compartment syndrome. I. Definitions. Intensive Care Med. 2006;32(11):1722–32.
18. Peduzzi P, Concato J, Kemper E, Holford TR, Feinstein AR. A simulation study of the number of events per variable in logistic regression analysis. J Clin Epidemiol. 1996;49(12):1373–9.
19. Epstein SK. Decision to extubate. Intensive Care Med. 2002;28(5):535–46.
20. Korpáš J. Tomori Zn: cough and other respiratory reflexes. Basel: S. Karger; 1979.
21. Tatar M, Hanacek J, Widdicombe J. The expiration reflex from the trachea and bronchi. Eur Respir J. 2008;31(2):385–90.
22. Widdicombe J, Fontana G. Cough: what's in a name? Eur Respir J. 2006;28(1):10–5.
23. Hermans G, Van den Berghe G. Clinical review: intensive care unit acquired weakness. Crit Care. 2015;19:274.

17

Severe atypical pneumonia in critically ill patients

S. Valade[1,2*], L. Biard[2,3], V. Lemiale[1,2], L. Argaud[4], F. Pène[5], L. Papazian[6], F. Bruneel[7], A. Seguin[8], A. Kouatchet[9], J. Oziel[10], S. Rouleau[11], N. Bele[12], K. Razazi[13], O. Lesieur[14], F. Boissier[15], B. Megarbane[16], N. Bigé[17], N. Brulé[18], A. S. Moreau[19], A. Lautrette[20], O. Peyrony[21], P. Perez[22], J. Mayaux[23] and E. Azoulay[1,2]

Abstract

Background: *Chlamydophila pneumoniae* (CP) and *Mycoplasma pneumoniae* (MP) patients could require intensive care unit (ICU) admission for acute respiratory failure.

Methods: Adults admitted between 2000 and 2015 to 20 French ICUs with proven atypical pneumonia were retrospectively described. Patients with MP were compared to *Streptococcus pneumoniae* (SP) pneumonia patients admitted to ICUs.

Results: A total of 104 patients were included, 71 men and 33 women, with a median age of 56 [44–67] years. MP was the causative agent for 76 (73%) patients and CP for 28 (27%) patients. Co-infection was documented for 18 patients (viruses for 8 [47%] patients). Median number of involved quadrants on chest X-ray was 2 [1–4], with alveolar opacities ($n=61$, 75%), interstitial opacities ($n=32$, 40%). Extra-pulmonary manifestations were present in 34 (33%) patients. Mechanical ventilation was required for 75 (72%) patients and vasopressors for 41 (39%) patients. ICU length of stay was 16.5 [9.5–30.5] days, and 11 (11%) patients died in the ICU. Compared with SP patients, MP patients had more extensive interstitial pneumonia, fewer pleural effusion, and a lower mortality rate [6 (8%) vs. 17 (22%), $p=0.013$]. According MCA analysis, some characteristics at admission could discriminate MP and SP. MP was more often associated with hemolytic anemia, abdominal manifestations, and extensive chest radiograph abnormalities. SP-P was associated with shock, confusion, focal crackles, and focal consolidation.

Conclusion: In this descriptive study of atypical bacterial pneumonia requiring ICU admission, mortality was 11%. The comparison with SP pneumonia identified clinical, laboratory, and radiographic features that may suggest MP or CP pneumonia.

Keywords: Pneumonia, Outcome, ICU, *Mycoplasma pneumoniae*, *Chlamydophila pneumoniae*

Background

Severe pneumonia remains the major reasons for admission to the intensive care unit (ICU), mainly related to *Streptococcus pneumoniae* (SP). Atypical pneumonia (AP) related, for instance, to *Chlamydophila pneumoniae* (CP) and *Mycoplasma pneumoniae* (MP) accounts for 1–30% of documented pneumonia in patients admitted to ICU [1–11]. Although AP is rarely severe, some patients with community-acquired AP require ICU admission. Several retrospective studies reported ICU admission for 2–16.3% of patients with AP [1–3, 8, 11–15]. In one study, even 38.8% of patients with AP, older than 65 years, were admitted to ICU [12]. Among ICU-admitted patients with AP, 0.3–11% required mechanical ventilation [4, 5], with acute respiratory distress syndrome (ARDS) for few patients [15, 16]. In previous studies, mortality rates were low, around 3% [5, 13, 14, 17], although a recent retrospective study found 29.4% mortality [12] in a population with high rates of co-infection and cardiac complications.

*Correspondence: sandrine.valade@aphp.fr
[1] AP-HP, Medical ICU, Hôpital Saint-Louis, 1 Avenue Claude Vellefaux, 75010 Paris, France
Full list of author information is available at the end of the article

In previous non-ICU studies, compared to bacterial pneumonia, AP was associated with younger age and fewer comorbidities, a lower risk of severe respiratory failure, and better outcome [4, 6, 13, 14, 18]. For patients admitted to ICU, studies remained rare.

The main objective of the study was to describe AP in patients admitted to ICU. Our secondary objective was to compare the diagnostic strategy and outcomes between *Mycoplasma pneumoniae*-related pneumonia (MP) and *Streptococcus pneumoniae*-related pneumonia (SP) admitted to ICU.

Methods

Patients with atypical pneumonia (AP)

This is a retrospective chart review of adults admitted to 20 ICUs in France with a diagnosis of AP over the 16-year period from 2000 to 2015 (Additional file 1: Figure S1). Inclusion criteria were pneumonia defined with sepsis and a new pulmonary infiltrate on the chest radiograph and either a positive specific polymerase chain reaction (PCR) test for MP or CP on respiratory specimens (noninvasive samples or bronchoalveolar lavage) or blood serologic tests suggesting acute MP or CP infection (elevated specific IgM or fourfold increase in IgG level between two time points or elevated anti-MP IgG combined with presence of cold agglutinins) [19].

This study was approved by a local ethic committee (Société de Réanimation de Langue Française, CE SRLF 18-01).

Data collection

Clinical and laboratory data at ICU admission were collected, as well as organ failure during ICU stay. The SAPS II score [20] was used to assess severity at ICU admission. We also collected extra-pulmonary symptoms; arthritis was defined as new inflammation with one or more joints, myocarditis with cardiac dysfunction and troponin elevation and cutaneous involvement with the onset of skin rash. Bacterial and/or viral co-infections at diagnosis were recorded.

Patients with *Streptococcus pneumoniae* pneumonia (SP-P)

Patients with MP-AP were compared to a group of consecutive patients with proven SP-P admitted to one of the study ICUs (Saint Louis Hospital, Paris) during the same period. SP-P was diagnosed based on sepsis with a new pulmonary infiltrate and identification of SP in at least one microbiological specimen (blood culture, respiratory specimen, or urinary antigen with no alternative diagnosis).

Statistical analysis

Categorical variables were described as *n* (%) and quantitative variables as median [25th–75th percentiles]. We first described the features in the patients with AP at ICU admission. Then, we conducted univariate analyses with a nonparametric test to compare the groups with MP-AP and SP-P. Finally, multiple correspondence analysis (MCA) was performed to identify the dimensions associated with the parameters at ICU admission (HIV, symptom duration, shock, confusion, diarrhea, physical chest findings, chest radiograph abnormalities, bilirubin level, and hemolytic anemia) and the causative organism, using the FactoMineR library in the R software platform. MCA is an extension of simple correspondence analysis designed to analyze relations among categorical variables. The aim is to redefine the principal dimensions or axes of the space in a way that captures the highest possible percentage of the inertia (which can be likened to the explained variance).

All tests were two-tailed. p values < 0.05 were considered significant. All statistical analyses were carried out using the R 2.13.1 statistical platform (http://www.R-project.org).

Results

Clinical findings in the patients with atypical pneumonia (AP)

We included 104 patients, 71 men and 33 women, with a median age of 56 [44–67] years (Additional file 2: Table S2). Acute respiratory failure was the main reason for ICU admission ($n=96$; 92%); other reasons were cardiovascular failure ($n=2$), neurological disorders ($n=3$), and miscellaneous reasons ($n=3$).

AP was more common in the fall and winter (Fig. 1). Furthermore, AP became more common over time, suggesting improved diagnosis after the introduction of PCR testing.

Table 1 and Additional file 3: Table S1 report the main features of the patients with AP. The most common comorbidity was chronic respiratory disease, which was present in 32 (31%) patients including 9 patients with chronic obstructive lung disease, 4 patients with asthma, and 4 patients with interstitial lung disease; of these 32 patients, 7 patients were on long-term oxygen therapy before ICU admission. Immunosuppression was noted in 21 patients including 10 (48%) with hematological malignancies (lymphoma, $n=6$), 7 with solid cancer, and 2 with HIV infection. Delay from respiratory symptoms onset to ICU admission was 5 [3–8] days. A fever defined with a body temperature above 38.5 °C was present in 77 patients (74%). At ICU admission, all patients were tachypneic (respiratory rate, 32 [26–37]/min) and

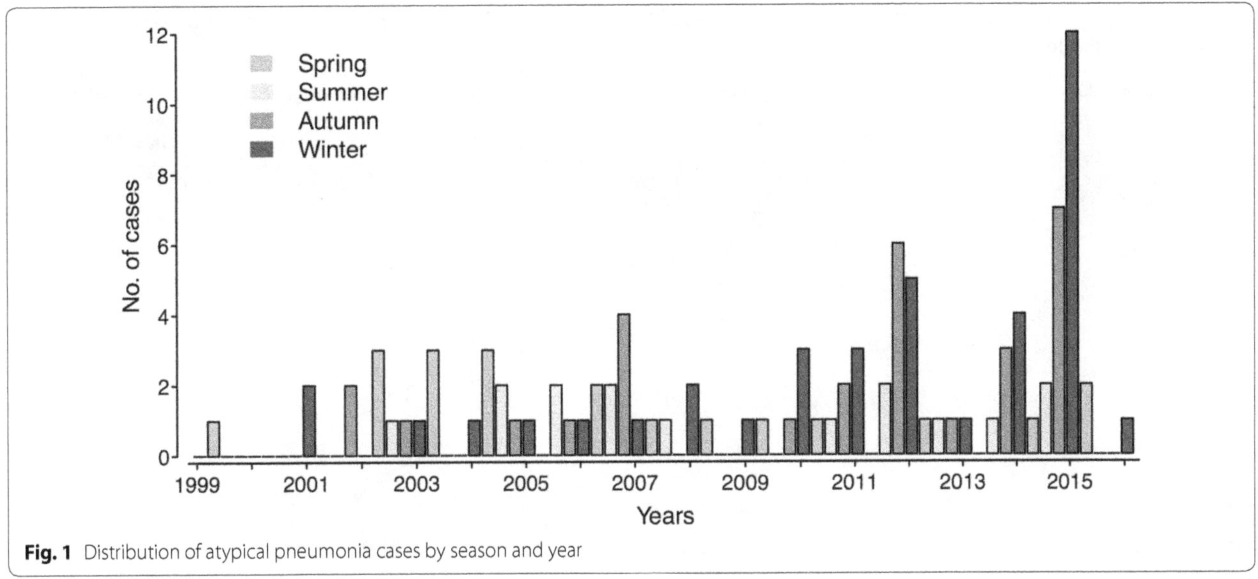

Fig. 1 Distribution of atypical pneumonia cases by season and year

48 (46%) had severe respiratory symptoms. Physical chest examination included crackles ($n=54$; 52%), rhonchi ($n=15$; 14%), wheezing ($n=12$; 11%), and signs of consolidation ($n=7$; 7%). No squeaks were reported. Extra-pulmonary symptoms concerned 34 (33%) patients and included arthritis ($n=2$), myocarditis ($n=4$), and skin rash ($n=6$). Almost one-third of the patients ($n=32$; 31%) had neurological symptoms at ICU admission, mostly with an altered level of consciousness related to severity of sepsis or to hypoxemia. Confusion was the main symptom for 3 (3%) patients, and meningo-encephalitis was diagnosed in 1 patient. Cold agglutinins assessed in case of hemolytic anemia were positive in 9 (9%) MP patients, cytolysis occurred in 11 (10%) patients, and rhabdomyolysis was present in 3 (3%) patients. At ICU admission, 10 (10%) patients had shock, the SOFA score was 5 [2–7], and the SAPS II was 33 [25–44].

Other findings in patients with atypical pneumonia (AP)

The most common findings by chest radiography were alveolar opacities ($n=61$, 59%), and interstitial opacities ($n=32$, 31%) in 2 [1–4] quadrants. Pleural effusion was rare ($n=6$, 6%).

The causative organism was MP in 76 (73%) patients and CP in 28 (27%) patients and was identified by serological testing (positive IgM or elevated IgG) in 71 patients, positive PCR on respiratory samples in 33 patients (18 on bronchoalveolar lavage, 10 on naso-pharyngeal aspirate, 2 on tracheal aspirate and 4 on nasal swab) and by both diagnostic methods in 5 patients. None of the collected variables differed between patients diagnosed with PCR, serology or both (Additional file 4: Table S3). Co-infection was found in 18 (20%) patients and was related to viruses ($n=9$; influenza, rhinovirus, respiratory syncytial virus, coronavirus) or bacteria ($n=6$; *Haemophilus influenzae, Proteus mirabilis, Staphylococcus aureus, Serratia marcescens*) or *Pneumocystis jirovecii* ($n=3$). None of MP patients had co-infection with CP or SP.

ICU management of atypical pneumonia (AP)

Mechanical ventilation was required for 75 (72%) patients and lasted 13 [8–19] days. Of the 34 (45%) patients meeting criteria for ARDS, 4 required extracorporeal membrane oxygenation. Vasoactive agents were required for 41 (39%) patients, and renal replacement therapy was started for 10 (10%) patients.

The first-line antibiotics were active on MP and CP in 62 (60%) patients. Time from ICU admission to antibiotic initiation was 1 [0–4] day. Combination therapy was used in 61 (59%) patients and consisted to a third-generation cephalosporin (C3G) and a macrolide in 24 (39%) patients, a C3G and a quinolone in 13 (21%) patients, another betalactam and a macrolide in 16 (26%) patients, another betalactam and a quinolone in 6 (9%) patients, or another antibiotic and a macrolide in 2 (3%) patients. Antibiotics was adapted according to microbiology results with a macrolide ($n=72$), a quinolone ($n=24$) or a cycline ($n=3$).

Outcomes of atypical pneumonia (AP)

Eleven (11%) patients died in the ICU. ICU stay length was 16.5 [9.5–30.5] days. Persistent hypoxemia was present at ICU discharge in 60 (58%) patients. By univariate analysis, factors associated with mortality were age ≥ 65 years ($p=0.033$), signs of respiratory distress ($p=0.017$), and interstitial opacities on the chest

Table 1 Clinical characteristics of patients with atypical pneumonia at ICU admission and outcome according to the causative agent

N (%) or median [IQR]	Total (*N* = 104)	*Mycoplasma pneumoniae* (*N* = 76)	*Chlamydophila pneumoniae* (*N* = 28)
Demographics			
Age	56 [44–67]	54 [41–69]	64 [52–75]
Female gender	33 (32%)	26 (34%)	7 (25%)
Comorbidities			
Chronic respiratory disease	32 (31%)	22 (29%)	10 (36%)
Current smoker	30 (29%)	20 (38%)	10 (36%)
Immunosuppression	21 (20%)	17 (22%)	4 (14%)
HIV infection	2 (2%)	2 (3%)	0
Hematological malignancy	10 (10%)	9 (12%)	1 (3.5%)
Cancer	7 (7%)	4 (5%)	3 (11%)
Hypertension	32 (31%)	24 (32%)	8 (28%)
Reason for ICU admission			
Acute respiratory distress	96 (92%)	70 (92%)	26 (93%)
Cardiovascular failure	2 (2%)	2 (3%)	0
Neurological disorders	3 3%)	2 (3%)	1 (3.6%)
Other	3 (3%)	2 (3%)	1 (3.6%)
Clinical respiratory findings			
Respiratory rate	32 [26–37]	33 [27–38]	30 [26–33]
Signs of respiratory failure	48 (46%)	33 (49%)	15 (54%)
Rhonchi	15 (14%)	9 (15%)	6 (21%)
Crackles	54 (52%)	36 (47%)	18 (64%)
Signs of consolidation	7 (7%)	5 (9%)	2 (7%)
Decreased vesicular breath sounds	14 (13%)	10 (17%)	4 (14%)
Clinical presentation			
Time since symptom onset (days)	5 [3–8]	6 [4–9]	4 [2–7]
Fever	77 (74%)	58 (83%)	19 (68%)
Shock	10 (10%)	6 (8%)	4 (14%)
Neurological symptoms	32 (31%)	19 (25%)	13 (46%)
Gastrointestinal symptoms	1 (1%)	1 (1%)	0
Extra-pulmonary signs			
≥ 1 extra-pulmonary symptom	34 (33%)	27 (36%)	7 (25%)
Arthritis	2 (2%)	1 (1%)	1 (3.5%)
Myocarditis	4 (4%)	4 (5%)	0
Treatments in the ICU			
Mechanical ventilation	75 (72%)	50 (66%)	25 (89%)
Duration of ventilation	13 [8–19]	12.5 [8–22.5]	13.5 [8.5–19]
Vasopressors	41 (39%)	26 (34%)	15 (54%)
Renal replacement therapy	10 (9.5%)	7 (9%)	3 (11%)
Outcomes			
Death in the ICU	11 (10%)	6 (8%)	5 (18%)
Length of ICU stay (days)			
Discharged alive	15 [8–26]	15 [8–27]	19 [12–24]
ICU death	39 [25–49]	37 [26–47]	39 [25–90]

HIV human immunodeficiency virus, *ICU* intensive care unit

radiograph ($p=0.017$). For MP patients, 26 (34%) did not receive adequate antibiotic at ICU admission. Among them 2 patients died.

Comparison to *Streptococcus pneumoniae* pneumonia (SP-P)

Tables 2 and 3 reports univariate analysis comparing patients with MP-AP and SP-P. Factors significantly associated with SP-P were HIV infection [12 (16%) vs. 2 (3%), $p=0.009$], neurological symptoms [20 (26%) vs. 1 (1%), $p<0.0001$], and gastrointestinal symptoms [15 (20%) vs. 1 (1%), $p=0.0003$]. Factors significantly associated with MP were hemolytic anemia or cold agglutinins [0 (0%) vs. 9 (12%), $p=0.003$]. Also, 6 patients with SP-P had co-infection (influenza A, $n=3$; *Haemophilus influenzae*, $n=2$; *Streptococcus constellatus*, $n=1$).

SP-P was associated with a shorter length of respiratory symptoms before ICU admission (3 days [2–7] vs. 6 days [4–9], $p=0.0008$). At ICU admission SAPS II score was higher for SP-P (42 [30–55] vs. 32 [22–41], $p=0.005$), shock was more frequent (32% vs. 8%; $p=0.0004$), creatinine level was higher (101 [69.5–168.8] μmol/L vs. 77 [57.5–108] μmol/L, $p=0.008$), and lactate level was high (2.3 [1.8–3.4] mmol/l vs. 1 [0.07–2.7] mmol/l; $p=0.003$).

Signs of consolidation and decreased breath sounds were more common in SP-P than in MP-AP (30% vs. 9% and 38% vs. 17%, respectively). MP-AP involved 4 quadrants on chest X-ray (26% vs. 8%, $p=0.013$) but less frequently pleural space (5% vs. 11%, $p=0.007$). The bilirubin level was higher in the patients with SP-P (15 [9.2–24.5] μmol/L vs. 8.4 [5.8–13] μmol/L, $p=0.0006$). MP-AP was associated with the use of mechanical ventilation (66% vs. 50%, $p=0.049$). ICU length of stay (LOS) seemed prolonged in case of MP-AP regardless of the ICU outcome (median LOS 37 vs. 5 days and 15 vs. 5 days, respectively, in patients who died in the ICU and in patients who were discharged alive). However, 28-day mortality was lower in the MP-AP group (5% vs. 20%, $p=0.005$).

Figure 2 shows the MCA results for the clinical and radiological characteristics at admission. Several characteristics discriminated between MP and CP. MP was more often associated with hemolytic anemia, abdominal manifestations and extensive chest radiograph abnormalities. SP-P was associated with shock, confusion, focal crackles, and focal consolidation.

Discussion

This multicenter study is the largest one analyzing 104 AP patients admitted to ICU. Extra-pulmonary symptoms were seen for one-third of patients, corresponding to data on previous study for patients not admitted to ICU [21]. However, AP in non-ICU patients was described as mild [6], whereas a substantial proportion of our patients had severe acute pneumonia, with shock at ICU admission for 10% of patients and mechanical ventilation required for 72% of patients including 45% of patients with ARDS.

In previous studies, patients with MP-AP were younger and had fewer comorbidities, lower respiratory disease severity and better outcomes [4, 6, 13, 14, 18]. In our study, with ICU patients, age was similar for patients with MP-AP and SP-P.

Previous studies also compared clinical and radiological features according to the causative organism of pneumonia [8, 15, 18]. In a Japanese cohort, among patients with pneumonia and audible crackles, these were more often heard only in late inspiration in patients with AP and throughout inspiration in patients with other bacteria [22]. In our study, patients with MP-AP had no specific clinical findings, except signs of consolidation which were associated with SP-P. On radiological findings, compared to SP-P, MP-AP was more often responsible for ground-glass opacification, centrilobular nodules, bronchial wall thickening, and diffuse radiological abnormalities [1, 15, 18]. In our study, extensive interstitial pneumonia was more common in MP-AP than in SP-P.

The Japanese Respiratory Society published guidelines for identifying MP-AP [17] and established a scoring system based on six parameters: age < 60 years, minor or no comorbidities, stubborn cough, abnormal chest auscultation, the absence of sputum and of an etiological agent identifiable by rapid diagnostic testing, and peripheral white blood cell count < 10,000/μL. A score ≥ 4 indicates a high probability of MP-AP (sensitivity, 88.7%; and specificity, 77.5%). Another scoring system performed well in separating patients with pneumonia into three groups: pyogenic bacteria; MP, CP, or virus; and unknown agent [23]. Nevertheless, neither scoring system had been assessed in ICU patients. In our study, MCA provided insights into differences between MP-AP and SP-P. Hemolytic anemia, diffuse chest radiograph abnormalities, and interstitial opacities were associated with MP-AP. On the contrary, HIV infection, shock, neurological symptoms, gastrointestinal symptoms, signs of consolidation, shorter symptom duration, higher bilirubin level, and radiological alveolar opacities were strongly linked to SP-P.

Compared to patients with SP-P, those with MP-AP more often required mechanical ventilation and spent more time in the ICU yet had a lower risk of death. This lower mortality may be ascribable to the smaller number of MP-AP patients with extra-pulmonary organ failure (shock, neurological manifestations, acute renal failure) and to the lower SAPS II severity score in the MP-AP group (32 [22–41] vs. 42 [30–55], $p=0.005$).

Table 2 Univariate analysis comparing clinical characteristics and outcomes of patients with *Mycoplasma pneumoniae* versus *Streptococcus pneumoniae* pneumonia

N (%) or median (IQR)	Total (*N* = 152)	*Mycoplasma pneumoniae* (*N* = 76)	*Streptococcus pneumoniae* (*N* = 76)	*p* value
Demographics				
Age	55 [43–69]	54 [41–69]	57 [44–73]	0.058
Female gender	51 (34%)	26 (34%)	25 (33%)	1
Comorbidities				
Chronic respiratory disease	36 (24%)	22 (29%)	14 (18%)	0.18
Current smoker	49 (41%)	20 (38%)	29 (43%)	
Immunosuppression	44 (29%)	17 (22%)	27 (36%)	0.11
HIV infection	14 (9%)	2 (3%)	12 (16%)	*0.009*
Hematological malignancy	18 (12%)	9 (12%)	9 (12%)	1
Cancer	12 (8%)	4 (5%)	8 (11%)	0.37
Hypertension	50 (33%)	24 (32%)	26 (34%)	0.86
Reason for ICU admission				
Acute respiratory distress	140 (92%)	70 (92%)	70 (92%)	0.59
Shock	6 (4%)	2 (3%)	4 (5%)	
Neurological symptoms	4 (3%)	2 (3%)	2 (3%)	
Other	2 (1%)	2 (3%)	0	
Clinical respiratory findings				
Respiratory rate	31 [26–38]	33 [27–38]	30 [26–36]	0.43
Signs of respiratory distress	67 (47%)	33 (49%)	34 (45%)	0.74
Rhonchi	21 (16%)	9 (15%)	12 (16%)	1
Crackles	79 (59%)	36 (61%)	44 (59%)	1
Signs of consolidation	27 (21%)	5 (9%)	22 (30%)	*0.008*
Decreased vesicular breath sounds	38 (28%)	10 (17%)	28 (38%)	*0.007*
Clinical presentation				
Time since symptom onset (days)	4 [2–7]	6 [4–9]	3 [2–7]	*0.0008*
Fever	112 (77%)	58 (83%)	54 (71%)	0.12
Shock	30 (20%)	6 (8%)	24 (32%)	*0.0004*
Neurological symptoms	21 (14%)	1 (1%)	20 (26%)	*< 0.0001*
Gastrointestinal symptoms	16 (11%)	1 (1%)	15 (20%)	*0.0003*
Extra-pulmonary signs				
≥ 1 extra-pulmonary sign	66 (43%)	27 (36%)	39 (51%)	0.071
Arthritis	1 (1%)	1 (1%)	0	1
Myocarditis	4 (3%)	4 (5%)	0	0.12
Treatments in the ICU				
Mechanical ventilation	88 (58%)	50 (66%)	38 (50%)	*0.049*
Duration of ventilation (days)				
Discharged alive	11 [7–19]	13 [8–23]	9 [6–16]	
ICU death	11 [3–18]	18 [17–34]	5 [2–15]	
Vasopressors	60 (39%)	26 (34%)	34 (45%)	0.26
Renal replacement therapy	17 (11%)	7 (9%)	10 (13%)	0.49
SAPS II	36 [24–47]	32 [22–41]	42 [30–55]	*0.0005*
Outcomes				
ICU stay length (days)				
Discharged alive	9 [5–19]	15 [8–27]	5 [3–10]	
ICU death	13 [4–27]	37 [26–47]	5 [3–14]	
28-day mortality	23 (15%)	6 (8%)	17 (22%)	*0.013*

HIV human immunodeficiency virus, *ICU* intensive care unit, *SAPS II* Simplified Acute Physiology Score version II

Table 3 Univariate analysis comparing laboratory findings in patients with *Mycoplasma pneumoniae* versus *Streptococcus pneumoniae* pneumonia

N (%) or median (IQR)	Total (*N* = 152)	*Mycoplasma pneumoniae* patients (*N* = 76)	*Streptococcus pneumoniae* patients (*N* = 76)	p value
Laboratory features				
Lactate (mmol/l)	2.2 [1.6–3.3]	1 [0.7–2.7]	2.3 [1.8–3.4]	0.003
P/F ratio	163 [92–267]	120 [88–236]	178 [114–280]	0.051
Serum sodium (mmol/L)	136 [133–139]	137 [135–140]	136 [132–139]	*0.028*
Creatinine (µmol/L)	87 [65–139.5]	77 [57.5–108]	101 [69.5–168.8]	*0.008*
CPK (IU/l)	122 [40–309]	138 [89–608]	108 [36–202]	0.093
ASAT (IU/l)	38 [23–80]	44 [24–81]	38 [22–77]	0.45
Bilirubin (µmol/l)	12.8 [8–21.7]	8.4 [5.8–13]	15 [9.2–24.5]	*0.0006*
Leukocytes	11,400 [7200–16,300]	11,140 [8100–17,000]	11,200 [5112–16,142]	0.63
Hemoglobin (g/dL)	11.6 [10–12.9]	11.3 [9.6–13.1]	11.6 [10.2–12.8]	0.89
Platelets (Giga/L)	217 [138–287]	262.5 [179.5–311.25]	204 [138–252]	*0.009*
Cytolysis	21 (14%)	8 (11%)	13 (17%)	0.35
Hemolytic anemia/cold agglutinins	9 (6%)	9 (12%)	0	*0.003*
Rhabdomyolysis	5 (3%)	2 (3%)	3 (4%)	1
Radiological features				
Number of quadrants involved				*0.013*
≤2	103 (68%)	37 (49%)	66 (87%)	
>2	25 (16%)	16 (21%)	9 (12%)	
Alveolar opacities	111 (85%)	42 (75%)	19 (68%)	*0.013*
Interstitial opacities	26 (20%)	20 (36%)	12 (43%)	*0.0001*
Pleural effusion	20 (15%)	3 (5%)	3 (11%)	*0.007*

P/F ratio ratio of partial pressure of oxygen in arterial blood over fraction of inspired oxygen, *CPK* creatine phosphokinase, *ASAT* aspartate aminotransferase

Interestingly, intracellular pathogens are underdiagnosed like viruses, but under-covered despite the availability of therapeutic agents. These findings are in line with these from Menendez et al. [24] who reported a lack of antibiotic compliance in patients with CAP. Our descriptive data may be useful to help clinicians to discriminate SP-related pneumonia and MP-related pneumonia, even if a double antibiotherapy active against atypical pathogens is recommended in severe patients.

This study had several limitations. First, the study design was retrospective and patients were included within a 16-year period. ICU management may have changed over this period. ICU admissions criteria could be different according to the center and the year of admission. Atypical pneumonia remains rare, and the main objective of the study was to describe AP in the most severe patients. However, the study assessed mostly the clinical and radiological characteristics at admission which would be unlikely to change between the centers.

Secondarily, SP-P patients were included from only one single center, whereas AP patients were included from several centers. The main objective of the study was to describe patients at ICU admission. Although admission rules would be different between the centers, the clinical presentation would not be affected. Thirdly, only patients with proven AP based on positive microbiologic samples were included. Half of the patients with MP-AP had their diagnosis based on serological testing. More recently only PCR was used to diagnose *Mycoplasma pneumoniae* infection. Positivity of IgM anti-MP is considered as the gold standard, and PCR sensitivity is equal [25]. Although some of the patients had serological tests with fourfold increase in IgG level between two time points, we believe that we included only proven MP-AP patients. Although different diagnostic tests were used within the study period and among the centers, those tests were enough sensitive and specific to include real MP-AP pneumonia.

Fourth, we did not include patients with *Legionella pneumophila* pneumonia, a more frequent atypical pneumonia. Although *Legionella pneumophila* pneumonia was associated with higher risk of ICU admission comparing to MP-AP and CP-AP, our goal was to focus on AP that is usually non-severe and only occasionally leads to ICU admission. Moreover, several studies analyzed *Legionella pneumophila* pneumonia. Similarly, we did not include more rare etiology of pneumonia as Q fever.

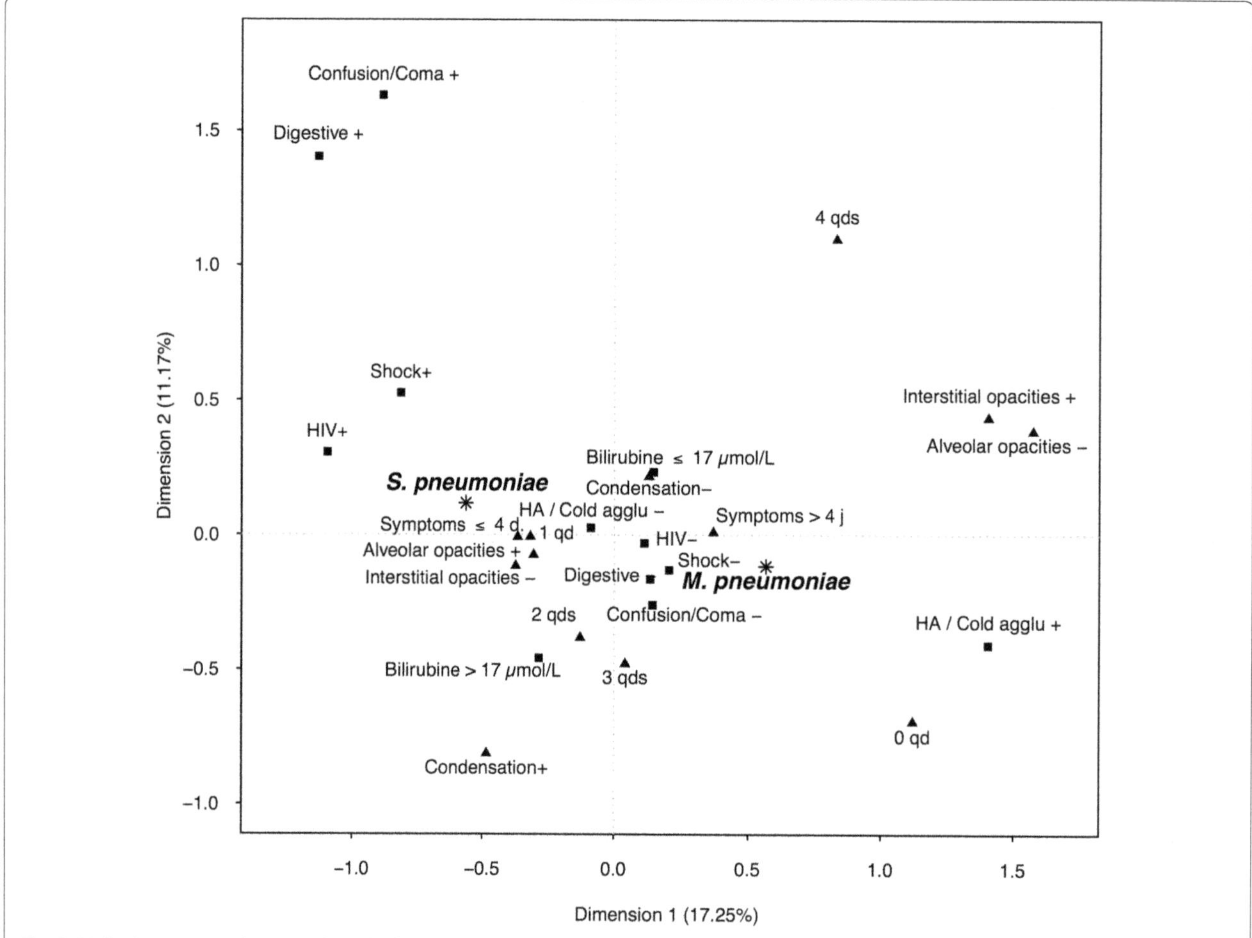

Fig. 2 Multiple correspondence analysis: the factors are mapped along two dimensions. Triangles indicate pulmonary signs and squares extra-pulmonary signs. *HA* hemolytic anemia, *Cold agglu+* presence of cold agglutinins, *QD* quadrants

Conclusion

Although considered as less severe pneumonia, atypical pneumonia requiring ICU admission remained associated with 11% mortality. At ICU admission, several clinical and radiological features could differ between MP-AP and SP-P, which may help physicians. Prospective studies are needed to validate clinical model to AP in ICU patients.

Abbreviations

AP: atypical pneumonia; ARDS: adult respiratory distress syndrome; CP: *Chlamydophila pneumoniae*; ICU: intensive care unit; MCA: multiple correspondence analysis; MP: *Mycoplasma pneumoniae*; MP-AP: atypical pneumonia due to *Mycoplasma pneumoniae*; PCR: polymerase chain reaction; SAPS II: Simplified Acute Physiology Score version II; SP: *Streptococcus pneumoniae*; SP-P: pneumonia due to *Streptococcus pneumoniae*.

Authors' contributions

EA is the guarantor for the content of the manuscript, including the data and analysis. SV, LB, VL, and EA contributed substantially to the study design, data analysis and interpretation, and the writing of the manuscript. SV, VL, LA, FP, LP, FB, AS, AK, JO, DS, NB, KR, OL, FB, BM, NB, NB, ASM, AL, OP, PP, JM, and EA contributed substantially to patients recruitment, collecting data, and manuscript revision. All authors read and approved the final manuscript.

Author details

[1] AP-HP, Medical ICU, Hôpital Saint-Louis, 1 Avenue Claude Vellefaux, 75010 Paris, France. [2] UFR de Médecine, University Paris-7 Paris-Diderot, Paris, France. [3] AP-HP, DBIM, Hôpital Saint-Louis, Paris, France. [4] Hôpital Edouard Herriot, Service de Réanimation Médicale, Hospices Civils de Lyon, Lyon, France. [5] AP-HP, Réanimation médicale, Hôpital Cochin, Paris, France. [6] Réanimation des Détresses Respiratoires et Infections Sévères, Assistance Publique-Hôpitaux de Marseille, Hôpital Nord, Marseille, France. [7] Service de Réanimation, Centre Hospitalier de Versailles, Le Chesnay, France. [8] Department of Medical Intensive Care, CHU de Caen, Caen, France. [9] Service de Réanimation Médicale et Médecine Hyperbare, Hôpital Angers, Angers, France. [10] AP-HP, Medical-Surgical Intensive Care Unit, Avicenne University Hospital, Bobigny, France. [11] Service de Réanimation polyvalente, Angoulême, France. [12] Intensive Care Unit, Draguignan Hospital, Draguignan, France. [13] AP-HP, Groupe Henri Mondor-Albert Chenevier, Service de Réanimation Médicale, Hôpital Henri Mondor, Créteil, France. [14] Service de Réanimation, CH Saint-Louis, La Rochelle, France. [15] AP-HP, Réanimation médicale, Hôpital Européen Georges Pompidou, Paris, France. [16] AP-HP, Department of Medical and Toxicological Critical Care, Lariboisière Hospital, Paris, France. [17] AP-HP, Medical Intensive Care Unit, Hôpital Saint-Antoine, Paris, France. [18] Medical Intensive Care Unit, Centre Hospitalier Universitaire de Nantes, Nantes, France. [19] Centre de réanimation, Hôpital Salengro, CHU-Lille, Lille, France. [20] Service de Réanimation Médicale Polyvalente, CHU Gabriel Montpied, Clermont-Ferrand, France. [21] AP-HP, Service des urgences, Hôpital Saint-Louis, Paris, France. [22] Service de Réanimation médicale, Hôpital Brabois, Nancy, France. [23] AP-HP, Pneumology and Critical Care Medicine Department, Universitary Hospital La Pitié Salpêtrière-Charles Foix, Paris, France.

Acknowledgements
None.

Competing interests
There is no financial or other competing interest in relation to this manuscript.

Funding
No part of the work presented has received financial support from any source.

References

1. Cillóniz C, Torres A, Niederman M, van der Eerden M, Chalmers J, Welte T, et al. Community-acquired pneumonia related to intracellular pathogens. Intensive Care Med. 2016;42(9):1374–86.
2. Ngeow Y-F, Suwanjutha S, Chantarojanasriri T, Wang F, Saniel M, Alejandria M, et al. An Asian study on the prevalence of atypical respiratory pathogens in community-acquired pneumonia. Int J Infect Dis. 2005;9(3):144–53.
3. Saraya T, Kurai D, Nakagaki K, Sasaki Y, Niwa S, Tsukagoshi H, et al. Novel aspects on the pathogenesis of *Mycoplasma pneumoniae* pneumonia and therapeutic implications. Front Microbiol. 2014 Aug 11. Cited 2015 Jun 24; 5. http://www.ncbi.nlm.nih.gov/pmc/articles/PMC4127663/.
4. von Baum H, Welte T, Marre R, Suttorp N, Lück C, Ewig S. *Mycoplasma pneumoniae* pneumonia revisited within the German Competence Network for Community-acquired pneumonia (CAPNETZ). BMC Infect Dis. 2009;9:62.
5. Marrie TJ. *Mycoplasma pneumoniae* pneumonia requiring hospitalization, with emphasis on infection in the elderly. Arch Intern Med. 1993;153(4):488–94.
6. Dumke R, Schnee C, Pletz MW, Rupp J, Jacobs E, Sachse K, et al. *Mycoplasma pneumoniae* and Chlamydia spp. infection in community-acquired pneumonia, Germany, 2011–2012. Emerg Infect Dis. 2015;21(3):426–34.
7. Spoorenberg SM, Bos WJW, Heijligenberg R, Voorn PG, Grutters JC, Rijkers GT, et al. Microbial aetiology, outcomes, and costs of hospitalisation for community-acquired pneumonia; an observational analysis. BMC Infect Dis. 2014;17(14):335.
8. Sohn JW, Park SC, Choi Y-H, Woo HJ, Cho YK, Lee JS, et al. Atypical pathogens as etiologic agents in hospitalized patients with community-acquired pneumonia in Korea: a prospective multi-center study. J Korean Med Sci. 2006;21(4):602–7.
9. Walden AP, Clarke GM, McKechnie S, Hutton P, Gordon AC, Rello J, et al. Patients with community acquired pneumonia admitted to European intensive care units: an epidemiological survey of the GenOSept cohort. Crit Care. 2014;18(2):R58.
10. Gaillat J, Flahault A, deBarbeyrac B, Orfila J, Portier H, Ducroix J-P, et al. Community epidemiology of Chlamydia and *Mycoplasma pneumoniae* in LRTI in France over 29 months. Eur J Epidemiol. 2005;20(7):643–51.
11. Sopena N, Sabrià M, Pedro-Botet ML, Manterola JM, Matas L, Domínguez J, et al. Prospective study of community-acquired pneumonia of bacterial etiology in adults. Eur J Clin Microbiol Infect Dis. 1999;18(12):852–8.
12. Khoury T, Sviri S, Rmeileh AA, Nubani A, Abutbul A, Hoss S, et al. Increased rates of intensive care unit admission in patients with *Mycoplasma pneumoniae*: a retrospective study. Clin Microbiol Infect. 2016;22(8):711–4.
13. Cillóniz C, Ewig S, Ferrer M, Polverino E, Gabarrús A, de la Bellacasa JP, et al. Community-acquired polymicrobial pneumonia in the intensive care unit: aetiology and prognosis. Crit Care. 2011;15(5):R209.
14. Lui G, Ip M, Lee N, Rainer TH, Man SY, Cockram CS, et al. Role of 'atypical pathogens' among adult hospitalized patients with community-acquired pneumonia. Respirol Carlton Vic. 2009;14(8):1098–105.
15. Miyashita N, Obase Y, Ouchi K, Kawasaki K, Kawai Y, Kobashi Y, et al. Clinical features of severe *Mycoplasma pneumoniae* pneumonia in adults admitted to an intensive care unit. J Med Microbiol. 2007;56(Pt 12):1625–9.
16. Chan ED, Welsh CH. Fulminant *Mycoplasma pneumoniae* pneumonia. West J Med. 1995;162(2):133–42.
17. Yin Y-D, Zhao F, Ren L-L, Song S-F, Liu Y-M, Zhang J-Z, et al. Evaluation of the Japanese Respiratory Society guidelines for the identification of *Mycoplasma pneumoniae* pneumonia. Respirol Carlton Vic. 2012;17(7):1131–6.
18. Guo Q, Li H-Y, Zhou Y-P, Li M, Chen X-K, Peng H-L, et al. Associations of radiological features in *Mycoplasma pneumoniae* pneumonia. Arch Med Sci AMS. 2014;10(4):725–32.
19. Daxboeck F, Krause R, Wenisch C. Laboratory diagnosis of *Mycoplasma pneumoniae* infection. Clin Microbiol Infect. 2003;9(4):263–73.
20. Le Gall JR, Lemeshow S, Saulnier F. A new Simplified Acute Physiology Score (SAPS II) based on a European/North American multicenter study. JAMA. 1993;270(24):2957–63.
21. Waites KB, Talkington DF. *Mycoplasma pneumoniae* and its role as a human pathogen. Clin Microbiol Rev. 2004;17(4):697–728.
22. Norisue Y, Tokuda Y, Koizumi M, Kishaba T, Miyagi S. Phasic characteristics of inspiratory crackles of bacterial and atypical pneumonia. Postgrad Med J. 2008;84(994):432–6.
23. Ruiz-González A, Falguera M, Vives M, Nogués A, Porcel JM, Rubio-Caballero M. Community-acquired pneumonia: development of a bedside predictive model and scoring system to identify the aetiology. Respir Med. 2000;94(5):505–10.
24. Menéndez R, Torres A, Reyes S, Zalacain R, Capelastegui A, Aspa J, et al. Initial management of pneumonia and sepsis: factors associated with improved outcome. Eur Respir J. 2012;39(1):156–62.
25. Medjo B, Atanaskovic-Markovic M, Radic S, Nikolic D, Lukac M, Djukic S. *Mycoplasma pneumoniae* as a causative agent of community-acquired pneumonia in children: clinical features and laboratory diagnosis. Ital J Pediatr. 2014;18(40):104.

Validation of a new WIND classification compared to ICC classification for weaning outcome

Byeong-Ho Jeong[1†], Kyeong Yoon Lee[2†], Jimyoung Nam[2], Myeong Gyun Ko[2], Soo Jin Na[3], Gee Young Suh[1,3] and Kyeongman Jeon[1,3*]

Abstract

Background: Although the WIND (Weaning according to a New Definition) classification based on duration of ventilation after the first separation attempt has been proposed, this new classification has not been tested in clinical practice. The objective of this cohort study was to evaluate the clinical relevance of WIND classification and its association with hospital mortality compared to the International Consensus Conference (ICC) classification.

Methods: All consecutive medical ICU patients who were mechanically ventilated for more than 24 h between July 2010 and September 2013 were prospectively registered. Patients were classified into simple, difficult, or prolonged weaning group according to ICC classification and Groups 1, 2, 3, or no weaning (NW) according to WIND classification.

Results: During the study period, a total of 1600 patients were eligible. These patients were classified by the WIND classification as follows: Group NW = 580 (36.3%), Group 1 = 617 (38.6%), Group 2 = 186 (11.6%), and Group 3 = 217 (13.6%). However, only 735 (45.9%) patients were classified by ICC classification as follows: simple weaning = 503 (68.4%), difficult weaning = 145 (19.7%), and prolonged weaning = 87 (11.8%). Clinical outcomes were significantly different across weaning groups by ICC classification and WIND classification. However, there were no statistical differences in successful weaning rate (96.6% vs. 95.2%) or hospital mortality (22.5% vs. 25.5%) between simple and difficult weaning groups by the ICC. Conversely, there were statistically significant differences in successful weaning rate (98.5% vs. 76.9%) and hospital mortality (21.2% vs. 33.9%) between Group 1 and Group 2 by WIND.

Conclusions: The WIND classification could be a better tool for predicting weaning outcomes than the ICC classification.

Keywords: Mechanical ventilation, Ventilator weaning, Treatment outcome, Classification

Introduction

Weaning from mechanical ventilation (MV) is a complex process involving daily assessment of readiness to wean and spontaneous breathing trial (SBT) to extubation [1]. The weaning process comprises at least 40% of the total duration of MV [2], and prolonged weaning is associated with higher mortality [3, 4]. A good understanding of the weaning process will reduce the duration of MV, lead to successful extubation, and eventually reduce the mortality rate and length of stay (LOS) in the intensive care unit (ICU) [1, 5].

In 2007, an International Consensus Conference (ICC) on weaning from MV proposed a classification into three different groups (simple, difficult, and prolonged weaning) according to the number, duration, and results of SBTs as well as extubation outcomes to simply classify

*Correspondence: kjeon@skku.edu
†Byeong-Ho Jeong and Kyeong Yoon Lee contributed equally to this study
[1] Division of Pulmonary and Critical Care Medicine, Department of Medicine, Samsung Medical Center, Sungkyunkwan University School of Medicine, 81 Irwon-ro, Gangnam-gu, Seoul 06351, Republic of Korea
Full list of author information is available at the end of the article

and deeply understand the weaning process [1]. However, ICC classification had some problems when applied in clinical practice: (a) it does not apply to patients without a weaning trial (unplanned extubation, death, or transfer out), (b) patients with tracheostomy tube before weaning trials are difficult to classify with ICC, and (c) ICC classification is based only on the successful results of SBT. Therefore, approximately half of mechanically ventilated patients could not be classified by the ICC classification [3, 4, 6, 7]. To overcome these limitations, the WIND (Weaning according to a New Definition) Study Group and the REVA (Réseau Européen de Recherche en Ventilation Artificielle) Network proposed a new classification using four different groups (Groups 1, 2, 3, and no weaning [NW]) [8]. However, WIND classification has not yet been fully validated and has not been sufficiently compared with ICC classification. Therefore, the objective of this cohort study was to evaluate the clinical relevance of WIND classification and its association with hospital mortality compared to ICC classification.

Methods

Study population

All consecutive patients admitted to the medical ICU and requiring MV for more than 24 h between July 2010 and September 2013 were prospectively registered at Samsung Medical Center, a 1989-bed tertiary referral hospital with tertiary-level ICU, in Seoul, South Korea [3, 9, 10]. If a patient was re-admitted to the ICU for MV support during the same hospital admission, only the first weaning episode was included in analysis. Multiple ICU visits during different hospital admissions were enrolled separately. Patients who were transferred from other hospitals after more than 48 h of intubation or were successfully treated by noninvasive ventilation (NIV) were excluded. The Institutional Review Board of Samsung Medical Center approved this study and allowed review and publication of information from patient records. Informed consent was waived because of the study's observational nature.

Standardized weaning process

Since 2010, the medical ICU of our hospital has utilized a specific protocol-based weaning program according to the recommendations by Boles et al. [1]. Details of our weaning program were described in previous reports [3, 9, 10] and an additional file provided. In short, respiratory care practitioners (RCP), who are registered nurses specializing in respiratory care, screened patients daily for weaning readiness and conducted SBTs according to the protocol. When a patient passed the SBT, extubation proceeded. If a patient failed the SBT, MV was resumed, and the team reviewed possible reversible etiologies for the failure. Again, when a patient proved ready for weaning, the SBT was repeated the following day.

Weaning classification by ICC and WIND

Patients were classified into simple, difficult, or prolonged weaning groups according to ICC classification [1] and Groups 1, 2, 3, or NW according to WIND classification [8]. The three weaning groups by ICC classification were defined as follows: simple weaning, patients who proceed from initiation of weaning to successful extubation (no need to reinstitute ventilator support within 48 h of extubation) on the first attempt without difficulty; difficult weaning, patients who failed initial weaning and required up to three SBTs or as long as 7 days from the first SBT to achieve successful extubation; or prolonged weaning, patients who required more than three SBTs or > 7 days of weaning after the first SBT. To apply the ICC classification, unclassifiable patients were excluded as follows: patients with tracheostomy prior to MV; patients who died, underwent tracheostomy, transferred out, or had unplanned extubation before weaning trial; and patients with unclassifiable weaning after SBT who died or were transferred to another hospital after failure of the first SBT and before the third SBT or 7 days (Fig. 1). The four weaning groups by WIND classification were defined as follows: Group NW, patients who never experienced any separation attempt (SA); Group 1, the first SA resulted in termination of the weaning process within 1 day (successful separation or early death); Group 2, weaning was completed after more than 1 day but in less than 1 week after the first SA (successful separation or death); and Group 3, weaning was not terminated by 7 days after the first SA (by successful separation or death). In WIND classification, SA is defined as SBT or extubation directly performed without SBT (including unplanned extubation) for intubated patients and as ≥ 24 h with spontaneous ventilation through tracheostomy without any mechanical ventilation for tracheostomized patients.

Weaning outcomes

To analyze differences in weaning outcomes among groups according to ICC and WIND classifications, clinical outcomes of MV days, ventilator-free days, tracheostomy rate, successful weaning rate, ICU mortality, LOS in ICU, hospital mortality, and LOS in hospital were investigated. Ventilator-free days were calculated as the number of days without invasive ventilation to day 28. Nonsurvivors were considered as patients with 0 ventilator-free days. Because there is no applicable definition for tracheostomized patients in ICC classification, successful weaning was defined according to WIND definitions as follows: for intubated patients,

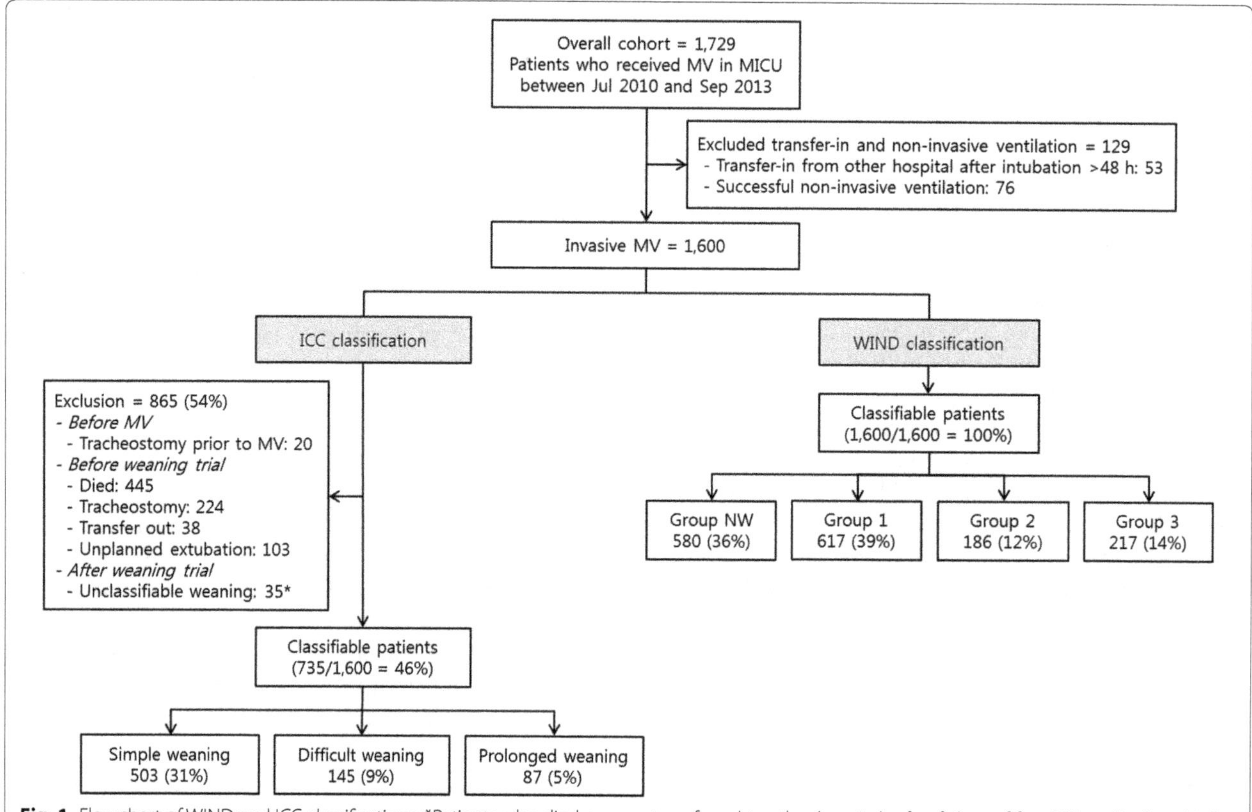

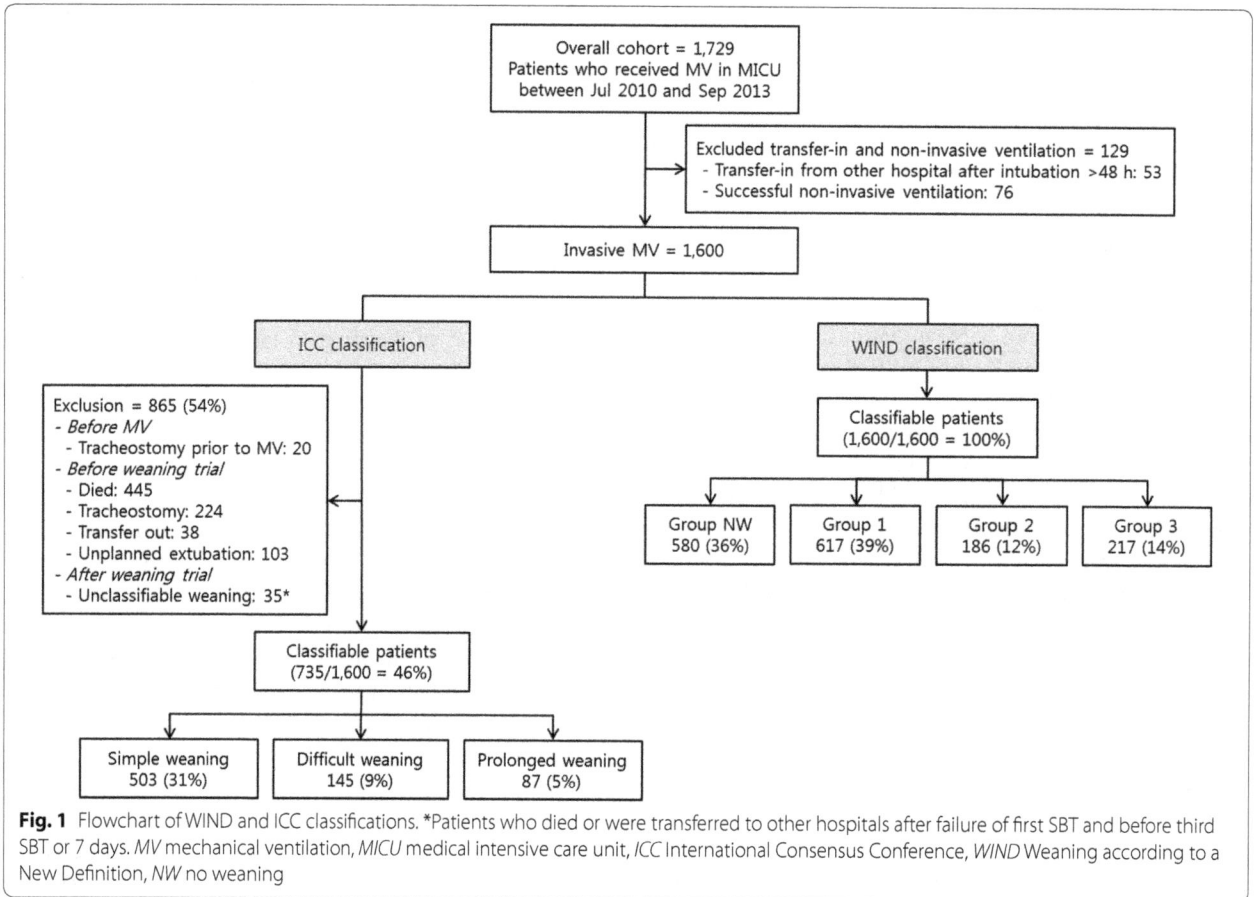

Fig. 1 Flowchart of WIND and ICC classifications. *Patients who died or were transferred to other hospitals after failure of first SBT and before third SBT or 7 days. *MV* mechanical ventilation, *MICU* medical intensive care unit, *ICC* International Consensus Conference, *WIND* Weaning according to a New Definition, *NW* no weaning

extubation without death or reintubation within the next 7 days whether postextubation NIV was used or not or ICU discharge without invasive MV within 7 days, whichever comes first; for tracheostomized patients, spontaneous ventilation through tracheostomy without any MV for 7 consecutive days or discharged with spontaneous breathing, whichever comes first. The date of successful weaning was counted to the actual day of extubation or spontaneous ventilation through tracheostomy after the patient had completed 7 days without reintubation or any MV through tracheostomy (or was alive and discharged earlier).

Statistical analysis

The data are presented as medians and interquartile ranges (IQR) for continuous variables and as numbers and percentages for categorical variables. The Jonckheere–Terpstra test for continuous variables [11] and the Mantel–Haenszel test for categorical variables [12] were used to analyze trends of baseline characteristics and outcomes across weaning groups. The Mann–Whitney *U* test was used for continuous variables, and Pearson's Chi-square test was used for categorical variables to identify statistical differences of main weaning outcomes between weaning groups according to the ICC and WIND classifications, respectively. All tests were two-tailed, and a P value < 0.05 was considered significant. The data were analyzed using PASW Statistics 18 (SPSS Inc., Chicago, IL, USA).

Results

Application of ICC and WIND classifications to the same cohort

During the study period, a total of 1600 patients were eligible after excluding patients who transferred from other hospitals after more than 48 h of intubation ($n = 53$) or underwent successful NIV ($n = 76$) (Fig. 1). All eligible patients were classified by the WIND classification as follows: Group NW = 580 (36.3%), Group 1 = 617 (38.6%), Group 2 = 186 (11.6%), and Group 3 = 217 (13.6%). However, only 735 (45.9%) patients could be classified by the ICC classification as follows: simple weaning = 503 (31.4%), difficult weaning = 145 (9.1%), and prolonged weaning = 87 (5.4%).

Baseline characteristics of the total cohort are presented in Table 1. Median age was 65 years, and 68.0% of patients were male. The most common comorbidity was malignant disease (59.5%), and the most common cause of respiratory failure was pneumonia (33.4%), followed by extrapulmonary sepsis (21.6%) and acute respiratory distress syndrome (9.8%).

Table 1 Baseline characteristics of the total cohort, excluded patients by ICC classification, and Group NW by WIND classification

Variables	Total ($n=1600$)	ICC Excluded ($n=865$)	WIND Group NW ($n=580$)
Age, years	65 (54–72)	63 (54–72)	63 (52–71)
Sex, male	1088 (68.0)	580 (67.1)	387 (66.7)
Underlying disease			
Malignancy	952 (59.5)	561 (64.9)	389 (67.1)
Respiratory	458 (28.6)	250 (28.9)	156 (26.9)
Neurologic	225 (14.1)	122 (14.1)	60 (10.3)
Gastrointestinal	209 (13.1)	135 (15.6)	108 (18.6)
Cardiovascular	202 (12.6)	99 (11.4)	65 (11.2)
Genitourinary	171 (10.7)	70 (8.1)	48 (8.3)
Interval between hospital admission and ICU admission, days	2 (0–11)	3 (0–14)	3 (0–14)
Cause of respiratory failure			
Pneumonia	535 (33.4)	270 (31.2)	165 (28.4)
Extrapulmonary sepsis	345 (21.6)	201 (23.2)	165 (28.4)
ARDS	157 (9.8)	93 (10.8)	66 (11.4)
CPR	114 (7.1)	73 (8.4)	55 (9.5)
Coma	88 (5.5)	51 (5.9)	29 (5.0)
Pulmonary edema	76 (4.8)	20 (2.3)	15 (2.6)
Ventilatory failure	63 (3.9)	24 (2.8)	12 (2.1)
Central airway obstruction	55 (3.4)	36 (4.2)	11 (1.9)
Exacerbation of ILD	35 (2.2)	18 (2.1)	14 (2.4)
Others	132 (8.3)	79 (9.1)	48 (8.3)
SAPS III on ICU admission	64 (53–77)	66 (55–79)	68 (58–83)
SOFA score on ICU admission	9 (6–13)	11 (8–14)	12 (8–15)
Interval between hospital admission and intubation, days	2 (0–12)	4 (0–16)	4 (0–16)

ICC International Consensus Conference, *NW* no weaning, *WIND* Weaning according to a New Definition, *ICU* intensive care unit, *ARDS* acute respiratory distress syndrome, *ILD* interstitial lung disease, *CPR* cardiopulmonary resuscitation, *SAPS III* Simplified Acute Physiology Score III, *SOFA* Sequential Organ Failure Assessment

Comparison of baseline characteristics among groups according to ICC and WIND classifications

Agreement of weaning results between ICC and WIND classifications is presented in Table 2. Although most patients in the simple weaning (462/503, 91.8%) or prolonged weaning groups (76/87, 87.4%) were classified as Group 1 or 3, respectively, only 59.3% (86/145) of patients in the difficult weaning group by ICC classification were classified as Group 2 by WIND classification. Of 865 patients whose weaning results could not be classified by ICC, 285 were classifiable to Group 1 ($n=109$), 2 ($n=68$), or 3 ($n=108$) by WIND.

In a comparison of baseline characteristics among weaning groups, there were statistically significant trends with more underlying malignancy and neurologic disorders, longer interval between hospital admission and ICU admission, more pneumonia as a cause of respiratory failure, less pulmonary edema as a cause of respiratory failure, and longer interval between hospital admission and intubation across the ICC classification from simple to prolonged weaning groups (Table 3). In addition to this trend, except for neurologic disorders, there were statistically significant trends with more respiratory disorders and less gastrointestinal and genitourinary disorders as underlying diseases across the WIND classification from Group 1 to Group 3.

Clinical outcomes among groups according to ICC and WIND classifications

Clinical outcomes of the total cohort are listed in Table 4. Median interval between intubation and first SA was 3 days (IQR, 2–6 days), and median MV requirement was 5 days (IQR 2–11 days). Tracheostomy was needed in 416/1580 (26.3%) patients after a median of 11 days (IQR, 6–15 days) of intubation. The successful weaning rate was 51.5%, and ICU and hospital mortality were 41.0% and 53.0%, respectively.

All of these clinical outcomes showed statistically significant trends across the ICC and WIND classifications (Table 5). However, there were no statistical differences in successful weaning rate (96.6% vs. 95.2%, $P=0.416$), ICU mortality (5.4% vs. 5.5%, $P=0.944$), and hospital mortality (22.5% vs. 25.5%, $P=0.443$) between simple and difficult weaning groups by ICC (Fig. 2). Conversely, there were statistically significant differences in successful weaning rate (98.5% vs. 76.9%, $P<0.001$), ICU mortality (3.6% vs. 16.7%, $P<0.001$), and hospital mortality (21.2% vs. 33.9%, $P<0.001$) between Group 1 and Group 2 by WIND. By the WIND classification, only the LOS between Group 1 and Group 2 had no statistically significant difference (median 25 days [IQR 15–51 days] versus median 29 days [IQR 16–52 days], $P=0.300$).

Discussion

To the best of our knowledge, this is the first validation study of WIND classification compared to ICC classification. Our study demonstrates that the WIND

Table 2 Agreement according to ICC and WIND classifications

ICC	Simple	Difficult	Prolonged	Not classified	Total	Agreement, %
WIND						
Group NW	0	0	0	580	580	NA
Group 1	462	46	0	109	617	74.9
Group 2	21	86	11	68	186	46.2
Group 3	20	13	76	108	217	35.0
Total	503	145	87	865	1600	
Agreement, %	91.8	59.3	87.4	NA		39.0

For each line and column, agreement was calculated as follows: (number of patients classified in the same group by 2 classifications)/(total number of patients in line or column)

ICC International Consensus Conference, *WIND* Weaning according to a New Definition, *NW* no weaning, *NA* not accessible

Table 3 Comparison of baseline characteristics according to ICC and WIND classifications

Variables	ICC classification				WIND classification			
	Simple (*n* = 503)	Difficult (*n* = 145)	Prolonged (*n* = 87)	*P* for trend	Group 1 (*n* = 617)	Group 2 (*n* = 186)	Group 3 (*n* = 217)	*P* for trend
Age, years	65 (53–72)	68 (55–75)	67 (55–75)	0.081	65 (54–73)	66 (56–74)	66 (54–73)	0.774
Sex, male	351 (69.8)	93 (64.1)	64 (73.6)	0.952	427 (69.2)	127 (68.3)	147 (67.7)	0.673
Underlying disease								
Malignancy	249 (49.5)	81 (55.9)	61 (70.1)	< 0.001	296 (48.0)	116 (62.4)	151 (69.6)	< 0.001
Respiratory	135 (26.8)	42 (29.0)	31 (35.6)	0.106	163 (26.4)	57 (30.6)	82 (37.8)	0.002
Neurologic	62 (12.3)	24 (16.6)	17 (19.5)	0.042	94 (15.2)	35 (18.8)	36 (16.6)	0.484
Gastrointestinal	54 (10.7)	17 (11.7)	3 (3.4)	0.108	68 (11.0)	20 (10.8)	13 (6.0)	0.048
Cardiovascular	76 (15.1)	17 (11.7)	10 (11.5)	0.239	92 (14.9)	21 (11.3)	24 (11.1)	0.108
Genitourinary	74 (14.7)	17 (11.7)	10 (11.5)	0.292	90 (14.6)	12 (6.5)	21 (9.7)	0.014
Interval between hospital admission and ICU admission, days	1 (0–6)	1 (0–7)	3 (1–11)	0.001	1 (0–7)	2 (0–8)	3 (1–14)	< 0.001
Cause of respiratory failure								
Pneumonia	170 (33.8)	49 (33.8)	46 (52.9)	0.004	211 (34.2)	62 (33.3)	97 (44.7)	0.013
Extrapulmonary sepsis	104 (20.7)	30 (20.7)	10 (11.5)	0.095	111 (18.0)	38 (20.4)	31 (14.3)	0.343
ARDS	40 (8.0)	15 (10.3)	9 (10.3)	0.326	50 (8.1)	14 (7.5)	27 (12.4)	0.087
CPR	31 (6.2)	8 (5.5)	2 (2.3)	0.204	39 (6.3)	11 (5.9)	9 (4.1)	0.259
Coma	23 (4.6)	8 (5.5)	6 (6.9)	0.396	35 (5.7)	10 (5.4)	14 (6.5)	0.725
Pulmonary edema	45 (8.9)	10 (6.9)	1 (1.1)	0.014	48 (7.8)	9 (4.8)	4 (1.8)	0.001
Ventilatory failure	28 (5.6)	9 (6.2)	2 (2.3)	0.409	34 (5.5)	11 (5.9)	6 (2.8)	0.159
Central airway obstruction	14 (2.8)	2 (1.4)	3 (3.4)	1.000	30 (4.9)	9 (4.8)	5 (2.3)	0.143
Exacerbation of ILD	12 (2.4)	3 (2.1)	2 (2.3)	1.000	13 (2.1)	4 (2.2)	4 (1.8)	0.894
Others	36 (7.2)	11 (7.6)	6 (6.9)	1.000	46 (7.5)	18 (9.7)	20 (9.2)	0.332
SAPS III on ICU admission	61 (50–73)	63 (54–76)	64 (53–77)	0.046	61 (50–73)	63 (54–76)	65 (55–76)	0.001
SOFA score on ICU admission	8 (5–11)	8 (5–11)	8 (5–11)	0.514	8 (5–11)	8 (5–11)	9 (5–12)	0.063
Interval between hospital admission and intubation, days	1 (0–8)	2 (0–8)	3 (1–14)	< 0.001	1 (0–8)	3 (1–10)	4 (1–16)	< 0.001

ICC International Consensus Conference, *WIND* Weaning according to a New Definition, *ICU* intensive care unit, *ARDS* acute respiratory distress syndrome, *ILD* interstitial lung disease, *CPR* cardiopulmonary resuscitation, *SAPS III* Simplified Acute Physiology Score III, *SOFA* Sequential Organ Failure Assessment

classification could be operational for every patient under MV and better discriminates clinical outcomes by weaning group compared to ICC classification.

In this study, only 46% of patients receiving invasive MV were classifiable by ICC. However, WIND classification was applicable to all patients, even in

Table 4 Clinical outcomes of total cohort, excluded patients by ICC classification, and Group NW by WIND classification

Variables	Total ($n=1600$)	ICC Excluded ($n=865$)	WIND Group NW ($n=580$)
Interval between intubation and the first SA, days[a]	3 (2–6)	4 (2–10)	–
SOFA score at the day of first SA[a]	5 (3–8)	7 (5–9)	–
MV days	5 (2–11)	6 (2–15)	5 (2–11)
Ventilator-free days[b]	2 (0–24)	0 (0–0)	0
Tracheostomy	436 (27.3)	277 (32.0)	101 (17.4)
No	1164 (72.8)	568 (65.7)	479 (82.6)
Before MV	20 (1.3)	20 (2.3)	6 (1.0)
Between MV and first SA	219 (13.7)	219 (25.3)	95 (16.4)
Between first SA and extubation	151 (9.4)	54 (6.2)	–
After the first extubation	46 (2.9)	4 (0.5)	–
Interval between intubation and tracheostomy, days[c]	11 (6–15)	9 (5–14)	10 (7–14)
Successful weaning from MV[d]	824 (51.5)	160 (18.5)	0
ICU mortality	656 (41.0)	588 (68.0)	511 (88.1)
LOS in ICU, days	7 (4–15)	8 (3–17)	6 (2–13)
Hospital mortality	848 (53.0)	643 (74.3)	520 (89.7)
LOS in hospital, days	24 (13–46)	20 (9–43)	15 (5–30)
Type of discharge			
Home	422 (26.4)	44 (5.1)	0
Other hospital	219 (13.7)	90 (10.4)	5 (0.9)
Other ICU	24 (1.5)	20 (2.3)	10 (1.7)
Hospice	87 (5.4)	68 (7.9)	45 (7.8)
Death	848 (53.0)	643 (74.3)	520 (89.7)

ICC International Consensus Conference, *NW* no weaning, *WIND* Weaning according to a New Definition, *SA* separation attempt, *SOFA* Sequential Organ Failure Assessment, *MV* mechanical ventilation, *ICU* intensive care unit, *LOS* length of stay

[a] Excluded patients who had no SA from MV. Therefore, total patients, excluded patients by ICC, and Group NW by WIND numbered 1020, 285, and 0, respectively

[b] Ventilator-free days are defined as 28 minus the total number of days with invasive MV. Nonsurvivors were considered as having 0 ventilator-free days

[c] Excluded patients with no tracheostomy or tracheostomy prior to mechanical ventilation

[d] Successful weaning is defined as in the WIND Study (Intubated patients: extubation without death or reintubation within 7 days after extubation [whether postextubation noninvasive ventilation was used or not] or ICU discharge without invasive mechanical ventilation within 7 days, whichever comes first. Tracheostomized patients: spontaneous ventilation through tracheostomy without any mechanical ventilation during 7 consecutive days or ICU discharge with spontaneous breathing, whichever comes first)

tracheostomized patients and patients not receiving the SBT. Our results are similar to those of the original study that proposed WIND classification, which classified only 1330/2709 (51%) patients by ICC and all patients by WIND [8]. In previous studies related to ICC classification, 40–60% of mechanically ventilated patients were excluded from studies because they died, had a tracheostomy, transferred to another hospital, had unplanned extubation before they were ready to wean or during weaning, or did not use SBT to wean [3, 4, 6, 7]. However, all patients could adopt the WIND classification because (a) the starting point of weaning in WIND classification was defined as SA including methods other than SBT, even unplanned extubation, (b) WIND classification provided clear criteria for the starting point of weaning and successful weaning in both intubated and tracheostomized patients, and (c) the WIND classification is based on duration of ventilation between the first SA and the end of weaning, regardless of the results, such as successful separation or death.

Although most previous studies have shown that prolonged weaning increases ICU and hospital mortality rates, there are no statistical differences between simple and difficult weaning [3, 4, 6, 7, 13]. As with previous studies, ICU and hospital mortality and successful weaning rates between simple and difficult weaning groups by ICC classification showed no differences in the present study. However, WIND classification had stepwise differences in Groups 1–3 for these weaning outcomes. In Table 4, successful weaning was noted in 18.5% (160/865) of the unclassifiable patients by ICC. In addition, their ICU survival rate was 32.0%, which was higher than that of Group NW (11.9%). Because these patients were

Table 5 Clinical outcomes according to ICC and WIND classifications

Variables	ICC classification				WIND classification			
	Simple (n = 503)	Difficult (n = 145)	Prolonged (n = 87)	P for trend	Group 1 (n = 617)	Group 2 (n = 186)	Group 3 (n = 217)	P for trend
Interval between intubation and the first SA, days	3 (2–5)	3 (2–6)	4 (2–7)	0.002	3 (2–5)	3 (2–6)	4 (2–9)	< 0.001
SOFA score at the day of first SA	5 (3–7)	6 (3–8)	5 (4–8)	< 0.001	5 (3–7)	6 (4–8)	7 (5–9)	< 0.001
MV days	3 (2–6)	7 (4–10)	19 (12–28)	< 0.001	3 (2–5)	7 (5–10)	21 (14–35)	< 0.001
Ventilator-free days[a]	25 (22–26)	21 (18–24)	0 (0–13)	< 0.001	25 (23–26)	19 (0–23)	0 (0–5)	< 0.001
Tracheostomy	40 (8.0)	37 (25.5)	62 (71.3)	< 0.001	109 (17.7)	64 (34.4)	162 (74.7)	< 0.001
No	463 (92.0)	108 (74.5)	25 (28.7)	–	508 (82.3)	122 (65.6)	55 (25.3)	–
Before MV	–	–	–	–	10 (1.6)	3 (1.6)	1 (0.5)	–
Between MV and first SA	–	–	–	–	63 (10.2)	21 (11.3)	40 (18.4)	–
Between first SA and extubation	12 (2.4)	25 (17.2)	60 (69.0)	–	0	32 (17.2)	119 (54.8)	–
After the first extubation	28 (5.6)	12 (8.3)	2 (2.3)	–	36 (5.8)	8 (4.3)	2 (0.9)	–
Interval between intubation and tracheostomy, days[b]	18 (13–33)	12 (5–19)	11 (9–15)	< 0.001	10 (2–17)	7 (4–12)	12 (9–15)	< 0.001
Successful weaning from MV[c]	486 (96.6)	138 (95.2)	40 (46.0)	< 0.001	608 (98.5)	143 (76.9)	73 (33.6)	< 0.001
ICU mortality	27 (5.4)	8 (5.5)	33 (37.9)	< 0.001	22 (3.6)	31 (16.7)	92 (42.4)	< 0.001
LOS in ICU, days	6 (3–9)	10 (6–14)	21 (14–30)	< 0.001	6 (4–9)	10 (7–14)	24 (17–35)	< 0.001
Hospital mortality	113 (22.5)	37 (25.5)	55 (63.2)	< 0.001	131 (21.2)	63 (33.9)	134 (61.8)	< 0.001
LOS in hospital, days	24 (14–45)	31 (19–57)	40 (27–74)	< 0.001	25 (15–51)	29 (16–52)	45 (29–78)	< 0.001
Type of discharge								
Home	296 (58.8)	72 (49.7)	10 (11.5)	–	343 (55.6)	62 (33.3)	17 (7.8)	–
Other hospital	82 (16.3)	30 (20.7)	17 (19.5)	–	129 (20.9)	45 (24.2)	40 (18.4)	–
Other ICU	0	1 (0.7)	3 (3.4)	–	0	4 (2.2)	10 (4.6)	–
Hospice	12 (2.4)	5 (3.4)	2 (2.3)	–	14 (2.3)	12 (6.5)	16 (7.4)	–
Death	113 (22.5)	37 (25.5)	55 (63.2)	–	131 (21.2)	63 (33.9)	134 (61.8)	–

ICC International Consensus Conference, *WIND* Weaning according to a New Definition, *SA* separation attempt, *SOFA* Sequential Organ Failure Assessment, *MV* mechanical ventilation, *ICU* intensive care unit, *LOS* length of stay

[a] Ventilator-free days are defined as 28 minus the total number of days with invasive MV. Nonsurvivors were considered as having 0 ventilator-free days

[b] Excluded patients with no tracheostomy and tracheostomy prior to mechanical ventilation

[c] Successful weaning is defined as in the WIND Study (Intubated patients: extubation without death or reintubation within 7 days after extubation [whether postextubation noninvasive ventilation was used or not] or ICU discharge without invasive mechanical ventilation within 7 days, whichever comes first. Tracheostomized patients: spontaneous ventilation through tracheostomy without any mechanical ventilation during 7 consecutive days or ICU discharge with spontaneous breathing, whichever comes first)

classified as Groups 1–3 by WIND, the WIND classification seems to show greater differences in weaning outcomes between groups than does the ICC classification.

Although this study provides new information on weaning outcome based on new definitions that allow classification of all mechanically ventilated patients, our study has some limitations that should be considered. First, given its observational nature in a single tertiary referral hospital, there could be a selection bias that might have influenced the significance of our results. However, the data were collected prospectively between July 2010 and September 2013 from all consecutive patients who were admitted to the medical ICU and mechanically ventilated for more than 24 h. The patients were screened daily for weaning readiness according to a protocol-based weaning program [3, 9]. Thus, our cohort is more likely to reflect the patients encountered in routine ICU practice, and our findings are therefore readily applicable in similar settings. Second, our cohort was weaned from MV according to a protocol-based program with SBT using a T-piece. In addition, tracheostomy was performed in a quarter of patients, which is higher than the rate of 11–15% in an international multicenter study [14]. Although SBT using a T-piece is a general method of withdrawal from MV [4] and tracheostomy may improve aspects of care of patients on MV [15], our findings have limitations in their generalizability to other groups that underwent methods such as SBT using low pressure support, continuous positive airway pressure, gradual reduction in support using pressure support

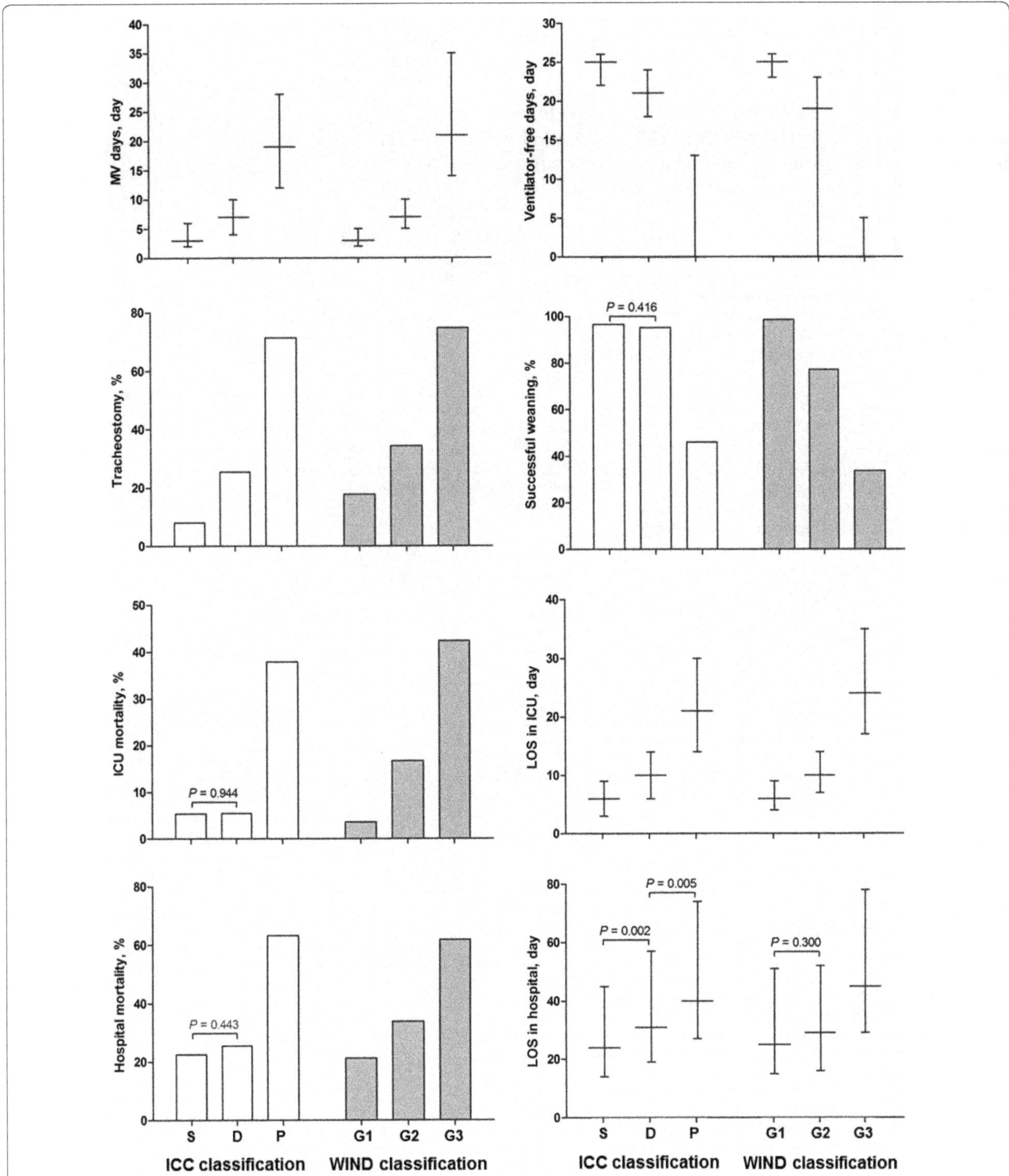

Fig. 2 Comparisons of weaning outcomes between groups according to ICC and WIND classifications. Data are presented as medians and interquartile ranges for continuous variables and as percentages for categorical variables. *P* values between groups are < 0.001 except where otherwise noted. *ICC* International Consensus Conference, *WIND* Weaning according to a New Definition, *MV* mechanical ventilation, *ICU* intensive care unit, *LOS* length of stay, *G1* Group 1, *G2* Group 2, *G3* Group 3, *S* simple weaning group, *D* difficult weaning group, *P* prolonged weaning group

mode, or synchronized intermittent mandatory ventilation, and that has lower rate of tracheostomy.

Conclusion

In conclusion, WIND classification could be a better tool for predicting weaning outcomes than ICC classification because WIND classification is applicable to all mechanically ventilated patients and has higher discriminatory power for weaning outcomes.

Abbreviations

ICC: International Consensus Conference; ICU: intensive care unit; IQR: interquartile range; LOS: length of stay; MV: mechanical ventilation; NIV: noninvasive ventilation; NW: no weaning; RCP: respiratory care practitioners; REVA: Réseau Européen de Recherche en Ventilation Artificielle; SA: separation attempt; SBT: spontaneous breathing trial; WIND: Weaning according to a New Definition.

Authors' contributions

BHJ, KYL, and KJ conceived and designed the study; BHJ, KYL, JN, MGK, SJN, GYS, and KJ analyzed and interpreted the data; BHJ, KYL, and KJ drafted the manuscript for intellectual content; BHJ, KYL, JN, MGK, SJN, GYS, and KJ revised the manuscript. All authors read and approved the final manuscript.

Author details

[1] Division of Pulmonary and Critical Care Medicine, Department of Medicine, Samsung Medical Center, Sungkyunkwan University School of Medicine, 81 Irwon-ro, Gangnam-gu, Seoul 06351, Republic of Korea. [2] Intensive Care Unit Nursing Department, Samsung Medical Center, Sungkyunkwan University School of Medicine, Seoul, Republic of Korea. [3] Department of Critical Care Medicine, Samsung Medical Center, Sungkyunkwan University School of Medicine, Seoul, Republic of Korea.

Acknowledgements

Not applicable.

Competing interests

The authors declare that they have no competing interests.

Funding

This work was supported by a Samsung Medical Center Grant (SMO1180151).

References

1. Boles JM, Bion J, Connors A, Herridge M, Marsh B, Melot C, et al. Weaning from mechanical ventilation. Eur Respir J. 2007;29:1033–56.
2. Esteban A, Ferguson ND, Meade MO, Frutos-Vivar F, Apezteguia C, Brochard L, et al. Evolution of mechanical ventilation in response to clinical research. Am J Respir Crit Care Med. 2008;177:170–7.
3. Jeong BH, Ko MG, Nam J, Yoo H, Chung CR, Suh GY, et al. Differences in clinical outcomes according to weaning classifications in medical intensive care units. PLoS ONE. 2015;10:e0122810.
4. Penuelas O, Frutos-Vivar F, Fernandez C, Anzueto A, Epstein SK, Apezteguia C, et al. Characteristics and outcomes of ventilated patients according to time to liberation from mechanical ventilation. Am J Respir Crit Care Med. 2011;184:430–7.
5. Blackwood B, Alderdice F, Burns K, Cardwell C, Lavery G, O'Halloran P. Use of weaning protocols for reducing duration of mechanical ventilation in critically ill adult patients: cochrane systematic review and meta-analysis. BMJ. 2011;342:c7237.
6. Funk GC, Anders S, Breyer MK, Burghuber OC, Edelmann G, Heindl W, et al. Incidence and outcome of weaning from mechanical ventilation according to new categories. Eur Respir J. 2010;35:88–94.
7. Pu L, Zhu B, Jiang L, Du B, Zhu X, Li A, et al. Weaning critically ill patients from mechanical ventilation: a prospective cohort study. J Crit Care. 2015;30(862):e7–13.
8. Beduneau G, Pham T, Schortgen F, Piquilloud L, Zogheib E, Jonas M, et al. Epidemiology of Weaning Outcome according to a New Definition. The WIND Study. Am J Respir Crit Care Med. 2017;195:772–83.
9. Jeon K, Jeong BH, Ko MG, Nam J, Yoo H, Chung CR, et al. Impact of delirium on weaning from mechanical ventilation in medical patients. Respirology. 2016;21:313–20.
10. Jeong BH, Nam J, Ko MG, Chung CR, Suh GY, Jeon K. Impact of limb weakness on extubation failure after planned extubation in medical patients. Respirology. 2018;23:842–50.
11. Bewick V, Cheek L, Ball J. Statistics review 10: further nonparametric methods. Crit Care. 2004;8:196–9.
12. Bewick V, Cheek L, Ball J. Statistics review 8: qualitative data: tests of association. Crit Care. 2004;8:46–53.
13. Tonnelier A, Tonnelier JM, Nowak E, Gut-Gobert C, Prat G, Renault A, et al. Clinical relevance of classification according to weaning difficulty. Respir Care. 2011;56:583–90.
14. Esteban A, Frutos-Vivar F, Muriel A, Ferguson ND, Penuelas O, Abraira V, et al. Evolution of mortality over time in patients receiving mechanical ventilation. Am J Respir Crit Care Med. 2013;188:220–30.
15. Nieszkowska A, Combes A, Luyt CE, Ksibi H, Trouillet JL, Gibert C, et al. Impact of tracheotomy on sedative administration, sedation level, and comfort of mechanically ventilated intensive care unit patients. Crit Care Med. 2005;33:2527–33.

19

Nasal high-flow bronchodilator nebulization

François Reminiac[1,2,3], Laurent Vecellio[2], Laetitia Bodet-Contentin[1,4,5], Valérie Gissot[4], Deborah Le Pennec[2], Charlotte Salmon Gandonnière[1,4,5], Maria Cabrera[2], Pierre-François Dequin[1,2,4,5], Laurent Plantier[2,6] and Stephan Ehrmann[1,2,4,5]*

Abstract

Background: There is an absence of controlled clinical data showing bronchodilation effectiveness after nebulization via nasal high-flow therapy circuits.

Results: Twenty-five patients with reversible airflow obstruction received, in a randomized order: (1) 2.5 mg albuterol delivered via a jet nebulizer with a facial mask; (2) 2.5 mg albuterol delivered via a vibrating mesh nebulizer placed downstream of a nasal high-flow humidification chamber (30 L/min and 37 °C); and (3) nasal high-flow therapy without nebulization. All three conditions induced significant individual increases in forced expiratory volume in one second (FEV_1) compared to baseline. The median change was similar after facial mask nebulization [+350 mL (+180; +550); +18% (+8; +30)] and nasal high flow with nebulization [+330 mL (+140; +390); +16% (+5; +24)], $p=0.11$. However, it was significantly lower after nasal high-flow therapy without nebulization [+50 mL (−10; +220); +3% (−1; +8)], $p=0.0009$. FEV_1 increases after facial mask and nasal high-flow nebulization as well as residual volume decreases were well correlated ($p<0.0001$ and $p=0.01$). Both techniques showed good agreement in terms of airflow obstruction reversibility (kappa 0.60).

Conclusion: Albuterol vibrating mesh nebulization within a nasal high-flow circuit induces similar bronchodilation to standard facial mask jet nebulization. Beyond pharmacological bronchodilation, nasal high flow by itself may induce small but significant bronchodilation.

Keywords: Albuterol, Respiratory function tests, Nebulizers and vaporizers, Chronic obstructive pulmonary disease

Background

Nasal high-flow (NHF) therapy consists of delivering heated and humidified gas through a nasal cannula, at high flow rates, frequently exceeding patients' inspiratory flow. This non-invasive respiratory support is increasingly used, particularly among hypoxemic critically ill patients as those high oxygen flow rates very efficiently improve oxygenation and reduce the rate of intubation [1, 2]. Nebulization is a technique used to deliver inhaled drugs directly acting on the respiratory tract. In critically ill patients, nebulization is very frequently used, in particular among patients undergoing non-invasive respiratory support [3]. The most frequently delivered inhaled drugs are bronchodilators, such as albuterol, provided to approximately 20% of patients in intensive care [3]. Thus, one may question the best way to combine the two therapies in order to deliver inhaled bronchodilators to patients undergoing NHF therapy. Indeed, NHF may be especially beneficial to patients suffering obstructive pulmonary disease for whom inhaled bronchodilator delivery is a cornerstone of therapy [4–6]. NHF washes out the anatomical dead space clearing exhaled carbon dioxide, and this may have benefit to patients with hypercapnia [7, 8]; it induces a positive end-expiratory pressure, a reduction in respiratory rate and increase in tidal volume, which all potentially lead to a reduction in the work of breathing among patients with dynamic

*Correspondence: stephanehrmann@gmail.com
[1] Médecine Intensive Réanimation, CHRU de Tours, 2, Bd Tonnellé, 37044 Tours Cedex 9, France
Full list of author information is available at the end of the article

hyperinflation [9, 10]; it enables precise control of the inspired fraction of oxygen to avoid excessive delivery among patients with chronic hypercapnia and altered respiratory drive; it ensures high humidification of inhaled gases favouring mucus hydration and thus clearance and is a very well-tolerated oxygen delivery method. Nevertheless, NHF merely represents an obstacle impeding inhaled drug delivery. Indeed, high gas flow rate and associated turbulent flow, high gas humidity, geometric angulation of the nasal cannula, and the nose anatomy physiologically retaining inhaled particles all represent hurdles to efficient inhaled drug delivery through an NHF circuit. In vitro data showed that when placing a vibrating mesh nebulizer close to the humidification chamber and limiting the system flow rate at 30 L/min, significant amounts of drug may be delivered to the respiratory tract [11–15]. That data have been confirmed by in vivo evaluation in a paediatric animal model and in adult radiolabelled deposition studies [16, 17]. Although uncontrolled case series are in favour of a clinically significant bronchodilation after delivery of albuterol through an NHF circuit, no controlled data are available in humans [18].

The objective of this study was to investigate the effect of vibrating mesh nebulized albuterol delivered through an NHF circuit on respiratory system mechanics as compared to Standard-nebulization using a jet nebulizer with a facial mask and NHF delivered without inhaled albuterol in a randomized controlled fashion.

Methods

The study was approved by the institutional review board (Comité de Protection des Personnes Ouest-1, 2016-R6-PHAO15-SE/Airvoneb-2016-A00064-47, NCT02812979). Adult patients with reversible obstructive lung disease defined as a baseline of forced expiratory volume in one second (FEV_1) over vital capacity ratio below 70% and a positive bronchodilator reversibility test (FEV_1 increase of at least 12% and 200 mL after inhaled albuterol delivery [19]) as assessed in the past month were included after written informed consent. Non-inclusion criteria were ongoing exacerbation, hemoptysis, uncontrolled asthma, recent pneumothorax, lung or pleural biopsy, broncho-alveolar lavage, pregnancy, breast feeding, trusteeship, guardianship and albuterol allergy or intolerance. Patients underwent, on three separate days within 1 week, in a randomized order: (1) albuterol nebulization through a facial aerosol mask (Standard-nebulization), (2) albuterol nebulization within an NHF circuit (NHF-nebulization) and (3) sham nebulization within an NHF circuit (Control-NHF). Patients were instructed not to smoke or to take short- or long-acting bronchodilators, respectively 4, 6 and 12 h prior to each procedure.

Standard-nebulization

2.5 mg albuterol (albuterol sulphate 2.5 mg/2.5 mL, Mylan N.V., Canonsburg, PA, USA) was placed in a jet nebulizer connected to a bucco-nasal facial mask positioned on the patient and driven with 6 L/min of non-heated and non-humidified pressurized air (Cirrus2 nebulizer and Adult EcoLite™ Aerosol Mask, both from Intersurgical, Wokingham, UK).

NHF-nebulization

2.5 mg albuterol was placed in a vibrating mesh nebulizer (Aerogen Solo®, Aerogen Ltd., Galway, Ireland) positioned immediately downstream of the humidification chamber of an NHF system (Airvo™2, Fisher & Paykel Healthcare, Auckland, New Zealand), using the Airvo™Neb connector (Fig. 1). NHF was set at 30 L/min of air with 100% relative humidity at 37 °C using medium size nasal cannula. The NHF session lasted 30 min, and nebulization was started after 10 min of NHF therapy.

Control-NHF

The patient was placed under NHF during 30 min in the same conditions as for NHF-nebulization with an empty nebulizer. The patient was kept blind between the NHF-nebulization and Control-NHF procedures.

The primary outcome was the relative increase in FEV_1 after NHF-nebulization as compared to Standard-nebulization. Pulmonary function tests (spirometry and plethysmography; calibrated Jaeger MasterScreen body plethysmograph, Spirometry SentrySuite v2.10, CareFusion, Rolle, Switzerland) were performed before and after each procedure, according to guidelines [19]. Spirometry was started immediately after the end of the 30 min NHF sessions, at least 10 min after the end of nebulization. Pulmonary function tests were performed following

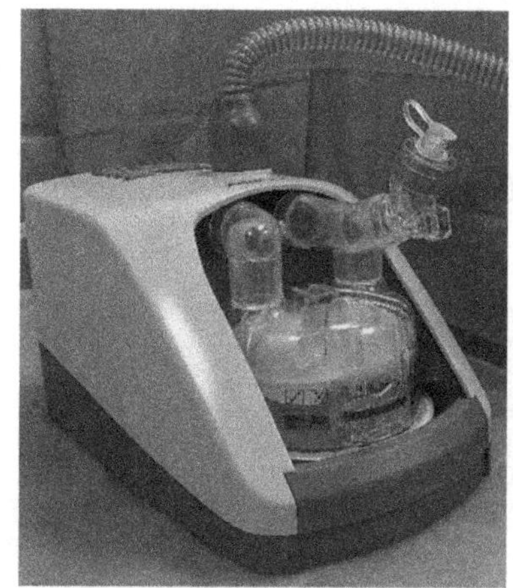

Fig. 1 Nasal high flow nebulization set-up

the same time span after the end of NHF therapy in both conditions comprising NHF (NHF-nebulization and Control-NHF) and following the same time span after the end of nebulization in both conditions comprising active nebulization (Standard-nebulization and NHF-nebulization).

Plethysmography loops were evaluated, and patients were classified as presenting expiratory flow limitation or not [20, 21]. Volumetric capnography was performed before and after each procedure (5 duplicate measurements, patients breathing out at slow and steady flow from maximal inspiration to maximal expiration) and the slope of the third phase of the capnogram measured. All pulmonary function tests were performed and interpreted by investigators and technicians blind to the procedure randomization. Patients' comfort was recorded using a visual analogical scale (range 0–100, with higher scores indicating higher comfort). The NHF-nebulization set-up and vibrating mesh nebulizer performance were tested in vitro prior to the clinical study (see Additional file 1).

Statistical analysis

The sample size calculation was based on previous data which showed a standard deviation of FEV_1 of 10% of the baseline value [22]. Taking into account the cross-over design, this non-inferiority trial, testing the hypothesis that NHF-nebulization is non-inferior to Control-nebulization in terms of FEV_1 relative increase, with a non-inferiority margin of 8%, a unilateral alpha risk of 2.5% and a beta risk of 10%, had to enrol 24 patients.

An association between the randomization order and primary outcome was assessed looking for interaction between the relative increase in FEV_1 and the procedure position to rule out a carry-over or learning effect on pulmonary function tests (nonparametric Kruskal–Wallis test). To partition the increase in FEV_1 potentially due to NHF alone from the pharmacological effect of albuterol nebulization, the FEV_1 increase attributable to albuterol nebulization was calculated individually, by subtracting Control-NHF-induced absolute FEV_1 increase from NHF-nebulization-induced absolute FEV_1 increase.

Quantitative variables were expressed as median and interquartile range and were compared before and after each procedure using a Wilcoxon signed rank test. Individual changes (before/after the procedure) were compared between procedures (Standard-nebulization, NHF-nebulization and Control-NHF) using the nonparametric Friedman test accounting for the cross-over design, and if significant, two-by-two comparisons were performed with the Wilcoxon signed rank test. Correlation between quantitative variables was evaluated with the Spearman correlation coefficient. Qualitative variables were expressed as counts and percentages. The agreement between Standard-nebulization and NHF-nebulization in terms of airway obstruction reversibility (200 mL absolute and 12% relative increase in FEV_1 [19]) was assessed using the kappa coefficient. A p value < 0.05 was considered significant.

Results

In vitro results are presented in the Additional file 1. From June 2016 to April 2018, 11,288 patients underwent pulmonary function tests, 4905 spirometry with plethysmography, and beta-2-adrenergic agonist-induced reversibility was tested in 3552 patients of which 25 were included (Table 1).

FEV_1 change

After Standard-nebulization, FEV_1 significantly increased from 1.77 L (1.43; 2.16) to 2.20 L (1.69; 2.47), $p < 0.0001$ (Table 2). Individual absolute and relative increases in FEV_1 were, respectively, 350 mL (180; 550) and 18% (8; 30). NHF-nebulization similarly induced a significant FEV_1 increase: 1.77 L (1.47; 2.27) to 2.14 L (1.71; 2.41), $p < 0.0001$, with individual absolute and relative increases of 330 mL (140; 390) and 16% (5; 24): Fig. 2.

After Control-NHF without bronchodilator delivery, FEV_1 increased from 1.83 L (1.36; 2.42) to 1.93 L (1.27; 2.52), $p = 0.044$: Fig. 2. Median individual absolute and

Table 1 Patients' baseline characteristics

Variable	$N = 25$
Female/male	10 (40%)/15 (60%)
Age (years)	60 (53; 68)
Main respiratory disease	
Asthma	9 (36%)
COPD	14 (56%)
Other	2 (8%)
Height (cm)	169 (165; 176)
Weight (kg)	75 (64; 80)
Body mass index (high/weight^2)	26 (23; 29)
FEV_1 (L)	1.83 (1,38; 2,03)
Percentage of predicted (%)	60 (53; 71)
FEV_1/vital capacity (%)	54 (45; 60)
Functional residual capacity (L)	5,0 (3,9; 6,0)
Percentage of predicted (%)	150 (139; 171)
Residual volume (L)	4,0 (2,9; 4,4)
Percentage of predicted (%)	172 (154; 184)
Presence of expiratory flow limitation	6 (24%)

Data are presented as count (percentage) and median (interquartile range)

COPD chronic obstructive pulmonary disease, *FEV_1* forced expiratory volume in one second

Table 2 Spirometry, plethysmography and volumetric capnography results

	Standard-nebulisation			NHF-nebulization			Control-NHF		
	Before	After	Individual change	Before	After	Individual change	Before	After	Individual change
FEV_1 (L)	1.77 (1.43; 2.16)	2.20 (1.69; 2.47)	0.350 (0.180; 0.550)* 18% (8; 30)*	1.77 (1.47; 2.27)	2.14 (1.71; 2.41)	0.330 (0.140; 0.390)* 16% (5; 24)*	1.83 (1.36; 2.42)	1.93 (1.27; 2.52)	0.050 (−0.010; 0.220)* 3% (−1; 8)*
Functional residual capacity (L)	4.58 (3.89; 5.22)	4.07 (3.42; 4.88)	−0.33 (−0.71; −0.17)*	4.42 (3.67; 5.35)	4.04 (3.45; 5.09)	−0.40 (−0.64; −0.12)*	4.58 (3.80; 5.38)	4.42 (3.72; 5.53)	−0.02 (−0.24; 0.10)
Residual volume (L)	3.42 (2.63; 4.22)	2.89 (2.42; 3.54)	−0.37 (−0.82; −0.12)*	3.22 (2.53; 4.29)	2.90 (2.52; 4.20)	−0.34 (−0.64; −0.06)*	3.27 (2.76; 3.99)	3.19 (2.72; 4.56)	−0.09 (−0.34; 0.16)
Forced vital capacity (L)	3.57 (2.66; 4.39)	3.65 (3.15; 4.59)	0.32 (0.08; 0.57)*	3.41 (2.79; 4.37)	3.51 (3.05; 4.47)	0.11 (0.00; 0.34)*	3.28 (2.74; 4.52)	3.58 (2.64; 4.42)	0.10 (−0.10; 0.25)
Plethysmographic airway resistances (raw)	5.31 (3.72; 6.94)	2.89 (2.54; 3.80)	−2.06 (−3.82; −0.96)*	4.62 (3.48; 7.27)	3.10 (2.39; 3.79)	−1.89 (−3.36; −0.69)*	4.71 (3.22; 7.02)	4.64 (2.86; 5.77)	−0.39 (−1.02; 0.04)*
Inspiratory capacity (L)	2.36 (2.03; 2.71)	2.63 (2.26; 3.34)	0.30 (0.14; 0.54)*	2.59 (2.12; 2.90)	2.72 (2.17; 3.17)	0.20 (0.05; 0.47)*	2.21 (1.78; 2.97)	2.61 (1.93; 2.91)	0.10 (−0.07; 0.20)
Part III of the volumetric capnography slope ($n = 16$)	0.56 (0.47; 0.74)	0.66 (0.51; 0.92)	0.04 (−0.03; 0.13)	0.67 (0.41; 0.94)	0.64 (0.40; 0.98)	0.03 (−0.11; 0.08)	0.62 (0.47; 0.89)	0.65 (0.45; 0.91)	0.01 (−0.05; 0.12)

Standard-nebulization consisted in 2.5 mg albuterol delivery with a jet nebulizer connected to an aerosol facial mask; NHF-nebulization: 2.5 mg albuterol delivered within a nasal high-flow (NHF) circuit; Control-NHF: nasal high flow without nebulization

FEV_1 forced expiratory volume in one second, *NHF* nasal high-flow

*$p < 0.05$ for individual changes before and after each session with one technique

relative increases were 50 mL (−10; 220) and 3% (−1; 8): Table 2.

No interaction was observed between the randomization order of the procedures and the absolute and relative increase in FEV_1 ($p = 0.66$ and $p = 0.59$, respectively). There was an overall statistically significant difference between procedures for the absolute and relative increase in FEV_1 ($p < 0.001$ and $p = 0.001$, respectively). In two-by-two comparisons, changes in FEV_1 after NHF-nebulization and Standard-nebulization were not significantly different (Fig. 2) and well correlated (Fig. 3) and exhibited low bias (Figure E3 of the Additional file 1). Changes in FEV_1 after Control-NHF were significantly lower (Fig. 2). Of note, when calculating changes attributable to albuterol nebulization during NHF-nebulization (subtracting Control-NHF-induced changes from NHF-nebulization-induced changes), the individual absolute increase in FEV_1 attributable to albuterol nebulization was 230 mL (−45; 385), a value significantly lower than the FEV_1 increase after Standard-nebulization ($p = 0.009$).

Airflow obstruction reversibility

Of the 18 patients with an increase in FEV_1 of more than 200 mL after Standard-nebulization during study measurements, 14/18 (78%) also showed such an increase after NHF-nebulization. Seventeen patients had an increase in FEV_1 of more than 12% after Standard-nebulization, of these 15/17 (88%) did so after NHF-nebulization. Combining both criteria according to guidelines (absolute and relative increase in FEV_1 [19]), 16 patients met the criteria for airway obstruction reversibility after albuterol Standard-nebulization during study measurements, all but two of these ($n = 14/16$, 88%) met the criteria after albuterol NHF-nebulization; conversely, all but one of the patients meeting the criteria after NHF-nebulization (13/14 93%) did so after Standard-nebulization (kappa 0.60, 95% confidence interval 0.29–0.90).

Of note, after Control-NHF, 8/25 patients (32%) had an FEV_1 increase of at least 200 mL and 5/25 (20%) of at least 12%. Five patients (20%) met the criteria for airway obstruction reversibility after Control-NHF without the addition of a bronchodilator drug [19]. See Additional file 1: Table E2 for details on those patients. No association was observed between expiratory flow limitation observed on plethysmographic loop inspection (observed in 6 patients) and positive response in terms of FEV_1

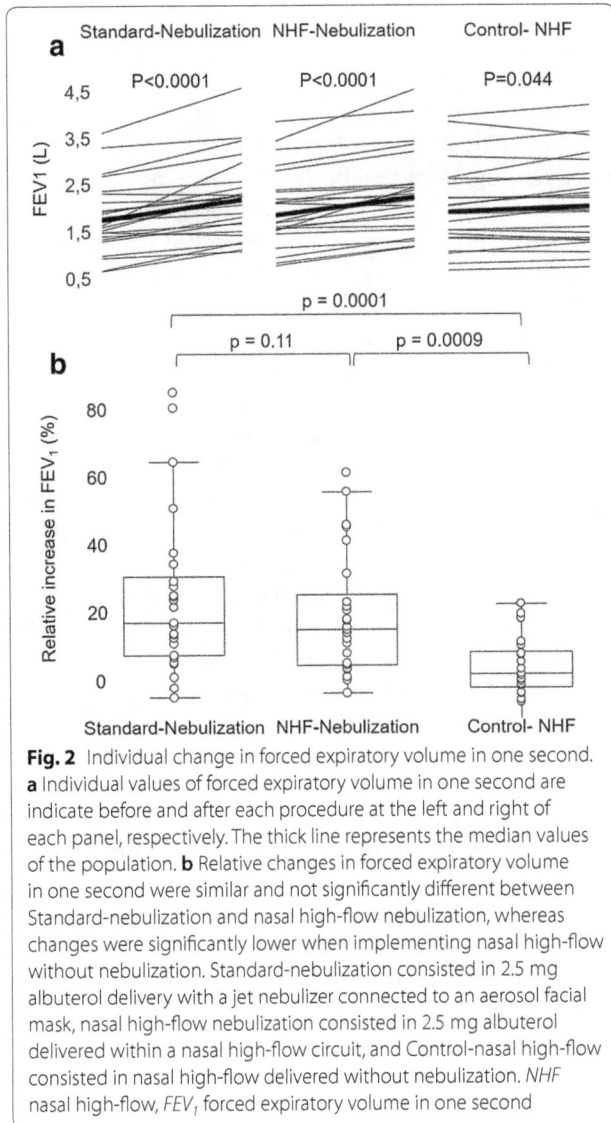

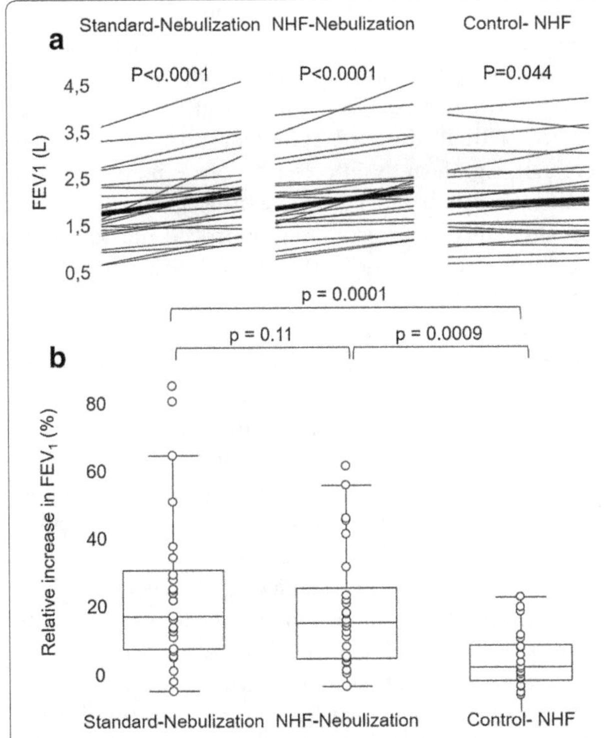

Fig. 2 Individual change in forced expiratory volume in one second. **a** Individual values of forced expiratory volume in one second are indicate before and after each procedure at the left and right of each panel, respectively. The thick line represents the median values of the population. **b** Relative changes in forced expiratory volume in one second were similar and not significantly different between Standard-nebulization and nasal high-flow nebulization, whereas changes were significantly lower when implementing nasal high-flow without nebulization. Standard-nebulization consisted in 2.5 mg albuterol delivery with a jet nebulizer connected to an aerosol facial mask, nasal high-flow nebulization consisted in 2.5 mg albuterol delivered within a nasal high-flow circuit, and Control-nasal high-flow consisted in nasal high-flow delivered without nebulization. *NHF* nasal high-flow, *FEV*$_1$ forced expiratory volume in one second

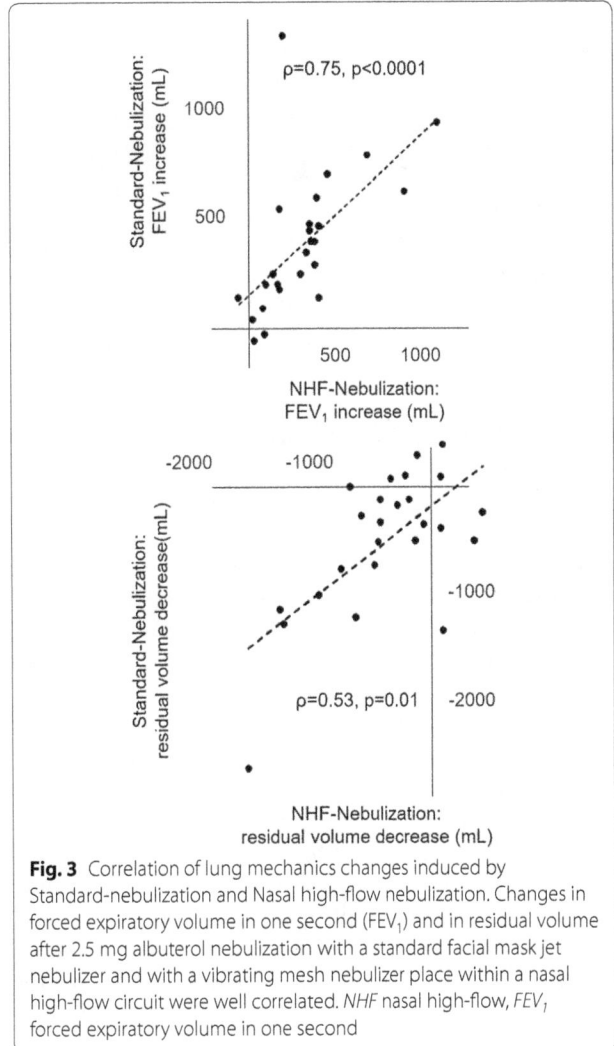

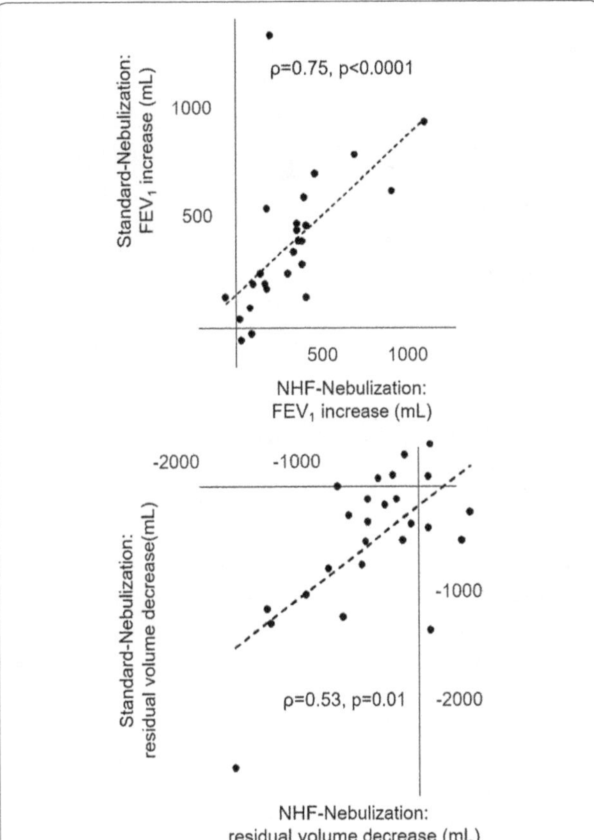

Fig. 3 Correlation of lung mechanics changes induced by Standard-nebulization and Nasal high-flow nebulization. Changes in forced expiratory volume in one second (FEV$_1$) and in residual volume after 2.5 mg albuterol nebulization with a standard facial mask jet nebulizer and with a vibrating mesh nebulizer place within a nasal high-flow circuit were well correlated. *NHF* nasal high-flow, *FEV*$_1$ forced expiratory volume in one second

increases after Control-NHF, as only one flow limited patient showed such a positive response.

Other pulmonary function tests

Plethysmography showed significant improvement in lung volumes after Standard-nebulization and NHF-nebulization (Table 2). Significant individual reduction in functional residual capacity was observed after NHF-nebulization: from 4.42 L (3.67; 5.35) to 4.04 L (3.45; 5.09)—individual changes −400 mL (−640; −120), $p=0.001$. This change was correlated with changes in residual volume observed after Standard-nebulization: Fig. 3. When NHF was delivered without albuterol nebulization, no such significant volume changes occurred (Table 2). Significant changes in plethysmography-measured airway resistances also occurred after Standard-nebulization, NHF-nebulization and Control-NHF (Table 2). The third part of the expired volumetric capnogram, which could be measured for all procedures in sixteen patients, did not show a significant change after either procedure, and individual changes were not significantly different between procedures ($p>0.05$).

Tolerance

Overall tolerance of the NHF therapy and nebulization was excellent. No side effects were recorded during NHF-nebulization; one patient complained of moderate reversible dyspnoea during Standard-nebulization and during Control-NHF. No clinically significant changes in heart rate and respiratory rate occurred; individual changes were not statistically different between procedures (data not shown). Comfort, as measured by the visual analogical scale, was not significantly different between procedures, 85 (77; 96), 85 (65; 93) and 82 (66; 92) for Standard-nebulization, NHF-nebulization and Control-NHF, respectively ($p = 0.34$).

Discussion

In patients with reversible obstructive pulmonary disease, away from an exacerbation, albuterol delivered by vibrating mesh nebulization through an NHF circuit appeared non-inferior to standard facial mask jet nebulization in terms of FEV_1 increase. This was in part due to a small but a significant increase in FEV_1 due to NHF without the addition of bronchodilator nebulization. To the best of our knowledge, this is the first controlled study in adults documenting clinical efficacy of nebulization within an NHF circuit adequately controlling for all confounding factors. These results have important clinical implications. As the use of NHF is expanding, physicians will increasingly be faced with patients undergoing NHF and requiring inhaled bronchodilator therapy [23]. Given the lack of controlled data, interrupting NHF therapy to deliver the inhaled medication may currently be the preferred option; these results show that albuterol can be delivered within the NHF circuit with the same efficacy and tolerance avoiding cumbersome equipment switches. These results are in line with the study of Bräunlich et al. who used a homecare NHF device to deliver a combination of albuterol and ipratropium bromide placing a jet nebulizer close to the nasal cannula but lacked a control group without nebulization [24]. Of note, positioning the nebulizer close to the nasal cannula may be suboptimal, as it favours aerosol deposition in the cannula. This deposition reduces drug delivery to the patient but was also associated with aerosol nasal dripping which may impact patients' comfort [11]. Our results provide controlled evidence supporting the observation made by Morgan et al. of efficient albuterol delivery after nebulization within a NHF circuit set-up similar to the present one among children with acute bronchiolitis [18].

Effects of NHF without bronchodilator nebulization on pulmonary function tests are of complex interpretation. We observed a statistically significant increase in FEV_1 after Control-NHF, albeit modest in magnitude (median increase of 50 mL and 3%, values below validated thresholds to define reversibility [19]); this result supports the hypothesis of an NHF-induced bronchodilation. Interestingly, 20% of the patients showed significant increases in FEV_1 after Control-NHF meeting guideline criteria for airflow obstruction reversibility without having received a bronchodilator. Of note, FEV_1 was measured after interruption of NHF in patients breathing spontaneously unlike other physiological studies which observed an increase in lung volumes measured during NHF therapy [25]. This may also explain the lack of association between flow limitation and FEV_1 increase after Control-NHF. Plethysmography-measured lung volumes were not significantly affected by NHF in the present study. One can speculate on potential mechanism such as positive airway pressure and improved mucus hydration during the 30-min NHF session leading to the significant increase in FEV_1 once the therapy is interrupted. Indeed, improved mucus clearance may lead to improved lung mechanics; however, no major cough and expectoration was observed among the included patients. NHF may also induce changes in respiratory pattern potentially leading to higher tidal volume and eventually to deeper inspiration during spirometry manoeuvres. Such mechanisms will need to be investigated in the future, particularly given the ongoing studies evaluating NHF among patients suffering obstructive pulmonary disease. This study has important limitations. Only stable patients were included; thus, extrapolation to the acute care setting of unstable decompensated patients warrants evaluation. Results cannot be extrapolated to other pharmacological classes, as the favourable results observe here in terms of nebulization efficiency during NHF are due in part to the large therapeutic index of albuterol [26]. Deposition studies performed in humans suggest other drugs like antibiotics are unlike effective when inhaled through an NHF circuit [17]. Clinical efficacy studies are required in intensive care unit, emergency department and pulmonology ward patients. Two different nebulizers were used in the study. We aimed to compare usual practice (facial mask jet nebulization) to the new modality of NHF-nebulization using a vibrating mesh nebulizer. Jet nebulization within the NHF circuit, albeit feasible, comes with important limitations as the gas driving the nebulizer interferes with the NHF oxygen content, humidity and temperature. Vibrating mesh facial mask nebulization is currently of uncommon practice. Thus, the potential limit of using different nebulizers represents a pragmatic choice favouring clinical applicability of the results. Using jet nebulization in combination with nasal high-flow therapy would need further evaluation. Of note, the study did not comprise a condition of sham jet nebulization to delineate individual effect of beta-2-adrenergic agonist nebulization per se. Only one NHF setting (temperature, flow rate, cannula size) and one dose of albuterol were evaluated clinically. However, results in other conditions, tested in the bench study, can give indications of potential dose adjustments, in case of nebulization with higher flow rates for example. The significantly improved delivery observed in vitro with non-humidified settings allows for new innovation in NHF devices to improve combined inhaled drug delivery.

In conclusion, the present work shows that albuterol vibrating mesh nebulization within an NHF circuit induces similar FEV_1 increases and patient comfort and tolerance compared to standard facial mask jet nebulization and can be implemented in clinical practice. Beyond pharmacologically induced bronchodilation, NHF by itself may induce a small but significant increase in FEV_1 which deserves further evaluation.

Abbreviations

NHF: nasal high-flow; FEV_1: forced expiratory volume in one second; Standard-nebulization: albuterol nebulization through a facial aerosol mask; NHF-nebulization: albuterol nebulization within a nasal high-flow circuit; Control-NHF: sham nebulization within a nasal high-flow circuit.

Authors' contributions

FR, LV, VG, LP and SE were involved in study design and conception. FR, LV, LBC, DLP, CSG, MC, PFD, LP and SE contributed to in vitro and clinical data acquisition. FR, LV, LP and SE analysed and interpreted the data. SE drafted the manuscript. FR, LV, LBC, VG, DLP, CSG, MC, PFD, LP and SE reviewed the manuscript for important intellectual content. All authors read and approved the final manuscript.

Author details

[1] Médecine Intensive Réanimation, CHRU de Tours, 2, Bd Tonnellé, 37044 Tours Cedex 9, France. [2] Centre d'étude des pathologies respiratoires, INSERM U1100, Faculté de médecine, Université de Tours, Tours, France. [3] Clinique du Mail, La Rochelle, France. [4] Centre d'investigation clinique, INSERM CIC 1415, CHRU de Tours, Tours, France. [5] CRICS-TRIGGERSEP Network, Tours, France. [6] Service de pneumologie et d'explorations fonctionnelles respiratoires, CHRU de Tours, Tours, France.

Acknowledgements

The authors sincerely thank Helene BANSARD and Lysiane BRICK from the Centre d'Investigation Clinique, INSERM CIC 1415, CHRU de Tours, Tours, France, for their invaluable help to carry out the study, gathering data and organizing study logistics, Sylvie ANGELLIAUME, Agnes BAUGE, Nathalie ROUILLARD and Nathalie JEAN from the Service de pneumologie et d'explorations fonctionnelles respiratoires, CHRU de Tours, Tours, France, for performing patients screening and carrying out pulmonary function tests, Annouck BAROUGIER and Lucas FISCHER from Service de Médecine Intensive Réanimation, and Marie LECLERC from Délégation à la Recherche Clinique et à l'Innovation, CHRU de Tours, Tours, France, for data management.

Competing interests

SE declares consultancies fees from Aerogen, Baxter healthcare and La Diffusion Technique Française, research support from Aerogen, Fisher & Paykel and Hamilton, travel expenses reimbursement from Aerogen and Fisher & Paykel. Others authors declare that they have no competing interests. LV is an employee of Nemera.

Funding

The study was funded by an unrestricted grant from Fisher & Paykel Healthcare Limited, Auckland, New Zealand. Nebulizers were provided free of charge by Aerogen Limited, Galway, Ireland.

References

1. Frat JP, Thille AX, Mercat A, Girault C, Ragot S, Perbet S, et al. High-flow oxygen through nasal cannula in acute hypoxemic respiratory failure. N Engl J Med. 2015;372:2185–96.
2. Zhu Y, Yin H, Zhang R, Wei J. High-flow nasal cannula oxygen therapy versus conventional oxygen therapy in patients with acute respiratory failure: a systematic review and metaanalysis of randomized controlled trials. BMC Pulm Med. 2017;17:201.
3. Ehrmann S, Roche-Campo F, Bodet-Contentin L, Razazi K, Dugernier J, Trenado-Alvarez J, et al. Aerosol therapy in intensive and intermediate care units: prospective observation of 2808 critically ill patients. Intensive Care Med. 2016;42:192–201.
4. Pisani L, Vega ML. Use of nasal high flow in stable COPD: rational and physiology. COPD. 2017;14:346–50.
5. Spoletini G, Alotaibi M, Blasi F, Hill NS. Heated humidified high-flow nasal oxygen in adults: mechanisms of action and clinical implications. Chest. 2015;148:253–61.
6. Pisani L, Fasano L, Corcione N, Comellini V, Musti MA, Brandao M, et al. Change in pulmonary mechanics and the effect on breathing pattern of high flow oxygen therapy in stable hypercapnic COPD. Thorax. 2017;72:373–5.
7. Onodera Y, Akimoto R, Suzuki H, Okada M, Nakane M, Kawamae K. A high-flow nasal cannula system with relatively low flow effectively washes out CO_2 from the anatomical dead space in a sophisticated respiratory model made by a 3D printer. Intensive Care Med Exp. 2018;6:7.
8. Möller W, Feng S, Domanski U, Franke KJ, Celik G, Bartenstein P, et al. Nasal high flow reduces dead space. J Appl Physiol. 2017;122:191–7.
9. Vargas F, Saint-Leger M, Boyer A, Bui NH, Hilbert G. Physiologic effects of high-flow nasal cannula oxygen in critical care subjects. Respir Care. 2015;60:1369–76.
10. Fraser JF, Spooner AJ, Dunster KR, Anstey CM, Corley A. Nasal high flow oxygen therapy in patients with COPD reduces respiratory rate and tissue carbon dioxide while increasing tidal and end-expiratory lung volumes: a randomised crossover trial. Thorax. 2016;71:759–61.
11. Réminiac F, Vecellio L, Heuzé-Vourc'h N, Petitcollin A, Respaud R, Cabrera M, et al. Aerosol therapy in adults receiving high flow nasal cannula oxygen therapy. J Aerosol Med Pulm Drug Deliv. 2016;29:134–41.
12. Bhashyam AR, Wolf MT, Marcinkowski AL, Saville A, Thomas K, Carcillo JA, et al. Aerosol delivery through nasal cannulas: an in vitro study. J Aerosol Med Pulm Drug Deliv. 2008;21:181–8.
13. Ari A, Harwood R, Sheard M, Dailey P, Fink JB. In vitro comparison of heliox and oxygen in aerosol delivery using pediatric high flow nasal cannula. Pediatr Pulmonol. 2011;46:795–801.
14. Sunbul FS, Fink JB, Harwood R, Sheard MM, Zimmerman RD, Ari A. Comparison of HFNC, bubble CPAP and SiPAP on aerosol delivery in neonates: an in vitro study. Pediatr Pulmonol. 2015;50:1099–106.
15. Dailey PA, Harwood R, Walsh K, Fink JB, Thayer T, Gagnon G, Ari A. Aerosol delivery through adult high flow nasal cannula with heliox and oxygen. Respir Care. 2017;62:1186–92.
16. Réminiac F, Vecellio L, Loughlin RM, Le Pennec D, Cabrera M, Heuzé-Vourc'h N, et al. Nasal high flow nebulization in infants and toddlers: an in vitro and in vivo scintigraphic study. Pediatr Pulmonol. 2017;52:337–44.
17. Dugernier J, Hesse M, Jumetz T, Bialais E, Roeseler J, Depoortere V, et al. Aerosol delivery with two nebulizers through high-flow nasal cannula: a randomized cross-over single-photon emission computed tomography study. J Aerosol Med Pulm Drug Deliv. 2017;30:349–558.
18. Morgan SE, Mosakowski S, Solano P, Hall JB, Tung A. High-flow nasal cannula and aerosolized β agonists for rescue therapy in children with bronchiolitis: a case series. Respir Care. 2015;60:e161–5.
19. Miller MR, Hankinson J, Brusasco V, Burgos F, Casaburi R, Coates A, et al. Standardisation of spirometry. Eur Respir J. 2005;26:319–38.
20. Radovanovic D, Pecchiari M, Pirracchio F, Zilianti C, D'Angerlo E, Santus P. Plethysmographic loops: a window on the lung pathophysiology of COPD patients. Front Physiol. 2018;9:484.
21. Tantucci C. Expiratory flow limitation definition, mechanisms, methods, and significance. Pulm Med. 2013;2013:749860. https://doi.org/10.1155/2013/749860.

22. Nava S, Karakurt S, Rampulla C, Braschi A, Fanfulla F. Salbutamol delivery during non-invasive mechanical ventilation in patients with chronic obstructive pulmonary disease: a randomized, controlled study. Intensive Care Med. 2001;27:1627–35.
23. Stefan MS, Eckert P, Tiru B, Friderici J, Lindenauer PK, Steingrub JS. High flow nasal oxygen therapy utilization: 7-year experience at a community teaching hospital. Hosp Pract. 2018;46:73–6.
24. Bräunlich J, Wirtz H. Oral versus nasal high-flow bronchodilator inhalation in chronic obstructive pulmonary disease. J Aerosol Med Pulm Drug Deliv. 2018;31:248–54.
25. Mauri T, Turrini C, Eronia N, Grasselli G, Volta CA, Bellani G, et al. Physiologic effects of high-flow nasal cannula in acute hypoxemic respiratory failure. Am J Respir Crit Care Med. 2017;195:1207–15.
26. Dhand R, Duarte AG, Jubran A, Jenne JW, Fink JB, Fahey PJ, et al. Dose response to bronchodilator delivered by metered dose inhaler in ventilator-supported patients. Am J Respir Crit Care Med. 1996;154:388–93.

20

Assessment of fluid responsiveness in spontaneously breathing patients

Renato Carneiro de Freitas Chaves[1*], Thiago Domingos Corrêa[1,2], Ary Serpa Neto[1,3], Bruno de Arruda Bravim[1], Ricardo Luiz Cordioli[1], Fabio Tanzillo Moreira[1], Karina Tavares Timenetsky[1] and Murillo Santucci Cesar de Assunção[1]

Abstract

Patients who increase stoke volume or cardiac index more than 10 or 15% after a fluid challenge are usually considered fluid responders. Assessment of fluid responsiveness prior to volume expansion is critical to avoid fluid overload, which has been associated with poor outcomes. Maneuvers to assess fluid responsiveness are well established in mechanically ventilated patients; however, few studies evaluated maneuvers to predict fluid responsiveness in spontaneously breathing patients. Our objective was to perform a systematic review of literature addressing the available methods to assess fluid responsiveness in spontaneously breathing patients. Studies were identified through electronic literature search of PubMed from 01/08/2009 to 01/08/2016 by two independent authors. No restrictions on language were adopted. Quality of included studies was evaluated with Quality Assessment of Diagnostic Accuracy Studies tool. Our search strategy identified 537 studies, and 9 studies were added through manual search. Of those, 15 studies (12 intensive care unit patients; 1 emergency department patients; 1 intensive care unit and emergency department patients; 1 operating room) were included in this analysis. In total, 649 spontaneously breathing patients were assessed for fluid responsiveness. Of those, 340 (52%) were deemed fluid responsive. Pulse pressure variation during the Valsalva maneuver (ΔPPV) of 52% (AUC $\pm$ SD: 0.98 $\pm$ 0.03) and passive leg raising-induced change in stroke volume (ΔSV-PLR) > 13% (AUC $\pm$ SD: 0.96 $\pm$ 0.03) showed the highest accuracy to predict fluid responsiveness in spontaneously breathing patients. Our systematic review indicates that regardless of the limitations of each maneuver, fluid responsiveness can be assessed in spontaneously breathing patients. Further well-designed studies, with adequate simple size and power, are necessary to confirm the real accuracy of the different methods used to assess fluid responsiveness in this population of patients.

Keywords: Fluid responsiveness, Spontaneously breathing, Echocardiography, Stroke volume, Pulse pressure, Intensive care, Critical care

Background

Intravascular volume expansion is a common intervention in critically ill patients [1]. Patients who will benefit from intravascular volume expansion, i.e., will boost stroke volume (SV) after a volume expansion, have both ventricles in the ascending portion of the Frank–Starling curve, characterizing a preload dependency [1, 2]. Nevertheless, nearly 50% of critically ill patients will not benefit from an intravascular volume expansion [2, 3]. Conversely, an accurate assessment of fluid responsiveness prior to volume expansion is critical to avoid fluid overload, which has been associated with increased morbidity and mortality in critically ill patients [4–6].

The concept of predicting fluid responsiveness was initially reported in deeply sedated patients under volume-controlled mechanical ventilation with tidal volume

*Correspondence: chavesrcf@hotmail.com
[1] Intensive Care Unit, Hospital Israelita Albert Einstein, Av. Albert Einstein, 627/701, 5th Floor, São Paulo, SP 05651-901, Brazil
Full list of author information is available at the end of the article

(VT) of at least 8 ml/Kg and positive end-expiratory pressure (PEEP) lower than 10 cm H_2O [7]. Nonetheless, since many patients in the intensive care unit (ICU) are not under such conditions, for many years the presence of spontaneous breathing or inspiratory efforts, with or without an endotracheal tube, was considered a major limitation to assess fluid responsiveness in critically ill patients [8].

Knowledge on the interaction between heart, lung and abdominal compartment is critical to understanding the concept of fluid responsiveness [9, 10]. In spontaneous breathing patients without mechanical ventilation, intrathoracic pressure decreases, while venous return and stroke volume increases during inspiration [10]. On the other hand, at expiration, intrathoracic pressure increases, while venous return and stroke volume decreases [10]. Thus, quantifying stroke volume variation, between respiratory cycles could be used to assess fluid responsiveness [1].

Static [11, 12] and dynamic [8, 13] parameters have been proposed to assess fluid responsiveness in critically ill patients. The available evidence clearly shows that dynamic parameters exhibited a higher accuracy than static parameters to predict fluid responsiveness [13, 14]. Pulse pressure variation, [15–20] echocardiography maneuvers [21–28] and passive leg raising [18, 21–23, 25, 27, 29] are tools that could be used to assess fluid responsiveness in spontaneously breathing patients.

Thus, our primary objective was to perform a systematic review addressing the available methods for fluid responsiveness assessment in spontaneously breathing patients. A secondary objective was to summarize the performance of available methods to assess fluid responsiveness in spontaneously breathing patients.

Methods

This systematic review was reported following the PRISMA (Preferred Reporting Items for Systematic Reviews and Meta-Analyses) guidelines [30].

Eligibility criteria

Articles were selected for inclusion if they evaluated fluid responsiveness in spontaneous breathing adult patients. Articles were assessed for eligibility if one of the following standard definitions of fluid responsiveness and fluid challenge was adopted: increase in stroke volume (SV) $\geq$ 10% and/or cardiac output (CO) $\geq$ 10% and/or cardiac index (CI) [31] $\geq$ 10% and/or aortic velocity–time integral (VTI) $\geq$ 10% after a fluid challenge [2, 32]. Fluid challenge was considered adequate if at least 250 ml over 30 min of intravenous (I.V.) fluid was infused [2, 33]. Spontaneously breathing was defined as patients without any ventilatory support, patients on noninvasive mechanical ventilation or patients on invasive mechanical ventilation in a spontaneous mode. Patients in the following clinical scenarios were included: ICU, emergency department (ED) and operating room.

Identifying studies

An electronic literature search was carried out by two authors through a computerized blinded search on PubMed. The following search strategy was applied: ((("hemodynamics"[MeSH Terms] OR "hemodynamics"[All Fields]) AND ("respiration"[MeSH Terms] OR "respiration"[All Fields] OR "cell respiration"[MeSH Terms] OR ("cell"[All Fields] AND "respiration"[All Fields]) OR "cell respiration"[All Fields]) AND ("cardiac output"[MeSH Terms] OR ("cardiac"[All Fields] AND "output"[All Fields]) OR "cardiac output"[All Fields]))). Literature search was limited to a period of time (01/08/2009 to 01/08/2016) and to "human." No restrictions on language were adopted. Additionally, we hand-searched the reference lists of the included studies to identify other relevant studies.

Study selection

Prospective studies that reported sensitivity, specificity, cutoff value of each maneuver to assess fluid responsiveness, number of patients included and frequency of fluid responsiveness and non-fluid responsiveness patients were included in this systematic review. Review articles, editorials, studies assessing fluid responsiveness during mechanical ventilation and studies that did not report outcomes of interest were excluded.

Data extraction

Two authors independently screened all retrieved citations by reviewing their titles and abstracts (RCFC and FTM). Then, the reviewers independently evaluated the full-text manuscripts for eligibility using a standardized form. Reviewers independently extracted the relevant data from the full-text manuscripts and assessed the risk of bias using a standardized form. Any disagreement between the authors was resolved by a third author (ASN).

Quality assessment

The quality of each study was evaluated by the Quality Assessment of Diagnostic Accuracy Studies tool (QUADAS) [34]. Details of the quality assessment are reported in Additional file 1.

Primary objective

The primary objective was to report the available methods to assess fluid responsiveness in spontaneously breathing patients.

Secondary objectives

Secondary objectives were to assess diagnostic performance and build a receiver operating characteristics curve (ROC curve) of methods available to assess fluid responsiveness in spontaneously breathing patients.

Methods for fluid responsiveness assessment

Assessed methods to predict fluid responsiveness were pulse pressure variation (ΔPP); [15, 17, 19] systolic pressure variation (ΔSP); [15] ΔPP during forced inspiratory effort (ΔPPf); [15] ΔSP during forced inspiratory effort (ΔSPf); [15] ΔPP during the Valsalva maneuver (ΔPPV); [16] ΔSP during the Valsalva maneuver (ΔVSP); [16] lowest pulse pressure (PPmin); [16] stroke volume variation (ΔSV); [17, 21, 26] passive leg raising (PLR)-induced change in stroke volume (ΔSV-PLR); [18, 23, 29] PLR-induced change in radial pulse pressure (ΔPP-PLR); [18] PLR-induced change in the velocity peak of femoral artery flow (ΔVF-PLR); [18] deep inspiration maneuver-induced change in pulse pressure (ΔPPdim); [19] respiratory change in velocity peak of femoral artery flow (ΔVF); [19] deep inspiration maneuver-induced change in velocity peak of femoral artery flow (ΔVFdim); [19] ΔPP during forced inspiratory breathing (ΔPP_{FB}); [20] PLR-induced change in stroke volume index (SVi-PLR); [21] change in cardiac output (ΔCO); [22] inferior vena cava collapsibility index (cIVC); [24, 26–28] E wave velocity; [24] aortic velocity time index (VTI) variations during PLR (ΔVTI-PLR); [25] VTI $\leq$ 21 cm; [25] aortic velocity variation (AoVV); [26] inferior vena cava maximum diameter (IVCmax); [27] ΔCO between baseline and after PLR (ΔCO-PLR) [27].

Pulse pressure variation was calculated as the difference in pulse pressure maximal (PPmax) and pulse pressure minimal (PPmin) over the respiratory cycle divided by the mean between PPmax and PPmin [$\Delta PP = (PPmax - PPmin)/(PPmax + PPmin)/2$] [16, 19, 20]. Passive leg raising consists in moving the patient from the 45° semirecumbent position to a horizontal position with the lower limbs lifted 30°–45° relative to the trunk [1, 18]. PLR was determined as the difference between baseline and the highest value induced during the PLR or after the PLR [21, 23, 27]. Inferior vena cava collapsibility index represents the difference in the vena cava maximum diameter (IVCmax) and vena cava minimum diameter (IVCmin) divided by the vena cava maximum diameter over the respiratory cycle [$cIVC = (IVCmax - IVCmin)/(IVCmax)$] [26, 27]. Valsalva maneuver consists of sustaining a forced expiration effort against a closed mouth [16]. Forced inspiratory breaths consist of three respiratory cycles of deep inspiration immediately followed by slow passive expiration [20]. Deep inspiration maneuver consists of slow continuous inspiration strain (5–8 s) followed by slow passive exhalation [19].

Statistical analysis

The number of patients included, study design, setting, inclusion and exclusion criteria, time and type of fluid infused, the best cutoff value of each maneuver and definition of fluid responders were extracted from published studies. The accuracy of each diagnostic test was assessed with sensitivity (Sens), specificity (Spec), positive predictive value (PPV), negative predictive value (NPV), positive likelihood ratio (LR +), negative likelihood ratio (LR −), AUC along with its standard deviation (SD) or 95% confidence interval (95% CI). Whenever not reported, accuracy, PPV, NPV, LR + and LR − were calculated using the Review Manager (RevMan) [computer program]—version 5.3—Copenhagen: The Nordic Cochrane Centre, The Cochrane Collaboration, 2014.

A receiver operator characteristics curve (ROC curve) was constructed using the sensitivity and specificity of each maneuver extracted from included study using Meta-DiSc version 1.4 (Universidad Complutense, Madrid, Spain) [35]. Methods for fluid responsiveness assessment were classified according to their accuracy [area under the receiver operating characteristics curve (AUC)]. AUC from 0.90 to 1.00 was considered excellent, from 0.80 to 0.89 adequate, from 0.70 to 0.79 fair, from 0.60 to 0.69 poor and from 0.50 to 0.59 failure [36].

Results

Search results

The initial search strategy identified 537 studies (Fig. 1). After screening the reference lists of the included studies, 9 potentially relevant articles were included and 546 potentially relevant articles were selected. Fifteen prospective studies (649 patients in total) were included in this systematic review after the exclusion of 531 studies

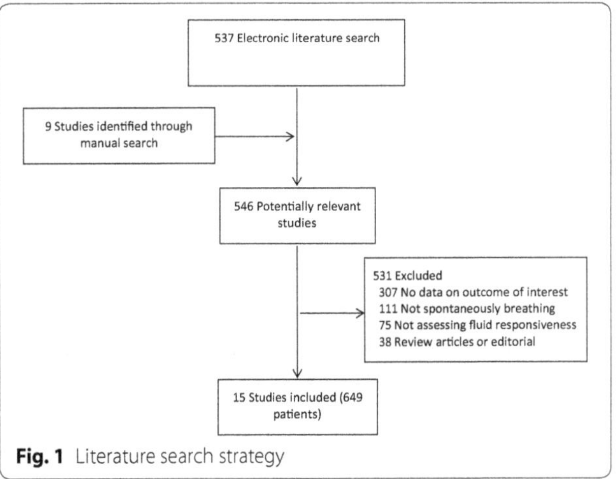

Fig. 1 Literature search strategy

(307 studies had no data on outcome of interest, 111 studies did not regard spontaneously breathing patients, 75 studies did not access fluid responsiveness, and 38 were review articles or editorials) (Fig. 1).

Characteristics of included studies

Characteristics of included studies are presented in Tables 1 [15–20] and 2 [21–29]. Out of fifteen studies included, twelve evaluated fluid responsiveness in ICU patients, [15–19, 21–27] one included ED patients, [29] one included ICU and ED patients [28] and one included operating room patients (elective thoracic surgery) [20] (Tables 1 and 2).

Out of 649 spontaneously breathing patients assessed for fluid responsiveness, 340 patients (52%) were responders. In 12 studies [12/15 (80%)], only spontaneous breathing patients without any type of ventilatory support were included (572 patients) [15, 16, 18–20, 22, 24–29]. Out of those, 51% (291/572) of patients without ventilatory support were considered fluid responsive (Tables 1 and 2). In 3 studies [3/15 (20%)], spontaneous breathing patient without any ventilatory support and patients under mechanical ventilation in a spontaneous mode were included (77 patients) [17, 21, 23]. Of those, 63% (49/77) patients were deemed responsive to a fluid challenge (Tables 1 and 2).

Table 1 Characteristics of included studies addressing pulse pressure variation for fluid responsiveness in spontaneously breathing patients

Author, year	*N*	Setting	Inclusion criteria	Exclusion criteria	Ventilation	Fluid challenge	Definition of responders	Maneuvers
Soubrier, 2007 [15]	32	ICU	1. Low blood pressure 2. Tachycardia 3. Oliguria 4. Mottled skin	1. Arrhythmia 2. Lack of cooperation	SB	500 ml I.V. 6% HES over 20 min	↑CI ≥ 15%	1. ΔPP 2. ΔSP 3. ΔPPf 4. ΔSPf
M. García, 2009 [16]	30	ICU	1. Hypotension 2. Tachycardia 3. Oliguria	1. Arrhythmia 2. History of syncope 3. Lack of cooperation	SB	500 ml I.V. 6% HES over 30 min	↑SVi > 15%	1. ΔPPV by PCA 2. ΔVSP by PCA 3. PPmin
Monnet, 2009 [17]	23	ICU	1. SBP < 90 mmHg 2. Tachycardia 3. UO < 0.5 ml/kg/h 4. Mottled skin	1. Not sustain an inspiration for over 15 seconds	SB and SBmv	500 ml I.V. saline over 10 min	↑CI > 15%	1. ΔPP by PCA 2. ΔSV by PCA
Préau, 2010 [18]	34	ICU	1. SBP < 90 mmHg 2. Tachycardia 3. UO < 0.5 mL/kg/h 4. Mottled skin	1. Arrhythmia 2. Aortic insufficiency 3. VNI was warranted	SB	500 mL I.V. 6% HES over 30 min	↑SV ≥ 15%	1. ΔSV-PLR by TE 2. ΔPP-PLR 3. ΔVF-PLR by Doppler
Préau, 2012 [19]	23	ICU	1. SBP < 90 mmHg 2. Tachycardia 3. Regular cardiac rhythm 4. UO < 0.5 mL/kg/h	1. RR > 30 2 Not sustain an inspiration for over 5 s 3. Aortic insufficiency 4. MV was warranted	SB	500 mL I.V. 6% HES over 30 min	↑SV > 15%	1. ΔPP 2 ΔPPdim 3. ΔVF by Doppler 4. ΔVFdim by Doppler
Hong, 2014 [20]	59	OP	1. Age 18–80 years 2. Elective thoracic surgery	1. Arrhythmia 2. Intracardiac shunt 3. Valvulopathy 4 Cardiac or pulmonary dysfunction	SB	6 ml/kg of I.V. HES for 10 min	↑CI ≥ 15%	1. ΔPP_{FB} by PCA

ICU intensive care unit, *OP* operating room, *SBP* systolic blood pressure, *UO* urine output, *VNI* ventilation noninvasive, *RR* respiratory rate, *MV* mechanical ventilation, *COPD* chronic obstructive pulmonary disease, *SB* spontaneous breathing without any ventilatory support, *SBmv* mechanical ventilation during spontaneous mode, *I.V.* intravenous, *HES* hydroxyethyl starch, ↑ = increase, *CI* cardiac index, *SV* stroke volume, *ΔPP* pulse pressure variation, *ΔSP* systolic pressure variation, *ΔPPf* ΔPP during forced inspiratory effort, *ΔSPf* ΔSP during forced inspiratory effort, *ΔPPV* ΔPP during the Valsalva maneuver, *PCA* pulse contour analysis, *ΔVSP* ΔSP during the Valsalva maneuver, *PPmin* lowest pulse pressure, *ΔSV* stroke volume variation, *PLR* passive leg raising, *ΔSV-PLR* PLR-induced change in stroke volume, *ΔPP-PLR* PLR-induced change in radial pulse pressure, *ΔVF-PLR* PLR-induced change in the velocity peak of femoral artery flow, *ΔPPdim* deep inspiration maneuver-induced change in pulse pressure, *ΔVF* respiratory change in velocity peak of femoral artery flow, *ΔVFdim* deep inspiration maneuver-induced change in velocity peak of femoral artery flow, ΔPP_{FB} ΔPP during forced inspiratory breathing

Table 2 Characteristics of included studies addressing echocardiography maneuvers, pulse contour analysis or noninvasive cardiac output monitor (NICOM®) for fluid responsiveness in spontaneously breathing patients

Author, year	N	Setting	Inclusion criteria	Exclusion criteria	Ventilation	Fluid challenge	Definition of responders	Maneuvers
Lamia, 2007 [21]	24	ICU	1. MAP < 60 mmHg 2. Tachycardia 3. UO < 0.5 ml/kg/h 4. Delayed CRT	1. Aortic valvulopathy 2. Mitral insufficiency or stenosis	SB and SBmv	500 ml I.V. saline for 15 min	↑SVi ≥ 15%	1. SVi-PLR by TE
Maizel, 2007 [22]	34	ICU	1. Hypotension 2. Acute renal failure 3. Dehydration	1. Hemorrhage 2. PLR contraindications 3. Arrhythmia	SB	500 ml I.V. saline over 15 min	↑CO ≥ 12%	1. ΔCO-PLR by TE 2. ΔSV-PLR by TE
Biais, 2009 [23]	30	ICU	1. SBP < 90 mmHg 2. Tachycardia 3. Acute renal failure 4 Mottled skin	1. ↑ intra-abdominal pressure 2. BMI < 15 or > 40 kg/m2 3. Valvulopathy 4 Intracardiac shunt	SB and SBmv	500 ml I.V. saline for 15 min	↑SV > 15%	1. $\Delta SV\text{-}PLR_{TE}$ by TE 2. $\Delta SV\text{-}PLR_{FloT}$ by PCA
Muller, 2012 [24]	40	ICU	1. MAP < 65 mmHg 2. Tachycardia 3. UO < 0.5 mL/Kg/h 4. Mottled skin	1. Pulmonary edema 2. Right ventricular failure 3. Elevated left atrial pressure	SB	500 mL I.V. 6% HES over 15 min	↑VTI ≥ 15%	1. cIVC by TE 2. E wave velocity by TE
Brun, 2013 [25]	23	ICU	1. Severe preeclampsia	1. Cardiac or renal disorders prior to pregnancy	SB	500 ml I.V. saline over 15 min	↑SVi ≥ 15%	1. ΔVTI-PLR 2. VTI
Lanspa, 2013 [26]	14	ICU	1. Age ≥ 14 years 2. Infection and SIRS 3. Refractory hypotension	1. Pregnancy 2. Aortic stenosis 3. Arrhythmia 4. COPD and asthma	SB	10 mL/kg of I.V. crystalloids over 20 min	↑CI ≥ 15%	1. cIVC by TE 2. ΔSV by PCA 3. AoVV by TE
Airapetian, 2015 [27]	59	ICU	1. Physician decided to perform fluid expansion	1. Hemorrhage 2. Arrhythmia 3. Compression stockings 4. PLR contraindications	SB	PLR and 500 ml I.V. saline over 15 min	↑CO ≥ 10%	1. cIVC by TE 2. IVCmax by TE 3. ΔCO-PLR by TE
Duus, 2015 [29]	100	ED	1. Age ≥ 18 years 2. Clinical team intended to administer IV fluid	1. Acuity precluding participation in research 2 PLR contraindications	SB	5 ml/kg I.V. saline	↑SV > 10%	1. ΔSV-PLR using NICOM®
Corl, 2017 [28]	124	ED and ICU	1. PAS < 90 mmHg 2. Tachycardia 3. UO < 0.5 ml/kg/h 4. Hypoperfusion	1. Cardiogenic, obstructive or neurogenic shock 2. Age < 18 years 3. Hospitalization for > 36 h	SB	500 ml I.V. saline	↑CI ≥ 10%	1. cIVC by TE

ICU intensive care unit, *ED* emergency department, *MAP* mean arterial pressure, *UO* urine output, *CRT* capillary refill time, *SBP* systolic blood pressure, *PLR* passive leg raising, ↑ = increase, *BMI* body mass index, *COPD* chronic obstructive pulmonary disease, *SB* spontaneous breathing without any ventilatory support, *SBmv* mechanical ventilation during spontaneous mode, *I.V.* intravenous, *HES* hydroxyethyl starch, *SV* stroke volume, *CO* cardiac output, *VTI* aortic velocity–time integral, *SVi* stroke volume index, *CI* cardiac index, *PLR* passive leg raising, *SVi-PLR* PLR-induced change in stroke volume index, *TE* transthoracic echocardiography, *ΔCO* change in cardiac output, *ΔCO-PLR* ΔCO between baseline and after PLR, *ΔSV* stroke volume variation, *ΔSV-PLR* PLR-induced change in stroke volume, *FloT* FloTrac™, *PCA* pulse contour analysis, *cIVC* inferior vena cava collapsibility index, *VTI* aortic velocity–time integral, *ΔVTI-PLR* VTI variations during PLR, *AoVV* aortic velocity variation, *NICOM®* noninvasive cardiac output monitor, *IVCmax* inferior vena cava maximum diameter

Fluid challenge characteristics

Fluid challenge was performed in seven (46.6%) studies through an I.V. infusion of 500 ml of saline; [17, 21–23, 25, 27, 28] five studies (33.3%) with 500 ml of hydroxyethyl starch (HES); [15, 16, 18, 19, 24] one (6.7%) study with 6 ml/kg of HES; [20] one (6.7%) study applied 10 mL/kg of crystalloid; [26] and one (6.7%) study used 5 ml/kg saline [29] (Tables 1 and 2).

Adopted definitions of fluid responsiveness were an increase in SV > 10% [29] or > 15%; [18, 19, 23] an increase in stroke volume index (SVi) ≥ 15%; [16, 21, 25] an increase in CI ≥ 10% [28] or ≥ 15%; [15, 17, 20, 26] an increase in CO ≥ 10% [27] or 12% [22] or an VTI ≥ 15% [24] (Tables 1 and 2). The triggers for intravascular volume expansion varied across the studies and are presented in Tables 1 and 2.

Methods for fluid responsiveness assessment

Thirty-four maneuvers for predicting fluid responsiveness in spontaneously breathing patients were reported (Tables 1 and 2). Studies that adopted pulse pressure variation to assess fluid responsiveness are summarized in Table 1. Studies that adopted echocardiography maneuvers, pulse contour analysis or noninvasive cardiac output monitor (NICOM®) are summarized in Table 2.

Performance of maneuvers for predicting fluid responsiveness

Pooled analysis (15 studies; 649 patients)

Out of 34 reported maneuvers for predicting fluid responsiveness in spontaneously breathing patients, 13 (38%) maneuvers had excellent accuracy (AUC from 0.9 to 1), 9 (26%) had adequate accuracy (AUC from 0.8 to 0.89), 6 (18%) had fair accuracy (AUC from 0.7 to 0.79), 5 (15%) had poor accuracy (AUC from 0.6 to 0.69) and 1 maneuver (3%) was classified as failure (AUC from 0.5 to 0.59) (Fig. 2) (Tables 3 and 4).

ΔPPV of 52% (AUC ± SD: 0.98 ± 0.03), [16] ΔSV-PLR > 13% (AUC ± SD: 0.96 ± 0.03), [23] ΔPPdim ≥ 12% (AUC ± SD: 0.95 ± 0.05), [19] ΔVFdim ≥ 12% (AUC ± SD: 0.95 ± 0.05) [19] and ΔSV-PLR ≥ 10% (AUC ± SD: 0.94 ± 0.04) [18] showed the highest accuracy to predict fluid responsiveness in spontaneously breathing patients (Fig. 2) (Tables 3 and 4). AoVV ≥ 25% [AUC (95% CI): 0.67 (0.32–1.00)], [26] cIVC > 42% [AUC (95% CI): 0.62 (0.66–0.88)], [27] IVCmax at baseline < 2.1 cm [AUC (95% CI): 0.07 (0.49–0.75)] [27] and ΔSV ≥ 10% [AUC (95% CI): 0.57(0.34-0.78) [17] showed the worst values of accuracy to predict fluid responsiveness (Fig. 2) (Tables 3 and 4).

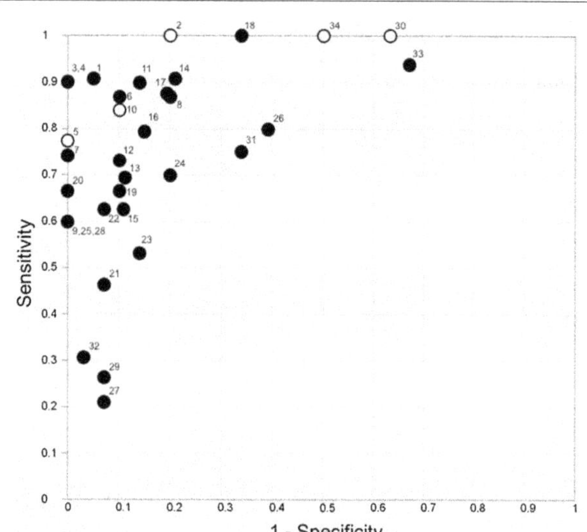

Fig. 2 Receiver operating characteristics curve with all methods found in the literature search of assessment volume responsiveness in spontaneous breathing patients. Closed circles represent studies including spontaneous breathing patients without ventilator support; open circles represent studies including patients under mechanical ventilation during spontaneous mode and spontaneous breathing without ventilator support. 1 = ΔPPV of 52%; 2 = ΔSV-PLR$_{TTE}$ >13%; 3 = ΔPPdim ≥12%; 4 = ΔVFdim ≥12%; 5 = SVi-PLR ≥12.5%; 6 = ΔSV-PLR ≥10%; 7 = ΔVTI-PLR >12%; 8 = ΔVF-PLR ≥8%; 9 = ΔSV ≥17%; 10 = ΔSV-PLR$_{FloT}$ >16%; 11 = ΔPP$_{FB}$ = 13.7%; 12 = ΔVSP of 30%; 13 = ΔSV >12%; 14 = PPmin of 45mmHg; 15 = ΔCO >12%; 16 = ΔPP-PLR ≥9%; 17 = cIVC of 25%; 18 = cIVC ≥15%; 19 = E wave velocity of 0.7; 20 = VTI ≤21cm; 21 = ΔSP of 9%; 22 = ΔPP of 12%; 23 = ΔCO-PLR >10%; 24 = cIVC =40%; 25 = ΔVF ≥10%; 26 = ΔSV-PLR; 27 = ΔPPf of 33%; 28 = ΔPP ≥10%; 29 = ΔSPf of 30%; 30 = ΔPP ≥11%; 31 = AoVV ≥25%; 32 = cIVC >42%, 33 = IVCmax <2.1cm, 34 = ΔSV≥10%

Spontaneous breathing patients without ventilatory support

ΔVSP of 52% [AUC ± SD: 0.98 ± 0.03] [16] had the highest accuracy and cIVC > 42% [AUC (95% CI): 0.62 (0.66–0.88)] and IVCmax < 2.1 cm [AUC (95% CI) 0.62 (0.49–0.75)] the worst accuracy to predict fluid responsiveness in spontaneous breathing patients without ventilatory support (12 studies totaling 572 patients) (Additional file 1: Figure S1).

Spontaneous breathing with ventilatory support

ΔSV-PLR$_{TE}$ > 13% [AUC ± SD: 0.96 ± 0.03] had the highest accuracy, while ΔSV ≥ 10% [AUC (95% CI) 0.57(0.34–0.78)] had the worst accuracy to predict fluid responsiveness in mechanically ventilated patients in a spontaneous mode (3 studies totaling 77 patients) (Additional file 1: Figure S2).

Table 3 Performance of included studies that addressed pulse pressure variation to predict fluid responsiveness in spontaneously breathing patients

Author, Year	Maneuver	Sens (%)	Spec (%)	PPV (%)	NPV (%)	LR +	LR−	AUC ± SD or (95% CI)
Soubrier, 2007 [15]	ΔPP of 12%	63	92	92	63	8.20	0.39	0.81. ± 0.08
	ΔSP of 9%	47	92	90	54	6.15	0.57	0.82 ± 0.08
	ΔPPf of 33%	21	92	80	44	3.01	0.85	0.72 ± 0.09
	ΔSPf of 30%	26	92	83	46	3.75	0.80	0.69 ± 0.10
M. García, 2009 [16]	ΔPPV of 52%	91	95	91	95	17,3	0.01	0.98 ± 0.03
	ΔVSP of 30%	73	90	80	85	6.91	0.30	0.90 ± 0.07
	PPmin of 45 mmHg	91	79	71	94	4.32	0.12	0.89 ± 0.06
Monnet, 2009 [17]	ΔPP ≥ 11%	100	37	80	100	1.75		0.68 (0.45–0.88)
	ΔSV ≥ 10%	100	50	84	100	2.00		0.57 (0.34–0.78)
Préau, 2010 [18]	ΔSV-PLR ≥ 10%	86	90	86	90	8.57	0.16	0.94 ± 0.04
	ΔPP-PLR ≥ 9%	79	85	79	85	5.24	0.25	0.86 ± 0.08
	ΔVF-PLR ≥ 8%	86	80	75	89	4.29	0.18	0.93 ± 0.04
Préau, 2012 [19]	ΔPP ≥ 10%	60	100	100	76		0.40	0.71. ± 0.12
	ΔPPdim ≥ 12%	90	100	100	93		0.10	0.95 ± 0.05
	ΔVF ≥ 10%	60	100	100	76		0.40	0.74 ± 0.11
	ΔVFdim ≥ 12%	90	100	100	93		0.10	0.95 ± 0.05
Hong, 2014 [20]	ΔPP_{FB} = 13.7%	90	87	87	90	6.72	0.12	0.91 (0.80–0.96)

Sens sensitivity, *Spec* specificity, *PPV* positive predictive value, *NPV* negative predictive value, *LR +* positive likelihood ratio, *LR −* negative likelihood ratio, *AUC* area under the receiver operating characteristics curve, *SD* standard deviation, *95% CI* 95% confidence intervals, *ΔPP* pulse pressure variation, *ΔSP* systolic pressure variation, *ΔPPf* ΔPP during forced inspiratory effort, *ΔSPf* ΔSP during forced inspiratory effort, *ΔPPV* ΔPP during the Valsalva maneuver, *ΔVSP* ΔSP during the Valsalva maneuver, *PPmin* lowest pulse pressure, *PLR* passive leg raising, *ΔSV-PLR* PLR-induced change in stroke volume, *ΔPP-PLR* PLR-induced change in radial pulse pressure, *ΔVF-PLR* PLR-induced change in the velocity peak of femoral artery flow, *ΔPPdim* deep inspiration maneuver-induced change in pulse pressure, *ΔVF* respiratory change in velocity peak of femoral artery flow, *ΔVFdim* deep inspiration maneuver-induced change in velocity peak of femoral artery flow, *ΔPP_{FB}* ΔPP during forced inspiratory breathing

Table 4 Performance of included studies that addressed echocardiography maneuvers, pulse contour analysis or noninvasive cardiac output monitor (NICOM®) to predict fluid responsiveness in spontaneously breathing patients

Author, year	Maneuver	Sens (%)	Spec (%)	PPV (%)	NPV (%)	LR+	LR−	AUC ± SD or (95% CI)
Lamia, 2007 [21]	SVi-PLR ≥ 12.5%	77	100	100	78		0.23	0.95 ± 0.04
Maizel, 2007 [22]	ΔCO > 12%	63	89	83	73	6.00	0.40	0.89 ± 0.06
	ΔSV > 12%	69	89	85	76	6.00	0.40	0.90 ± 0.06
Biais, 2009 [23]	$\Delta SV\text{-}PLR_{TE}$ > 13%	100	80	91	100	5.00		0.96 ± 0.03
	$\Delta SV\text{-}PLR_{FloT}$ > 16%	85	90	94	75	8.50	0.17	0.92 ± 0.05
Muller, 2012 [24]	cIVC = 40%	70	80	72	83	3.50	0.37	0.77 (0.60–0.88)
	E wave velocity of 0.7	67	90	84	83	6.67	0.37	0.83 (0.68–0.93)
Brun, 2013 [25]	ΔVTI-PLR > 12%	75	100	100	79		0.25	0.93 (0.83–1.00)
	VTI ≤ 21 cm	67	100	100	75		0.33	0.82 (0.64–1.00)
Lanspa, 2013 [26]	cIVC ≥ 15%	100	67	62	100	3.00		0.83 (0.58–1.00)
	ΔSV ≥ 17%	60	100	100	82		0.40	0.92 (0.73–1.00)
	AoVV ≥ 25%	75	67	50	85	2.25	0.37	0.67 (0.32–1.00)
Airapetian, 2015 [27]	cIVC > 42%	31	97	90	60	9.31	0.71	0.62 (0.66–0.88)
	IVCmax < 2.1 cm	93	33	57	83	1.40	0.21	0.62 (0.49–0.75)
	ΔCO-PLR > 10%	52	87	79	65	3.88	0.56	0.78 (0.66–0.88)
Duus, 2015 [29]	ΔSV-PLR	80	61	79	65	2.09	0.31	0.74 (0.65–0.83)
Corl, 2017 [28]	cIVC of 25%	87	81	81	87	4.56	0.16	0.84 (0.77–0.90)

Sens sensitivity, *Spec* specificity, *PPV* positive predictive value, *NPV* negative predictive value, *LR +* positive likelihood ratio, *LR −* negative likelihood ratio, *AUC* area under the receiver operating characteristics curve, *SD* standard deviation, *95% CI* 95% confidence intervals, *PLR* passive leg raising, *SVi-PLR* PLR-induced change in stroke volume index, *ΔCO* change in cardiac output, *ΔSV* stroke volume variation, *TE* transthoracic echocardiography, *FloT* FloTrac™, *cIVC* inferior vena cava collapsibility index, *VTI* aortic velocity–time integral, *ΔVTI-PLR* VTI variations during PLR, *AoVV* aortic velocity variation, *IVCmax* inferior vena cava maximum diameter, *ΔCO-PLR* change in cardiac output between baseline and after PLR

Discussion

The main finding of this systematic review is that, regardless of intrinsic limitations of each reported maneuver, fluid responsiveness can be assessed in spontaneously breathing patients with acceptable accuracy. Approximately two-thirds (19/29) of reported maneuvers were deemed adequate or excellent to predict fluid responsiveness in spontaneous breathing patients without ventilatory support and 60% (3/5) were deemed excellent in mechanically ventilated patients in a spontaneous mode. Moreover, approximately half of the patients included in this study were not fluid responsive. This finding reinforces the importance of assessing fluid responsiveness in critically ill patients prior to intravascular volume expansion, thus avoiding unnecessary exposure to additional fluids.

In patients with an invasive arterial line in place, dynamic parameters such as ΔPP in association with a maneuver that magnifies cyclic changes in intrathoracic pressures, i.e., deep inspiration or forced inspiratory breathing, represent important tools to assess fluid responsiveness continuously and with minimal inter-rater variability. [19, 20] Echocardiographic maneuvers such as ΔVF, ΔSV, cIVC represent important tools to assess fluid responsiveness in patients without availability of an invasive arterial line [19, 21, 23, 28]. Although it is operator-dependent, echocardiographic is a noninvasive technique that enables fluid responsiveness assessment with good accuracy in spontaneously breathing patients [19, 21, 23, 28]. The main disadvantages of echocardiographic measurements are non-continuous monitoring and high inter-rater variability [18, 24, 27].

Reversible and noninvasive maneuvers that magnify cyclic changes in intrathoracic pressures and on transpulmonary pressure, such as Valsalva or deep inspiration maneuver, in association with ΔPP or echocardiographic measurements, improve the accuracy of the maneuvers without adverse effects, allowing clinicians at the bedside to assess preload dependency [16, 19]. Nevertheless, it is important to emphasize that all reported methods to assess fluid responsiveness in spontaneously breathing patients have limitations [13, 14]. The need of patients cooperation, inability to sustain deep inspiration, presence of pain, intra-abdominal hypertension, major abdominal surgery, low diaphragm strength, higher respiratory rate, low reproducibility and lack of external validation are frequently reported limitations of available methods [16].

Furthermore, transforming a continuous diagnostic index, such as ΔPP and ΔSV, into binary variables (i.e., responders or non-responders) represents an important limitation of all methods to assess fluid responsiveness [37]. The decision of whether to support or avoid volume expansion in patients with intermediate values of continuous diagnostic index could be imprecise (gray zone) [37]. These patients may benefit from a reversible maneuver, such as PLR prior volume expansion to avoid unnecessary exposure to fluids [37].

Our study has limitations. First, it is important to emphasize that the results of this systematic review should be interpreted in the context of the included studies. Furthermore, studies with small sample size, carried out in different clinical scenarios and with a heterogeneous methodology, were included in this systematic review. Finally, systematic reviews are subject to publication bias, which may exaggerate the conclusion of the study if publication is related to the strengths of the results.

Conclusion

In conclusion, our systematic review suggests that regardless of the limitations of each maneuver, fluid responsiveness could be assessed in spontaneously breathing patients. Further research with adequate sample size and power are necessary to confirm the real accuracy of the different methods available to assess fluid responsiveness in this population of critically ill patients.

Abbreviations

95% CI: 95% confidence interval; ΔCO: change in cardiac output; ΔCO-PLR: change in cardiac output between baseline and after PLR; ΔPP: pulse pressure variation; ΔPPdim: deep inspiration maneuver-induced change in pulse pressure; ΔPP-PLR: PLR-induced change in radial pulse pressure; ΔPPf: ΔPP during forced inspiratory effort; ΔPP_{FB}: ΔPP during forced inspiratory breathing; ΔPPV: ΔPP during the Valsalva maneuver; ΔSP: systolic pressure variation; ΔSPf: ΔSP during forced inspiratory effort; ΔVSP: ΔSP during the Valsalva maneuver; ΔSV: stroke volume variation; ΔSV-PLR: passive leg raising-induced change in stroke volume; ΔVF: respiratory change in velocity peak of femoral artery flow; ΔVFdim: deep inspiration maneuver-induced change in velocity peak of femoral artery flow; ΔVF-PLR: PLR-induced change in the velocity peak of femoral artery flow; ΔVTI-PLR: VTI variations during PLR; AoVV: aortic velocity variation; AUC: area under the receiver operating characteristics curve; CI: cardiac index; cIVC: inferior vena cava collapsibility index; CO: cardiac output; CVP: central venous pressure; ED: emergency department; HES: hydroxyethyl starch; I.V.: intravenous; ICU: intensive care unit; ITBVI: intrathoracic blood volume index; IVCmax: inferior vena cava maximum diameter; IVCmin: vena cava minimum diameters; LR −: negative likelihood ratio; LR +: positive likelihood ratio; NICOM®: noninvasive cardiac output monitor; NPV: negative predictive value; PEEP: positive end-expiratory pressure; PLR: passive leg raising; PPmax: pulse pressure maximal; PPmin: lowest pulse pressure; PPV: positive predictive value; ROC curve: receiver operating characteristics curve; SD: standard deviation; Sens: sensitivity; Spec: specificity; SV: stroke volume; SVi: stroke volume index; SVi-PLR: PLR-induced change in stroke volume index; VTI: aortic velocity–time integral.

Authors' contributions

RCFC and MSCS conceived the study hypothesis and design. RCFC and FTM identified studies through electronic literature search. RCFC and TDC made the first manuscript draft. RCFC, TDC, ASN, BAB, RLC, FTM, KTT and MSCS critically revised the manuscript for important intellectual content. All authors approved the final manuscript and assumed responsibility for the integrity of the data and the accuracy of the data analysis. All authors read and approved the final manuscript.

Author details
[1] Intensive Care Unit, Hospital Israelita Albert Einstein, Av. Albert Einstein, 627/701, 5th Floor, São Paulo, SP 05651-901, Brazil. [2] Intensive Care Unit, Hospital Municipal Dr. Moysés Deutsch - M'Boi Mirim, São Paulo, SP, Brazil. [3] Department of Intensive Care, Academic Medical Center, University of Amsterdam, Amsterdam, The Netherlands.

Acknowledgements
We thank Helena Spalic for proofreading this manuscript. The work was performed in the intensive care unit of Hospital Israelita Albert Einstein.

Competing interests
The authors declare that they have no competing interests.

Funding
This research did not receive any specific grant from funding agencies in the public, commercial or not-for-profit sectors.

References

1. Monnet X, Teboul JL. Assessment of volume responsiveness during mechanical ventilation: recent advances. Crit Care. 2013;17(2):217.
2. Michard F, Teboul JL. Predicting fluid responsiveness in ICU patients: a critical analysis of the evidence. Chest. 2002;121(6):2000–8.
3. Cecconi M, Hofer C, Teboul JL, Pettila V, et al. Fluid challenges in intensive care: the FENICE study: a global inception cohort study. Intensive Care Med. 2015;41(9):1529–37.
4. Vincent JL, Sakr Y, Sprung CL, Ranieri VM, et al. Sepsis in European intensive care units: results of the SOAP study. Crit Care Med. 2006;34(2):344–53.
5. Payen D, de Pont AC, Sakr Y, Spies C, et al. A positive fluid balance is associated with a worse outcome in patients with acute renal failure. Crit Care. 2008;12(3):R74.
6. Sakr Y, Rubatto Birri PN, Kotfis K, Nanchal R, et al. Higher fluid balance increases the risk of death from sepsis: results from a large international audit. Crit Care Med. 2017;45(3):386–94.
7. Michard F, Boussat S, Chemla D, Anguel N, et al. Relation between respiratory changes in arterial pulse pressure and fluid responsiveness in septic patients with acute circulatory failure. Am J Respir Crit Care Med. 2000;162(1):134–8.
8. Yang X, Du B. Does pulse pressure variation predict fluid responsiveness in critically ill patients? A systematic review and meta-analysis. Crit Care. 2014;18(6):650.
9. Takata M, Wise RA, Robotham JL. Effects of abdominal pressure on venous return: abdominal vascular zone conditions. J Appl Physiol. 1990;69(6):1961–72.
10. Pinsky MR. Heart-lung interactions. Curr Opin Crit Care. 2007;13(5):528–31.
11. Muller L, Louart G, Bengler C, Fabbro-Peray P, et al. The intrathoracic blood volume index as an indicator of fluid responsiveness in critically ill patients with acute circulatory failure: a comparison with central venous pressure. Anesth Analg. 2008;107(2):607–13.
12. Eskesen TG, Wetterslev M, Perner A. Systematic review including re-analyses of 1148 individual data sets of central venous pressure as a predictor of fluid responsiveness. Intensive Care Med. 2016;42(3):324–32.
13. Cherpanath TG, Hirsch A, Geerts BF, Lagrand WK, et al. Predicting fluid responsiveness by passive leg raising: a systematic review and meta-analysis of 23 clinical trials. Crit Care Med. 2016;44(5):981–91.
14. Monnet X, Marik PE, Teboul JL. Prediction of fluid responsiveness: an update. Ann Intensive Care. 2016;6:111.
15. Soubrier S, Saulnier F, Hubert H, Delour P, et al. Can dynamic indicators help the prediction of fluid responsiveness in spontaneously breathing critically ill patients? Intensive Care Med. 2007;33(7):1117–24.
16. Monge García MI, Gil Cano A, Diaz Monrove JC. Arterial pressure changes during the Valsalva maneuver to predict fluid responsiveness in spontaneously breathing patients. Intensive Care Med. 2009;35(1):77–84.
17. Monnet X, Osman D, Ridel C, Lamia B, et al. Predicting volume responsiveness by using the end-expiratory occlusion in mechanically ventilated intensive care unit patients. Crit Care Med. 2009;37(3):951–6.
18. Preau S, Saulnier F, Dewavrin F, Durocher A, Chagnon JL. Passive leg raising is predictive of fluid responsiveness in spontaneously breathing patients with severe sepsis or acute pancreatitis. Crit Care Med. 2010;38(3):819–25.
19. Preau S, Dewavrin F, Soland V, Bortolotti P, et al. Hemodynamic changes during a deep inspiration maneuver predict fluid responsiveness in spontaneously breathing patients. Cardiol Res Pract. 2012;2012:191807.
20. Hong DM, Lee JM, Seo JH, Min JJ, et al. Pulse pressure variation to predict fluid responsiveness in spontaneously breathing patients: tidal vs. forced inspiratory breathing. Anaesthesia. 2014;69(7):717–22.
21. Lamia B, Ochagavia A, Monnet X, Chemla D, et al. Echocardiographic prediction of volume responsiveness in critically ill patients with spontaneously breathing activity. Intensive Care Med. 2007;33(7):1125–32.
22. Maizel J, Airapetian N, Lorne E, Tribouilloy C, et al. Diagnosis of central hypovolemia by using passive leg raising. Intensive Care Med. 2007;33(7):1133–8.
23. Biais M, Vidil L, Sarrabay P, Cottenceau V, et al. Changes in stroke volume induced by passive leg raising in spontaneously breathing patients: comparison between echocardiography and Vigileo/FloTrac device. Crit Care. 2009;13(6):R195.
24. Muller L, Bobbia X, Toumi M, Louart G, et al. Respiratory variations of inferior vena cava diameter to predict fluid responsiveness in spontaneously breathing patients with acute circulatory failure: need for a cautious use. Crit Care. 2012;16(5):R188.
25. Brun C, Zieleskiewicz L, Textoris J, Muller L, et al. Prediction of fluid responsiveness in severe preeclamptic patients with oliguria. Intensive Care Med. 2013;39(4):593–600.
26. Lanspa MJ, Grissom CK, Hirshberg EL, Jones JP, et al. Applying dynamic parameters to predict hemodynamic response to volume expansion in spontaneously breathing patients with septic shock. Shock. 2013;39(2):155–60.
27. Airapetian N, Maizel J, Alyamani O, Mahjoub Y, et al. Does inferior vena cava respiratory variability predict fluid responsiveness in spontaneously breathing patients? Crit Care. 2015;19:400.
28. Corl KA, George NR, Romanoff J, Levinson AT, et al. Inferior vena cava collapsibility detects fluid responsiveness among spontaneously breathing critically-ill patients. J Crit Care. 2017;41:130–7.
29. Duus N, Shogilev DJ, Skibsted S, Zijlstra HW, et al. The reliability and validity of passive leg raise and fluid bolus to assess fluid responsiveness in spontaneously breathing emergency department patients. J Crit Care. 2015;30(1):217.e1-5.
30. Stewart LA, Clarke M, Rovers M, Riley RD, et al. Preferred reporting items for systematic review and meta-analyses of individual participant data: the PRISMA-IPD statement. JAMA. 2015;313(16):1657–65.
31. Zarychanski R, Abou-Setta AM, Turgeon AF, Houston BL, et al. Association of hydroxyethyl starch administration with mortality and acute kidney injury in critically ill patients requiring volume resuscitation: a systematic review and meta-analysis. JAMA. 2013;309(7):678–88.
32. Zhang Z, Xu X, Ye S, Xu L. Ultrasonographic measurement of the respiratory variation in the inferior vena cava diameter is predictive of fluid responsiveness in critically ill patients: systematic review and meta-analysis. Ultrasound Med Biol. 2014;40(5):845–53.
33. Aya HD, Ster IC, Fletcher N, Grounds RM, et al. Pharmacodynamic analysis of a fluid challenge. Crit Care Med. 2016;44(5):880–91.

34. Whiting P, Rutjes AW, Reitsma JB, Bossuyt PM, et al. The development of QUADAS: a tool for the quality assessment of studies of diagnostic accuracy included in systematic reviews. BMC Med Res Methodol. 2003;3:25.
35. Zamora J, Abraira V, Muriel A, Khan K, et al. Meta-DiSc: a software for meta-analysis of test accuracy data. BMC Med Res Methodol. 2006;6:31.
36. Marik PE, Baram M, Vahid B. Does central venous pressure predict fluid responsiveness? A systematic review of the literature and the tale of seven mares. Chest. 2008;134(1):172–8.
37. Cannesson M. The "grey zone" or how to avoid the binary constraint of decision-making. Can J Anesth/J Can Anesth. 2015;62:1139–42.

21

Effect of high-frequency oscillatory ventilation on esophageal and transpulmonary pressures in moderate-to-severe acute respiratory distress syndrome

Christophe Guervilly[1*], Jean-Marie Forel[1], Sami Hraiech[1], Antoine Roch[1,2], Daniel Talmor[3] and Laurent Papazian[1]

Abstract

Background: High-frequency oscillatory ventilation (HFOV) has not been shown to be beneficial in the management of moderate-to-severe acute respiratory distress syndrome (ARDS). There is uncertainty about the actual pressure applied into the lung during HFOV. We therefore performed a study to compare the transpulmonary pressure (P_L) during conventional mechanical ventilation (CMV) and different levels of mean airway pressure (mPaw) during HFOV.

Methods: This is a prospective randomized crossover study in a university teaching hospital. An esophageal balloon catheter was used to measure esophageal pressures (Pes) at end inspiration and end expiration and to calculate P_L. Measurements were taken during ventilation with CMV (CMVpre) after which patients were switched to HFOV with three 1-h different levels of mPaw set at +5, +10 and +15 cm H_2O above the mean airway pressure measured during CMV. Patients were thereafter switched back to CMV (CMVpost).

Results: Ten patients with moderate-to-severe ARDS were included. We demonstrated a linear increase in Pes and P_L with the increase in mPaw during HFOV. Contrary to CMV, P_L was always positive during HFOV whatever the level of mPaw applied but not associated with improvement in oxygenation. We found significant correlations between mPaw and Pes.

Conclusion: HFOV with high level of mPaw increases transpulmonary pressures without improvement in oxygenation.

Background

Moderate or severe acute respiratory distress syndrome (ARDS) [1] is associated with substantial mortality. Use of a lung-protective strategy with low tidal volume (V_t) of 6 ml/kg of predicted body weight has been associated with improved outcomes [2]. High-frequency oscillatory ventilation (HFOV) is a non-conventional mode which has been proposed to achieve the targets of protective ventilation with very low V_t [3] and a greater alveolar stability due to relatively constant mean airway pressure (mPaw) [4]. However, two large recently published randomized clinical trials, OSCAR [5] and OSCILLATE [6], failed to prove any clinical benefit when HFOV was applied in adults with moderate-to-severe ARDS as compared with a strategy with low tidal volume, high positive expiratory pressure (PEEP) and limited plateau pressure (Pplat). In the latter study, side effects of HFOV were observed with more requirements for vasopressors, likely due to right ventricular failure secondary to high mPaw used [7, 8].

Another possible explanation of the lack of clinical benefit with HFOV in adults with ARDS may be due to the occurrence of pulmonary overdistension in non-dependant areas of the lung [9]. Because mPaw during HFOV does not reflect of the real pressure applied to the

*Correspondence: christophe.guervilly@ap-hm.fr
[1] Aix-Marseille Univ, APHM, URMITE UMR CNRS 7278, Hôpital Nord, Réanimation des Détresses Respiratoires et Infections Sévères, Marseille, France
Full list of author information is available at the end of the article

alveoli [10], with non-predictable attenuation all along the trachea–bronchial tree, it is not possible to know the true pulmonary distending pressure. Esophageal pressure (Pes) is an approximation of the pleural pressure, and its use has shown a possible clinical benefit when PEEP was set according to the value of Pes in moderate-to-severe ARDS [11]. Esophageal pressure measurement allows the calculation of the maximal and minimal transpulmonary pressures (P_L) applied during mechanical ventilation. Data reporting P_L during HFOV are scarce [12] and only describe the feasibility of the technique but not the comparison of range of P_L occurring during the switch from CMV to an HFOV trial. Therefore, we performed a prospective study of P_L determination in moderate-to-severe ARDS during and after an HFOV trial.

Methods

This is an ancillary study of a previously published study [7].

Patients

The study was approved by the ethics committee of the Marseille University Hospital (Comité de Protection des Personnes Sud Méditerranée, ID RCB:2008-A00077-48). Written informed consent was obtained from each patient's next of kin. Patients admitted in the intensive care unit of a university teaching hospital during a 10-month period were screened if they met inclusion criteria: moderate-to-severe ARDS with a PaO_2/FiO_2 ratio $\leq$150 mmHg at a PEEP $\geq$8 cm H_2O. Exclusion criteria were age <18 years, moribund status, risks associated with HFOV (head injury, pneumothorax or a chest tube in place with persistent air leak) and contraindications to the placement of a nasogastric probe. All patients were sedated and continuously paralyzed [13]. The severity of illness was determined according to the Simplified Acute Physiologic II Score, the Sepsis-related Organ Failure Assessment Score and the Lung Injury Score [14, 15].

Tested ventilatory strategies

Patients were submitted to a 6-h period of CMV (CMVpre) in volume-controlled, constant square flow, mode using the AVEA ventilator (VIASYS Healthcare, Palm Springs, CA, USA) with a tidal volume of 6 mL/kg of predicted body weight adjusted to obtain a plateau pressure <30 cm H_2O. PEEP and FiO_2 were adjusted according to the ARMA protocol [2]. Patients were then switched to HFOV using a 3100B ventilator (SensorMedics, Yorba Linda, CA, USA). After a recruitment maneuver was performed with a mPaw of 40 cm H_2O during 40 s with a pressure amplitude of oscillation of 0 cm H_2O [16], HFOV was set as follows: FiO_2 as during the CMVpre period; frequency of 5 Hz; inspiratory time of 33 %; and bias flow of 40 L/min. The pressure amplitude of oscillation and frequency were then adjusted to achieve a $PaCO_2$ close to the $PaCO_2$ measured during the CMVpre period. If pressure amplitude of oscillation of 110 cm H_2O was insufficient to achieve a pH $\geq$ 7.25, frequency was decreased at 4 Hz. The protocol consisted of three 1-h periods of HFOV (HFO + 5, HFO + 10, HFO + 15) in a randomized order, with a mPaw level calculated by adding 5, 10 or 15 cm H_2O to the mPaw measured during the CMVpre period (Fig. 1). A recruitment maneuver was performed at the beginning of each HFOV period and before switch back to CMV. Respiratory frequency and pressure amplitude of oscillation were adjusted to maintain $PaCO_2$ constant during the protocol. Measurements were taken at the end of each period of the protocol and 1 h after switch back to CMV. During the protocol, norepinephrine infusion was adjusted to maintain a mean arterial pressure above 65 mmHg.

Esophageal and transpulmonary pressure measurements

A specific nasogastric feeding probe (SmartCath®, VIASYS Healthcare, Palm Springs, CA, USA) equipped with an esophageal balloon was inserted after in vitro automatized test for leak search and compliance measurement, and then the balloon was filled with a volume of air between 0.5 and 2 mL as recommended by the manufacturer. Every 30 min, the ventilator evacuates and refills the balloon to maintain measurement accuracy. The correct positioning in the lower third of the esophagus was confirmed by the presence of cardiac artifacts, the changes in transpulmonary pressure during tidal ventilation and the parallelism of airway and esophageal curves after the interruption of a brief chest compression maneuver [17]. Finally, a chest X-ray excluded the misplacement of the probe into the airway. Esophageal pressures were recorded and monitored by the integrated system, CP-100 pulmonary monitor (Bicore Monitoring System Inc®, Irvine, CA, USA) present in the AVEA ventilator. An end-inspiratory occlusion of 2 s allowed the measurement of, respectively, Pplat and inspiratory Pes (Pes_{insp}), whereas an end-expiratory occlusion of 5 s allowed the measurement of, respectively, total PEEP (PEEPtot) and expiratory Pes (Pes_{exp}) during CMV. During HFOV periods, because interruption of ventilation is not possible, screen of the AVEA ventilator was frozen for measuring the peak and trough amplitude of oscillations for measurements of, respectively, the maximum and minimum Pes. The following formulas were computed as follows:

$$PEEP_{tot} = \text{external PEEP} + \text{intrinsic PEEP}$$

$$\text{Driving pressure} = \text{Pplat} - PEEP_{tot}$$

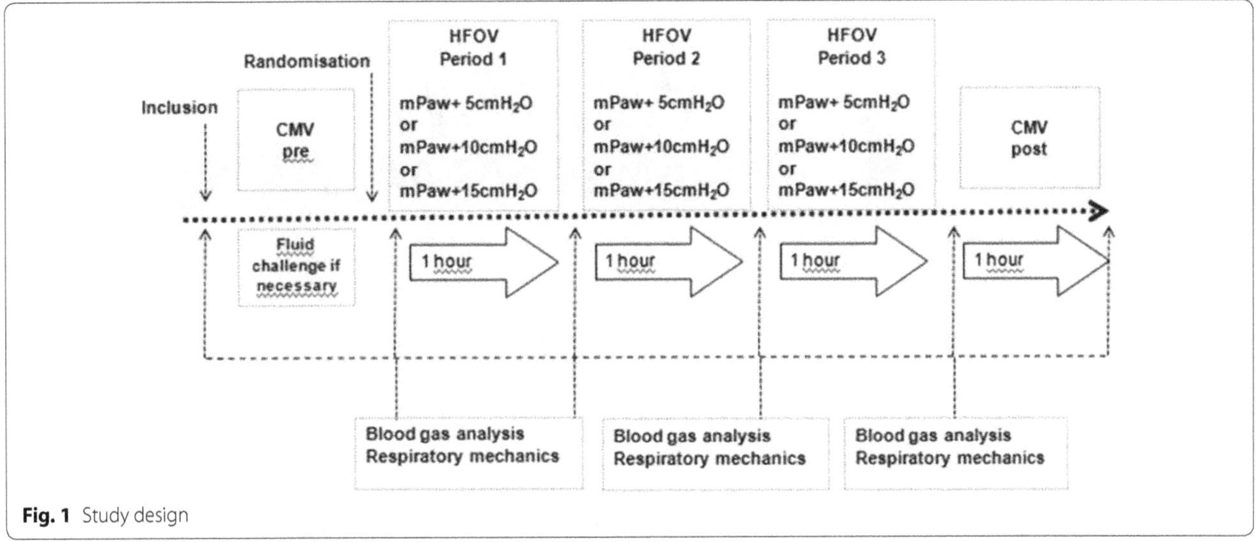

Fig. 1 Study design

During CMV,

P_{Linsp} = Pplat − Pes_{insp}

P_{Lexp} = $PEEP_{tot}$ − Pes_{exp}

Respiratory system elastance (EL_{RS}) = (Pplat−$PEEP_{tot}$)/V_t

Chest wall elastance (EL_{CW}) = (Pes_{insp} − Pes_{exp})/V_t

Pulmonary elastance (EL_L) = EL_{RS} − EL_{CW} = (P_{Lmax} − P_{Lmin})/V_t

During HFOV,

$$Pes_{mean} = (Pes_{max} + Pes_{min})/2$$

$$P_{Lmean} = mPaw - Pes_{mean}$$

An example of tracings in the two ventilatory modes with the airway, esophageal and transpulmonary pressures determinations and calculations is provided in Fig. 2.

Statistical analysis

Data are presented as mean ± SD or median (interquartile range) as required. Normality of variables was tested according the Kolmogorov–Smirnov test. Repeated-measures analysis of variance or Friedman's test was used to evaluate the effect of time and mPaw level. The Tukey test or the Wilcoxon test was used for intergroup comparisons. Bivariate correlations with Spearman's test for each period of ventilation were performed. All statistics and figures were performed with the SPSS 20.0 package (SPSS, Chicago, IL, USA).

Results

Among the 16 patients included in the princeps study [7], ten patients were monitored by the esophageal catheter and were used in this study.

Table 1 reports patient's characteristics at inclusion. Initial computed tomography scan or thoracic radiograph showed five lobar and five diffuse presentations. Causes of ARDS were bacterial pneumonia ($n = 4$), influenza A (H1N1), ($n = 2$), aspiration ($n = 2$), post-cardiopulmonary resuscitation (CPR) ($n = 1$) and acute pancreatitis ($n = 1$). Fluid loading was performed in three patients during the CMVpre period. At baseline, all except one received norepinephrine infusion to maintain mean arterial pressure (MAP) above 65 mmHg.

Respiratory parameters

During HFOV, mPaw was progressively increased from 18 ± 4 cm H_2O in CMVpre period to 33 ± 4 cm H_2O at HFO + 15 (Table 2). PaO_2/FiO_2 ratio did not significantly change under HFOV when compared with the CMVpre period. However, it increased by more than 20 % in three patients at HFO + 5, in four patients at HFO + 10 and in two patients at HFO + 15. FiO_2 was slightly lower at the end of the study. Worsening of oxygenation occurred in two patients at HFO + 5, in three patients at HFO + 10 and in four patients at HFO + 15. As required by the protocol, $PaCO_2$ and pH were kept constant throughout the study. Concerning respiratory mechanics, Pplat, driving pressure, respiratory system elastance, chest wall elastance and pulmonary elastance were similar during the CMVpre and CMVpost periods. These last parameters could not be calculated during the HFOV periods because of the lack of tidal volume monitoring.

At similar level of mPaw, during the volumetric periods of ventilation (CMVpre and CMV post), we did not find differences concerning esophageal and transpulmonary pressures. During HFOV periods, we observed a

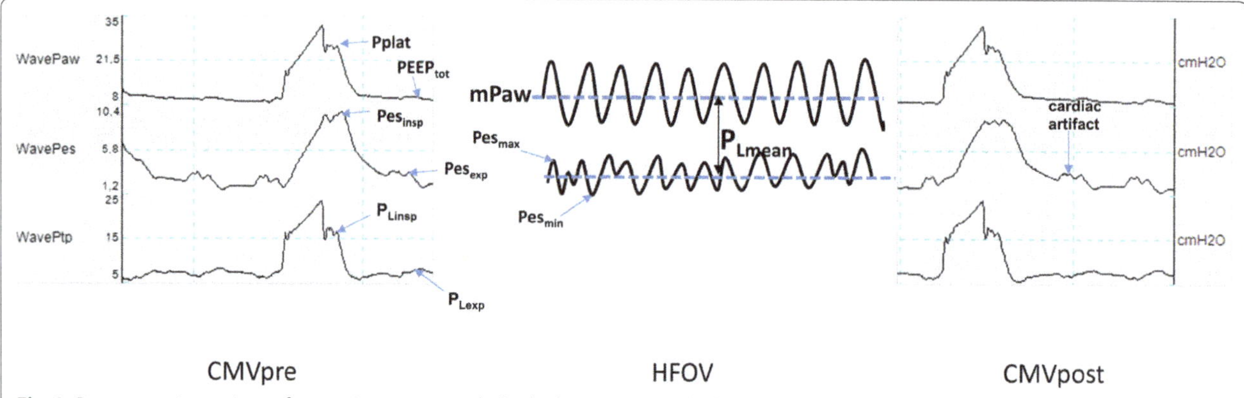

Fig. 2 Representative tracings of mean airway pressure (mPaw), plateau pressure (Pplat), total positive expiratory pressure ($PEEP_{tot}$), esophageal pressure (Pes) and transpulmonary pressure (P_L) during conventional mechanical ventilation (CMV) and high-frequency oscillatory ventilation

Table 1 Patient characteristics and respiratory data at inclusion

Age (years)	63 ± 15
Gender (male), n (%)	4 (40)
Body mass index (kg/m^2)	29 ± 8
SAPS II at the admission	49 ± 23
SOFA at the admission	11 ± 3
ICU mortality, *n* (%)	4(40)
Direct lung injury, *n* (%)	9 (90)
CT scan or X-ray presentation (lobar/diffuse), *n*	5/5
PaO_2/FiO_2 ratio (mmHg)	131 ± 51
FiO_2	0.74 ± 0.17
$PaCO_2$ (mmHg)	46 ± 7
PEEP (cm H_2O)	13 ± 3
V_t (mL)/(mL/kg/IPBW)	382 ± 41/6.6 ± 0.7
Respiratory rate (cycle/min)	26 ± 4
Plateau airway pressure (cm H_2O)	24 ± 4
Driving pressure (cm H_2O)	12 ± 3
mPaw (cm H_2O)	18 ± 3
Oxygenation index	17 ± 9
Lung Injury Score at the inclusion	3.0 ± 0.5
Time from ARDS to inclusion (*d*)	0 ± 0.5

Oxygenation index was calculated as mean airway pressure × FiO_2 × 100)/PaO_2. Results are provided as mean ± SD

FiO_2, inspired oxygen fraction; PEEP, positive end-expiratory pressure; mPaw, mean airway pressure; IPBW, ideal predicted body weight; SAPS II, Simplified Acute Physiology Score II; SOFA, Sepsis Organ Failure Assessment Score; V_t, tidal volume

linear increase in esophageal pressure from 12.4 [10.6; 16.7] to 19.1 [16.7; 23.3] cm of H_2O ($p = 0.001$) as mPaw increases from 23 ± 4 to 33 ± 4 cm of H_2O. As a consequence, mean P_L increased during HFOV periods from 10.5 [7.3; 13.8] to 14 [11.5; 16.3] cm of H_2O (Table 2; Fig. 3). Interestingly, there was no negative transpulmonary pressure whatever the period of HFOV ventilation. There were, however, seven (out of ten) patients with negative minimal P_L during the CMVpre period and only three (out of ten) patients during the CMVpost period ($p = 0.07, \chi^2$ test).

During HFO, mPaw was correlated with Pes_{mean} at HFO + 5 and HFO +15 periods (respectively, $\rho = 0.71$, $p = 0.02$ and $\rho = 0.84$, $p = 0.02$) but at no time with P_{Lmean}.

Discussion

The present study assessing the use of esophageal pressure measurements in patient with moderate-to-severe ARDS on whom a trial of HFOV is performed demonstrates (1) a linear increase in transpulmonary pressures with the increase in mPaw during HFOV, (2) a minimal transpulmonary pressure which was always >0 during HFOV and (3) a correlation between mean esophageal pressure and mPaw.

For decades, HFOV has been used for respiratory failure in both adults and children who were inadequately responsive to conventional mechanical ventilation. However, recently the results of the OSCAR [5] and OSCILLATE [6] studies performed on adults have not shown benefit to HFOV over conventional ventilation. A recent study in the pediatric population has also shown equivocal results with HFOV [18]. Indeed, positive studies on HFOV are limited [16, 19] and predate the era of low tidal volume conventional mechanical ventilation. During HFOV, there is uncertainty about the real pressure that is applied to the alveoli and therefore the distending pressure applied into the lung. Henderson et al. [12] have previously described the use of esophageal manometry to measure P_L during HFOV. With a mean airway pressure of 27 ± 5 cm H_2O during HFOV, they measured a mean esophageal pressure of 14 ± 4 cm H_2O and computed a mean P_L of 18 ± 4 cm H_2O. These data are

Table 2 Gas exchanges and respiratory mechanics

	CMVpre	HFO + 5	HFO + 10	HFO + 15	CMVpost	*p* value time
mPaw (cm of H_2O)	18 ± 4[a,b,c]	23 ± 4[b,c,d,e]	28 ± 4[a,c,d,e]	33 ± 4[a,b,d,e]	17 ± 4[a,b,c]	*<0.001*
PaO_2/inspired O_2 fraction (mmHg)	131 ± 51	132 ± 56	125 ± 23	138 ± 49	139 ± 34	0.9
Inspired O_2 fraction	74 ± 17	71 ± 16	72 ± 16	77 ± 18	67 ± 10[d]	*0.03*
Arterial pH	7.29 ± 0.04	7.31 ± 0.09	7.31 ± 0.01	7.29 ± 0.1	7.32 ± 0.06	0.3
$PaCO_2$ (mmHg)	46 ± 7	47 ± 12	46 ± 14	46 ± 9	42 ± 7	0.5
PEEP (cm of H_2O)	13 ± 3	NA	NA	NA	12 ± 3	0.4
V_t (ml/kg)	6.6 ± 0.7	NA	NA	NA	6.7 ± 0.8	0.2
Plateau airway pressure (cm of H_2O)	24.5 ± 4	NA	NA	NA	23.5 ± 4	0.06
Driving pressure (cm of H_2O)	11.8 ± 3.4	NA	NA	NA	11.5 ± 3.3	0.4
Power of oscillations, %	NA	73 ± 23	79 ± 29	81 ± 24	NA	0.1
Respiratory rate (cycle/min)	26 ± 4	NA	NA	NA	25 ± 6	1
Oscillatory frequency (Hz)	NA	4.8 ± 1	4.7 ± 0.7	4.6 ± 1	NA	0.2
Inspiratory esophageal pressure	15 [11.5; 21.2]	NA	NA	NA	14 [10.2; 17.2]	0.1
Expiratory esophageal pressure	12.5 [5.1; 13.5]	NA	NA	NA	9.1 [5.4; 13.5]	0.1
Mean esophageal pressure (cm of H_2O)	NA	12.4 [10.6; 16.7][b,c]	16.7 [12.5; 18.7][a,c]	19.1 [16.7; 23.3][a,b]	NA	*0.001*
Inspiratory P_L (cm of H_2O)	8.1 [5.7; 12.8]	NA	NA	NA	11.8 [5; 12.1]	1
Expiratory P_L (cm of H_2O)	−1 [−3; + 0.7)	NA	NA	NA	+3.5 [−3; + 6]	0.2
Mean P_L (cm of H_2O)	NA	10.5 [7.3; 13.8][c]	13.1 [9.2; 14.7]	14 [11.5; 16.3][a]	NA	*0.001*
Respiratory system elastance (cm of H_2O/L)	31.2 ± 9.7	NA	NA	NA	29.9 ± 8	0.2
Chest wall elastance (cm of H_2O/L)	15.7 ± 6	NA	NA	NA	11.1 ± 4.5	0.3
Pulmonary elastance (cm of H_2O/L)	15.9. ± 11	NA	NA	NA	18.9 ± 6	0.3

P_L transpulmonary pressure, *NA* not applicable

p values in italic are provided for < 0.05

[a] $p < .05$ vs. HFO + 5, [b] $p < .05$ vs. HFO + 10, [c] $p < .05$ vs. HFO + 15, [d] $p < .05$ vs. CMVpre, [e] $p < .05$ vs. CMVpost

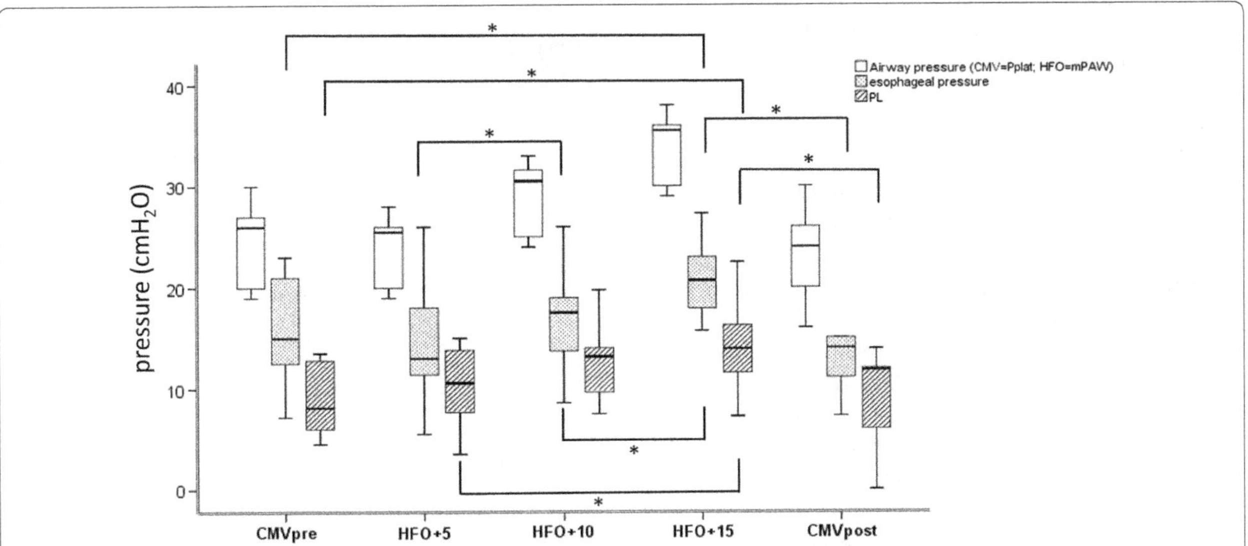

Fig. 3 Airway pressures, esophageal pressures and transpulmonary pressures (P_L) during conventional mechanical ventilation (CMV) before and after three levels of mean airway pressure (mPaw) during high-frequency oscillatory ventilation (HFO). Airway pressure is plateau pressure (Pplat) during CMV and mPaw during HFO. Esophageal pressure is the inspiratory pressure during CMV and the mean esophageal pressure during HFO. P_L is computed by Pplat minus inspiratory esophageal pressure during CMV and mPaw minus mean esophageal pressure during HFO. *Means < 0.05

consistent with the present results, namely a mPaw of 28 ± 4 cm H_2O, results in a median of 16.7 IQR [12.5; 18.7] cm H_2O range of Pes and a median of 13.1 IQR [9.2; 14.7] cm H_2O range of P_L. The safe range of P_L during HFO is not known. However, during conventional mechanical ventilation for ARDS, a P_L > 27 cm H_2O is associated with an unacceptably high level of strain [20]. The P_L value recorded during HFO remains below this threshold whatever the level of mPaw.

One interesting result is the correlation between mPaw and esophageal pressure that we obtained; the more mPaw is set, the more Pes is measured. In clinical practice, levels of mPaw in the OSCAR and OSCILLATE trials [5, 6] were not exactly the same. During the first 2 days of the studies, mPaw was set at 5 cm H_2O higher in the Canadian trial than in the UK trial. These differences could have led to more pulmonary overdistension and side effects that could explain the deleterious outcomes observed with HFOV in the OSCILLATE trial.

An ongoing study, the EPOCH study [21], which aim is to compare a strategy of preventing atelectrauma with a P_L of 0 cm H_2O at end expiration to a strategy of lung recruitment to target P_L of 15 cm H_2O at end-inspiratory volume in a crossover design either with CMV and either with HFOV will clarify the protective or deleterious roles of HFOV as compared to CMV.

Limitations

First, as measurements of esophageal pressure could not be taken in static conditions during HFO periods, we cannot rule out a possible bias of measurements due to cardiac artifacts. However, the use of mean esophageal pressure reduces this bias. Second, during HFOV, due to the lack of V_t monitoring, we use the calculation of P_L derived from Pes measurements [22] and not the elastance-derived measurements of P_L [23] which could lead to different results [24]. Indeed, experimental data have shown that although recorded value of Pes is a quite accurate approximation of measured pleural pressure in the middle part of the lungs, Pes can overestimate or underestimate the value of pleural pressure whether in the non-dependant part and whether in the dependant part of the lungs [25]. The more convincing results are that the variations of Peso reflect those in pleural pressure whatever the parts of the lung [26]. There is still a matter of controversy on the use of the former or the latter method. A prospective ongoing study could bring a response to the clinical utility of the method used [27]. Third, because we have not performed the registration of airway pressure during HFO, we cannot exclude negative P_L during the active expiratory phase, and further studies are needed to conclude. And fourth, from a technical point of view, we also cannot exclude that larger inflation volume as demonstrated by Mojoli et al. [28] could have led to different results. However, our study precedes the one from Mojoli, and we used the volume and the proceeding recommended by the manufacturer.

We cannot speculate whether lower mPaw during HFOV, the same range as recorded in CMV, could lead to lower esophageal and transpulmonary pressures recorded. A level of <+10 cm H_2O of mPaw during HFO does not increase significantly Peso and P_L. Only a level of ≥+15 cm H_2O of mPaw increases significantly both Peso and P_L.

Conclusion

The use of high mean airway pressures during HFOV leads to increase in transpulmonary pressures. Contrary to CMV, during HFOV, transpulmonary pressure remains always positive.

Authors' contributions

CG, JMF and LP designed the study. CG and JMF coordinated the study. CG, JMF, SH, AR and LP were responsible for patient enrolment and measurements of esophageal pressures. CG and JMF performed statistical analysis. CG, JMF, DT and LP analysed the data and wrote the manuscript. All authors read and approved the final manuscript.

Author details

[1] Aix-Marseille Univ, APHM, URMITE UMR CNRS 7278, Hôpital Nord, Réanimation des Détresses Respiratoires et Infections Sévères, Marseille, France.
[2] Service d'Accueil des Urgences, APHM, Hôpital Nord, Marseille, France.
[3] Department of Anesthesia, Critical Care, and Pain Medicine, Beth Israel Deaconess Medical Center, 330 Brookline Ave, Boston, MA, USA.

Competing interests

The authors declare that they have no competing interests.

References

1. ARDS Definition Task Force, Ranieri VM, Rubenfeld GD, Thompson BT, Ferguson ND, Caldwell E, et al. Acute respiratory distress syndrome: the Berlin Definition. JAMA. 2012;307:2526–33.
2. Ventilation with lower tidal volumes as compared with traditional tidal volumes for acute lung injury and the acute respiratory distress syndrome. The Acute Respiratory Distress Syndrome Network. N Engl J Med. 2000;342:1301–08.
3. Hager DN, Fuld M, Kaczka DW, Fessler HE, Brower RG, Simon BA. Four methods of measuring tidal volume during high-frequency oscillatory ventilation. Crit Care Med. 2006;34:751–7.
4. McCulloch PR, Forkert PG, Froese AB. Lung volume maintenance prevents lung injury during high frequency oscillatory ventilation in surfactant-deficient rabbits. Am Rev Respir Dis. 1988;137:1185–92.
5. Young D, Lamb SE, Shah S, MacKenzie I, Tunnicliffe W, Lall R, et al. High-frequency oscillation for acute respiratory distress syndrome. N Engl J Med. 2013;368:806–13.
6. Ferguson ND, Cook DJ, Guyatt GH, Mehta S, Hand L, Austin P, et al. High-frequency oscillation in early acute respiratory distress syndrome. N Engl J Med. 2013;368:795–805.
7. Guervilly C, Forel JM, Hraiech S, Demory D, Allardet-Servent J, Adda M, et al. Right ventricular function during high-frequency oscillatory ventilation in adults with acute respiratory distress syndrome. Crit Care Med. 2012;40:1539–45.

8. Ursulet L, Roussiaux A, Belcour D, Ferdynus C, Gauzere BA, Vandroux D, et al. Right over left ventricular end-diastolic area relevance to predict hemodynamic intolerance of high-frequency oscillatory ventilation in patients with severe ARDS. Ann Intensive Care. 2015;5:25. doi:10.1186/s13613-015-0068-6.
9. Dreyfuss D, Ricard JD, Gaudry S. Did studies on HFOV fail to improve ARDS survival because they did not decrease VILI? On the potential validity of a physiological concept enounced several decades ago. Intensive Care Med. 2015;41:2076–786.
10. Hirayama T, Nagano O, Shiba N, Yumoto T, Sato K, Terado M, et al. Mean lung pressure during adult high-frequency oscillatory ventilation: an experimental study using a lung model. Acta Med Okayama. 2014;68:323–9.
11. Talmor D, Sarge T, Malhotra A, O'Donnell CR, Ritz R, Lisbon A, et al. Mechanical ventilation guided by esophageal pressure in acute lung injury. N Engl J Med. 2008;359:2095–104.
12. Henderson WR, Dominelli PB, Griesdale DE, Talmor D, Sheel AW. Airway pressure and transpulmonary pressure during high-frequency oscillation for acute respiratory distress syndrome. Can Respir J. 2014;21:107–11.
13. Papazian L, Forel JM, Gacouin A, Penot-Ragon C, Perrin G, Loundou A, et al. Neuromuscular blockers in early acute respiratory distress syndrome. N Engl J Med. 2010;363:1107–3116.
14. Le Gall JR, Lemeshow S, Saulnier F. A new Simplified Acute Physiology Score (SAPS II) based on a European/North American multicenter study. JAMA. 1993;270:2957–63.
15. Vincent JL, Moreno R, Takala J, Willatts S, De Mendonça A, Bruining H, et al. The SOFA (Sepsis-related Organ Failure Assessment) score to describe organ dysfunction/failure. On behalf of the Working Group on Sepsis-Related Problems of the European Society of Intensive Care Medicine. Intensive Care Med. 1996;22:707–10.
16. Ferguson ND, Chiche JD, Kacmarek RM, Hallett DC, Mehta S, Findlay GP, et al. Combining high-frequency oscillatory ventilation and recruitment maneuvers in adults with early acute respiratory distress syndrome: the Treatment with Oscillation and an Open Lung Strategy (TOOLS) Trial pilot study. Crit Care Med. 2005;33:479–86.
17. Higgs BD, Behrakis PK, Bevan DR, Milic-Emili J. Measurement of pleural pressure with esophageal balloon in anesthetized humans. Anesthesiology. 1983;59:340–3.
18. Bateman ST, Borasino S, Asaro LA, Cheifetz IM, Diane S, Wypij D, et al. Early high-frequency oscillatory ventilation in pediatric acute respiratory failure: a propensity score analysis. Am J Respir Crit Care Med. 2016;193:495–503. doi:10.1164/rccm.201507-1381OC.
19. Derdak S, Mehta S, Stewart TE, Smith T, Rogers M, Buchman TG, et al. High-frequency oscillatory ventilation for acute respiratory distress syndrome in adults: a randomized, controlled trial. Am J Respir Crit Care Med. 2002;166:801–8.
20. Chiumello D, Carlesso E, Cadringher P, Caironi P, Valenza F, Polli F, et al. Lung stress and strain during mechanical ventilation for acute respiratory distress syndrome. Am J Respir Crit Care Med. 2008;178:346–55. doi:10.1164/rccm.200710-1589OC.
21. https://www.clinicaltrials.gov/ct2/show/NCT02342756.
22. Knowles JH, Hong SK, Rahn H. Possible errors using esophageal balloon in determination of pressure-volume characteristics of the lung and thoracic cage. J Appl Physiol. 1959;14:525–30.
23. Gattinoni L, Chiumello D, Carlesso E, Valenza F. Bench-to-bedside review: chest wall elastance in acute lung injury/acute respiratory distress syndrome patients. Crit Care. 2004;8:350–855.
24. Gulati G, Novero A, Loring SH, Talmor D. Pleural pressure and optimal positive end-expiratory pressure based on esophageal pressure versus chest wall elastance: incompatible results. Crit Care Med. 2013;41:1951–7.
25. Pelosi P, Goldner M, McKibben A, Adams A, Eccher G, Caironi P, et al. Recruitment and derecruitment during acute respiratory failure: an experimental study. Am J Respir Crit Care Med. 2001;164:122–30.
26. Chiumello D, Cressoni M, Colombo A, Babini G, Brioni M, Crimella F, et al. The assessment of transpulmonary pressure in mechanically ventilated ARDS patients. Intensive Care Med. 2014;40:1670–8.
27. https://www.clinicaltrials.gov/ct2/show/NCT01681225.
28. Mojoli F, Chiumello D, Pozzi M, Algieri I, Bianzina S, Luoni S, et al. Esophageal pressure measurements under different conditions of intrathoracic pressure. An in vitro study of second generation balloon catheters. Minerva Anestesiol. 2015;81:855–64.

High-flow nasal cannula oxygen therapy versus noninvasive ventilation in immunocompromised patients with acute respiratory failure

Rémi Coudroy[1,2*], Angéline Jamet[1], Philippe Petua[1], René Robert[1,2], Jean-Pierre Frat[1,2] and Arnaud W. Thille[1,2]

Abstract

Background: Acute respiratory failure is the main cause of admission to intensive care unit in immunocompromised patients. In this subset of patients, the beneficial effects of noninvasive ventilation (NIV) as compared to standard oxygen remain debated. High-flow nasal cannula oxygen therapy (HFNC) is an alternative to standard oxygen or NIV, and its use in hypoxemic patients has been growing. Therefore, we aimed to compare outcomes of immunocompromised patients treated using HFNC alone or NIV as a first-line therapy for acute respiratory failure in an observational cohort study over an 8-year period. Patients with acute-on-chronic respiratory failure, those treated with standard oxygen alone or needing immediate intubation, and those with a do-not-intubate order were excluded.

Results: Among the 115 patients analyzed, 60 (52 %) were treated with HFNC alone and 55 (48 %) with NIV as first-line therapy with 30 patients (55 %) receiving HFNC and 25 patients (45 %) standard oxygen between NIV sessions. The rates of intubation and 28-day mortality were higher in patients treated with NIV than with HFNC (55 vs. 35 %, $p = 0.04$, and 40 vs. 20 %, $p = 0.02$ log-rank test, respectively). Using propensity score-matched analysis, NIV was associated with mortality. Using multivariate analysis, NIV was independently associated with intubation and mortality.

Conclusions: Based on this observational cohort study including immunocompromised patients admitted to intensive care unit for acute respiratory failure, intubation and mortality rates could be lower in patients treated with HFNC alone than with NIV. The use of NIV remained independently associated with poor outcomes.

Keywords: Acute respiratory failure, Immunosuppression, Noninvasive positive pressure ventilation, Acute lung injury, Mechanical ventilation, High-flow oxygen therapy

Background

Acute respiratory failure is the main cause of admission to intensive care unit (ICU) in immunocompromised patients [1]. In this subset of patients, the need for intubation and invasive mechanical ventilation is associated with particularly high mortality rates, reaching 70 % of cases [2–4]. In the early 2000s, two randomized controlled trials reported lower rates of intubation and mortality with the use of noninvasive ventilation (NIV) as compared to standard oxygen [5, 6]. However, given the small samples of patients included in these studies, experts suggested that NIV could be used in immunocompromised patients with acute respiratory failure, but the strength of recommendation was assessed as weak [7]. As a consequence, so far NIV has been used as a first-line therapy in only 25–40 % of immunocompromised patients admitted to ICU for acute respiratory

*Correspondence: remi.coudroy@chu-poitiers.fr
[1] Service de Réanimation Médicale, CHU de Poitiers, 2, rue de la Milétrie, 86021 Poitiers, France
Full list of author information is available at the end of the article

failure [1, 8–10]. Recently, a large randomized controlled trial did not confirm the potential benefits of NIV and in fact found similar outcomes in immunocompromised patients with acute respiratory failure treated with NIV or oxygen alone [11]. It is important to note that, in this study, oxygen therapy could be delivered using either standard oxygen or high-flow oxygen through nasal cannula (HFNC).

HFNC is a recent technique that delivers heated and humidified oxygen at high-flow rates [12]. Several physiological studies have shown HFNC to be better tolerated than standard oxygen delivered through a mask [13–15]. High-flow rates of fresh gas help to increase the fraction of inspired oxygen (FiO_2) [16], to generate low levels of positive end-expiratory pressure [17], and to decrease physiological dead space by flushing expired carbon dioxide in the upper airways [18]. The result is a decrease in work of breathing [19] and dyspnea [14] while the heating and humidification of inspired gases may prevent thick secretions and atelectasis. HFNC could not only offer an alternative to standard oxygen in hypoxemic patients, but also avoid the need for NIV. In a recent multicenter randomized controlled trial, the mortality rate in patients with acute respiratory failure treated with HFNC alone was significantly lower in both those treated with standard oxygen and in those treated with NIV [20]. In this study, patients treated with NIV also received HFNC between NIV sessions, thereby suggesting a direct deleterious effect of NIV compared to the group receiving HFNC alone. That said, as patients with neutropenia were excluded from the trial, these results could not be extrapolated to all immunocompromised patients.

Given the fact that use of HFNC in patients with acute respiratory failure has been increasing in our unit over recent years, we aimed to compare the outcomes of immunocompromised patients treated with HFNC alone or with NIV as first-line therapy.

Some of the results of this study were reported in the form of an abstract at the 2016 meeting of the French Intensive Care Society in Paris, France.

Methods

Study design

Between 1 January 2007 and 31 December 2014, discharge reports from all patients admitted to our 15-bed medical ICU in a tertiary hospital were retrospectively reviewed. This study was approved by the Ethics Committee of the French Intensive Care Society (*Société de Réanimation de Langue Française*, SRLF, CE no. 14-27), and given its observational nature, informed consent was waived.

Screening of patients

We screened all patients admitted for acute respiratory failure defined by the following criteria: a respiratory rate $\geq$25 breaths/min or clinical signs of respiratory distress, and a calculated PaO_2-to-FiO_2 ratio $\leq$300 mmHg, FiO_2 being estimated as follows: (oxygen flow in liters per minute $\times$ 0.03) + 0.21 [20]. Among them, we included those who had immunosuppression caused by hematologic or solid cancer, stem cell or solid organ transplantation, a steroid dose of more than 0.5 mg/kg for at least 1 month, or cytotoxic drugs for non-malignant disease or acquired immune deficiency syndrome. Patients with acute-on-chronic respiratory failure, those treated with standard oxygen alone or needing immediate intubation, and those with a do-not-intubate order were excluded from the analysis.

Classification of patients

Patients were classified according to the time from the onset of acute respiratory failure and the start of the first-line strategy of ventilatory support including NIV or HFNC. All patients in whom NIV was started within the first 6 h after the onset of acute respiratory failure were included in the NIV group if they received at least 2 h of NIV within the first 24 h. Those who were treated with HFNC within the first 6 h after the onset of acute respiratory failure were included in the HFNC group, even if they received late NIV as a rescue therapy beyond the first 6 h. Therefore, patients initially treated with HFNC and who received late NIV as rescue therapy, i.e., the most severe patients, remained classified in the HFNC group. We excluded patients treated with standard oxygen during the first 6 h and who received short NIV (<2 h) considered as preoxygenation in case of frank respiratory worsening leading to intubation, and those treated with standard oxygen during the first 6 h and who received late NIV as rescue therapy. Each patient was classified by consensus of three senior intensivists (RC, JPF, and AWT) blinded to outcomes up to full agreement.

In our unit, the criteria to decide intubation were the same as those used in our previous studies [15, 20]: uncontrolled shock defined by mean arterial pressure $\leq$65 mm Hg despite a 30 ml/kg crystalloid fluid challenge and increasing doses of vasopressors, neurological impairment defined by a Glasgow score $\leq$12, or signs of persisting or worsening respiratory failure as defined by at least two of the following criteria: respiratory rate >40 breaths per minute, lack of improvement in signs of high respiratory muscle workload, development of copious tracheal secretions, acidosis with pH <7.35, an SpO_2 <90 % for more than 5 min without technical dysfunction, or a poor response to oxygenation techniques.

Data collection

For all included patients, we collected age, gender, functional status before ICU admission using the Knaus chronic health status score [21], Mac Cabe score reflecting the severity of underlying disease [22], severity scores including the Simplified Acute Physiology Score II [23], and the modified Sequential Organ Failure Assessment (excluding respiratory item) [24], type of immunosuppression, and year of ICU admission. Clinical, radiological, and biological parameters at inclusion such as heart rate, systolic blood pressure, respiratory rate, SpO_2, body temperature, bilateral lung infiltrates on chest X-ray, arterial pH, sodium bicarbonate, and PaO_2-to-FiO_2 ratio were recorded. Two senior physicians reviewed all charts to assess the reason for acute respiratory failure (AJ and PP). Initial settings during NIV or HFNC and ventilation characteristics during the ICU stay were collected.

Outcomes

Primary end-point was the mortality rate at day 28. Secondary outcomes included intubation rate, length of mechanical ventilation and ICU stay, in-ICU mortality, and variables associated with intubation and mortality at day 28.

Statistical analysis

Continuous variables were expressed as mean ± standard deviation (SD) or as median [interquartile range, from 25th to 75th percentiles] according to their distribution using the Kolmogorov–Smirnov test and compared using the Mann–Whitney or the Student's *t* test as appropriate. Dichotomous variables were expressed in percentage and compared using the Fischer's exact test or the Chi-square test as appropriate. We performed two multivariate analyses using a backward step-down logistic regression model including early clinical and biological variables associated first with mortality at day 28 and second with intubation, with a p value <0.15 using univariate analysis. As the year of ICU admission was different between the 2 groups, this variable was forced in the logistical regression model. Kaplan–Meier curves were plotted to assess time from the onset of acute respiratory failure to mortality within the first 28 days in the 2 groups and compared by the log-rank test. Given the baseline differences between groups, a propensity score was computed by using logistic regression with the dependent variables associated with mortality at day 28 (age and use of vasopressors within 24 h after ICU admission) to estimate the effect of NIV on mortality at day 28 [25]. A matching algorithm was performed according to the propensity score. Adjusted outcomes between patients who were or were not treated with NIV were compared using the paired t test or the Wilcoxon matched paired test as appropriate to compare adjusted outcomes. We considered two-tailed p values <0.05 as significant. Statistical analyses were performed using the statistical software package XLstat® (Addinsoft, Paris, France), GraphPadPrism 5® (La Jolla, CA, USA) and R statistical package (online at http://www.R-project.org).

Results

Of the 5244 patients admitted to our unit over an 8-year period, 1299 (25 %) were admitted for acute respiratory failure. Among them, 267 (21 %) were immunocompromised (Fig. 1). Baseline characteristics of the 115 patients (43 %) included in the analysis are given in Table 1. In the NIV group, patients were more likely to be male, to have hypercapnia and alkalemia at admission, whereas in the HFNC group they tended to be older. In the first half of the study period, patients were more likely to be treated with NIV as first-line therapy than in the second half: 68 % (26 of 38 patients) received NIV from 2007 versus 2010 versus 38 % (22 of the 77 patients) from 2011 to 2014, $p = 0.003$. Intubation rates in the NIV group did not differ between the 2 periods: 57 % (15/26 patients) in the first period versus 52 % (15/29) in the second one ($p = 0.66$).

In the NIV group, initial FiO_2 was 0.6 [0.5–0.9], whereas levels of pressure support and positive end-expiratory pressure were 10 cm H_2O [8–12] and 4 cm H_2O [4–5], respectively. Mean expiratory tidal volume delivered during the first 24 h after NIV initiation was 9.0 ± 2.4 ml/kg of predicted body weight. NIV was applied during 2.0 days [1.0–4.0] in median for a duration of 8 h [4–11] during the first 24 h. Among the 55 patients treated with NIV, 25 patients (45 %) received standard oxygen between NIV sessions, whereas the 30 other patients (55 %) received HFNC.

In the HFNC group, FiO_2 was 0.6 [0.5–1], whereas gas flow was 50 l/min [40–50]. HFNC was applied continuously for a total duration of 2.0 days [1.0–4.0] in median. Eight patients in the HFNC group (13 %) received NIV as rescue therapy during their ICU stay.

Overall intubation rate was 44 % (51 of 115 patients), and overall mortality at day 28 was 30 % (34 of 115 patients). The rates of intubation and of mortality in ICU and at day 28 were significantly lower in the HFNC group than in the NIV group (Table 1 and Fig. 2). Mortality of patients who needed intubation tended to be significantly lower in the HFNC group (9/21 patients, 43 %) than in the NIV group (21/30 patients, 70 %, $p = 0.05$).

In the NIV group, outcomes did not significantly differ between the patients who received HFNC between

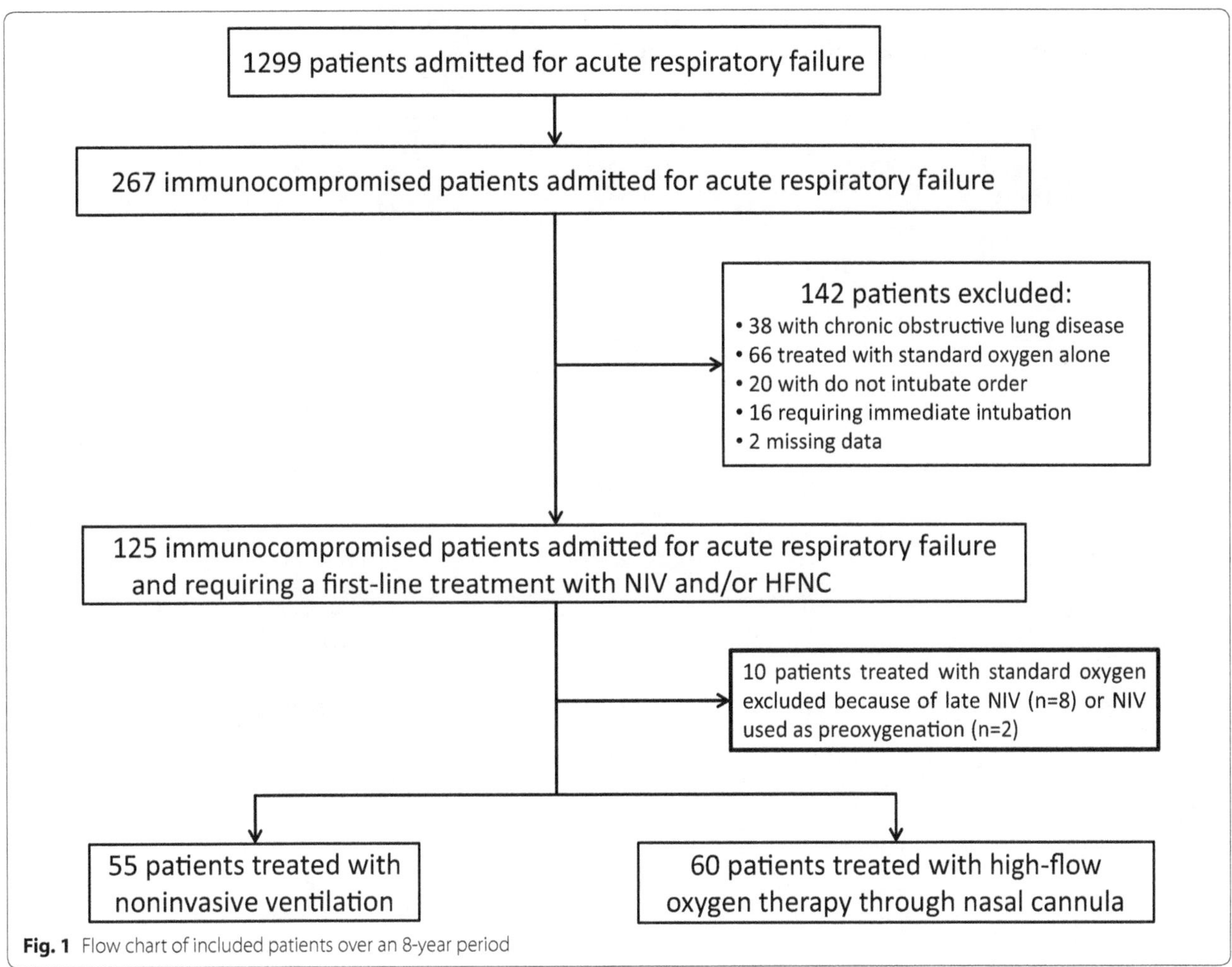

Fig. 1 Flow chart of included patients over an 8-year period

NIV sessions and those who received standard oxygen: the rates of intubation were 47 % (14/30) versus 64 % (16/25), respectively, $p = 0.28$; the rates of mortality at day 28 were 36 % (11/30) versus 44 % (11/25), respectively, $p = 0.59$.

Variables associated with intubation and mortality at day 28 in the overall population are given in Additional file 1 and Table 2, respectively. Using multivariate analysis, the 3 variables independently associated with intubation were severity at admission in the ICU as indicated by a high SAPS II, need for vasopressor within the 24 h after ICU admission, and use of NIV (Table 3). Use of NIV remained associated with mortality at day 28 independently from age and the need for vasopressor within 24 h after ICU admission (Table 3), even after forcing the year of admission in the model.

Baseline characteristics and outcomes of the 57 patients included in the propensity score-matched cohort are displayed in Table 4. In-ICU mortality at day 28 remained significantly lower in the HFNC than in the NIV group after matching on age and need for vasopressors within 24 h after ICU admission (Table 4). Using multivariate analysis in the matched cohort, NIV as a first-line therapy was the only factor independently associated with mortality at day 28 with and adjusted odds ratio of 4.03 and a 95 % confidence interval of [1.09–14.93], even after forcing the year of ICU admission.

Discussion

Our main finding is that immunocompromised patients admitted to ICU for acute respiratory failure had higher mortality when treated with NIV than those treated with HFNC alone. Moreover, they were more likely to be intubated and to have prolonged ICU length of stay. After adjustment, NIV remained independently associated with intubation and mortality at day 28.

In our study, intubation and mortality rates in the NIV group of the overall cohort were 55 and 40 %, respectively. These results are in keeping with the intubation and mortality rates reported in recent cohort studies [2,

Table 1 Comparison of baseline characteristics and outcomes between patients treated by noninvasive positive pressure ventilation (NIV) or high-flow nasal cannula (HFNC) oxygen therapy alone

	NIV ($n = 55$)	HFNC ($n = 60$)	p value
Age (years)	58 (44–66)	62 (50–70)	0.06
Gender (male)	42 (76 %)	35 (58 %)	0.048
Knaus chronic health status score			0.46
A	15 (27 %)	19 (32 %)	
B	17 (31 %)	22 (37 %)	
C	21 (38 %)	15 (25 %)	
D	2 (3.6 %)	4 (6.7 %)	
Mac Cabe classification			0.20
1	20 (36 %)	19 (32 %)	
2	19 (35 %)	30 (50 %)	
3	16 (29 %)	11 (18 %)	
SAPS II at ICU admission (points)	42 ± 11	46 ± 13	0.10
Modified SOFA score at inclusion (points)	3 (1–6)	4 (1–6)	0.28
Type of immunosuppression			0.30
Hematologic cancer or neutropenia	33 (60 %)	31 (52 %)	
Solid cancer	11 (20 %)	8 (13 %)	
Drug-induced immunosuppression	10 (18 %)	20 (33 %)	
Acquired immune deficiency syndrome	1 (2 %)	1 (2 %)	
Cause of respiratory failure			0.38
Documented infection	24 (44 %)	31 (52 %)	
Cardiogenic pulmonary edema	5 (9 %)	5 (8 %)	
Specific	13 (24 %)	6 (10 %)	
Other identified causes	7 (13 %)	11 (18 %)	
Not identified cause	6 (11 %)	7 (12 %)	
Clinical and biological parameters at inclusion			
Heart rate (beats/min)	111 ± 22	113 ± 23	0.71
Systolic blood pressure (mmHg)	130 (113–150)	119 (110–147)	0.28
Respiratory rate (breaths/min)	30 (26–33)	29 (26–32)	0.75
SpO_2 (%)	94 (91–98)	96 (94–99)	0.02
Body temperature (°C)	37.8 ± 1.1	38.0 ± 1.1	0.47
Bilateral lung infiltrates on chest X-ray	46 (84 %)	50 (83 %)	>0.99
Arterial pH	7.44 (7.40–7.47)	7.46 (7.43–7.50)	0.02
PaO_2-to-FiO_2 ratio (mmHg)	141 (111–177)	149 (107–204)	0.19
PaO_2-to-FiO_2 ratio $\leq$ 200 mmHg	47 (85 %)	44 (73 %)	0.17
$PaCO_2$ (mmHg)	37 (32–45)	32 (29–38)	<0.0001
$PaCO_2$ > 45 mmHg	12 (22 %)	2 (3 %)	0.003
Sodium bicarbonate (mmol/l)	25 (22–28)	21 (24–26)	0.04
Vasopressors within 24 h after ICU admission	9 (16 %)	14 (23 %)	0.35
Time from admission to ventilatory support initiation (h)	1 (0–1)	1 (0–1)	0.62
Need for immunosuppressive drug during ICU stay	13 (24 %)	15 (25 %)	>0.99
Admission before 2011	26 (47 %)	12 (20 %)	<0.0001
Primary outcome			
28-day mortality	22 (40 %)	12 (20 %)	0.02
Secondary outcomes			
Intubation	30 (55 %)	21 (35 %)	0.04
Time from admission to intubation (h)	28 (18–49)	35 (9–49)	0.99
Length of invasive mechanical ventilation (days)	8 (4–11)	7 (4–12)	0.63
Length of ICU stay (days)	8 (5–13)	7 (4–9)	0.08
In-ICU mortality	20 (36 %)	9 (15 %)	0.01

Nominal variables are given as number (%), and continuous data are given as median (25th–75th percentile) or mean ± standard deviation (SD) according to their distribution using the Kolmogorov–Smirnov test

SAPS Simplified Acute Physiology Score, *SOFA* Sequential Organ Failure Assessment

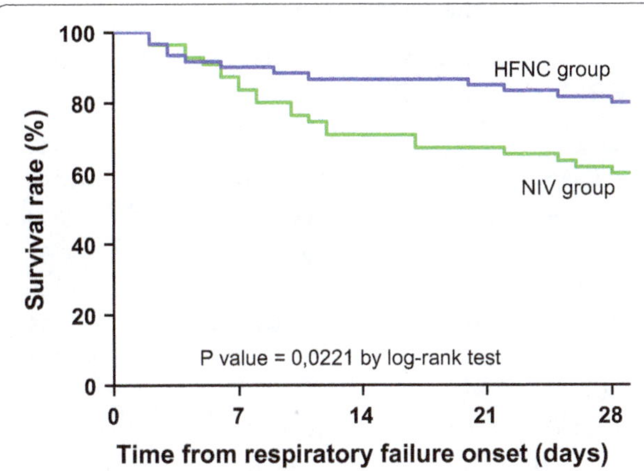

Fig. 2 Figure showing the Kaplan–Meier plots of the cumulative survival rates within the 28 days following the onset of acute respiratory failure in ICU in the overall population. The rate of mortality was significantly lower in patients treated with high-flow nasal cannula (HFNC) oxygen therapy alone (*blue line*) than in patients treated with noninvasive ventilation (NIV) as first-line therapy (*green line*), decreasing from 40 % (22/55) to 20 % (12/60) $p = 0.0221$ by log-rank test

26–28], reinforcing the external validation of our results. Conversely, the rates of intubation and mortality in our patients treated with HFNC alone were 35 and 20 %, respectively, which are markedly lower than the rates reported in the above-mentioned studies [2, 26–28]. Therefore, these differences seem more likely due to a decrease in intubation or mortality rates observed in the HFNC group rather than an excess of intubation or mortality in the NIV group.

In contrast to patients with chronic obstructive pulmonary disease [29, 30] or cardiogenic pulmonary edema [31], the benefits of NIV remain unclear in immunocompromised patients with acute respiratory failure. To date, three randomized controlled trials have compared the use of NIV versus standard oxygen in immunocompromised patients with acute respiratory failure [5, 6, 11]. In a first trial including 40 patients with solid organ transplantation, the rate of intubation was significantly reduced in patients treated with NIV [5]. However, nearly one quarter of the patients had cardiogenic pulmonary edema [5], a condition for which the benefits of NIV are supported by a strong level of evidence [31]. In a second trial including 52 patients, the rates of intubation and mortality were significantly lower in patients treated with NIV [6]. However, these beneficial effects were observed only in patients with hematologic cancer or neutropenia, which accounted only for 15 patients per group [6]. In the most recent trial including 374 patients, intubation and mortality rates did not differ between the two groups [11]. However, respiratory rate and oxygen requirement at inclusion were lower than in our study and in the two previous trials [5, 6], perhaps illustrating a lower severity of respiratory failure, which may have attenuated the impact of NIV on outcomes.

The case volume of patients treated with first-line NIV may also have influence on outcomes, with lower expected intubation rates in highly skilled centers. These findings have already been suggested in patients treated with NIV for cardiogenic pulmonary edema or acute-on-chronic respiratory failure [9, 32–35]. In our high case-volume center, this would have favoured the NIV group and attenuated the outcome difference between the 2 groups, which was not the case.

A recent retrospective study including 178 immunocompromised patients with acute respiratory failure suggested that the best strategy consisted in use of NIV associated with HFNC between NIV sessions [28]. The 37 % mortality rate recorded in the group treated by NIV and HFNC was almost the same as that of our patients treated by NIV (40 %). Once again, this mortality rate remained markedly higher than the 20 % rate we report herein in our patients treated with HFNC alone. Therefore, use of HFNC alone without NIV could be the treatment of choice in immunocompromised patients admitted to ICU for acute respiratory failure.

Although use of HFNC alone has been poorly evaluated in immunocompromised patients with acute respiratory failure, our results are in line with those found recently in a large multicenter randomized controlled trial [20]. Indeed, this study showed a significantly reduced mortality rate in patients treated with HFNC alone as compared to those treated by NIV with HFNC between NIV sessions [20]. In this trial, about one-third of included patients were immunocompromised, and the rates of intubation and in-ICU mortality in the HFNC group were 38 and 11 %, respectively, which are in line with those we report.

The beneficial effects of HFNC could be largely due to tolerance. HFNC seems better tolerated than NIV in patients with acute respiratory failure with a higher degree of comfort, a reduction in the severity of dyspnea and a decreased respiratory rate [15, 20]. Although these criteria were not assessed in our study, we believe that our findings may be extrapolated to immunocompromised patients. By contrast, NIV could be harmful due to potential ventilator-induced lung injury generated by pressure support that increases tidal volumes [36] and leads to high transpulmonary pressure [37]. Indeed, it

Table 2 Univariate analysis of variables associated with mortality at day 28 in the overall population

	Survivors ($n = 81$)	Non-survivors ($n = 34$)	Odds ratio (95 % CI)	p value
Demographic variables				
Age (years)	56 ± 15	60 ± 15	1.02 (0.99–1.05)	0.13
Gender (male)	54 (67 %)	23 (68 %)	0.96 (0.41–2.25)	0.92
ICU admission before 2011	24 (30 %)	14 (41 %)	1.66 (0.72–3.82)	0.23
Noninvasive ventilation as a first-line therapy	34 (42 %)	22 (65 %)	2.67 (1.16–6.12)	0.03
SAPS II score	42 ± 12	47 ± 13	1.036 (1.00–1.07)	0.04
Modified SOFA score excluding respiratory item	3 (1–6)	4 (1–7)	1.06 (0.93–1.21)	0.44
Knaus chronic health status score				0.32
A	24 (30 %)	10 (29 %)	1	
B	31 (38 %)	8 (24 %)	0.62 (0.21–1.81)	
C	23 (28 %)	13 (38 %)	1.36 (0.50–3.70)	
D	3 (3.7 %)	3 (8.8 %)	2.40 (0.41–13.98)	
Mac Cabe classification				0.32
1	28 (35 %)	11 (32 %)	1	
2	37 (46 %)	12 (35 %)	0.83 (0.32–2.14)	
3	16 (20 %)	11 (32 %)	1.75 (0.62–4.94)	
Type of immunosuppression				0.08
Hematologic cancer or neutropenia	49 (60 %)	15 (44 %)	1	
Solid cancer	9 (11 %)	10 (29 %)	3.53 (1.21–10.27)	
Drug-induced immunosuppression	21 (26 %)	9 (26 %)	1.41 (0.54–3.70)	
Acquired immune deficiency syndrome	2 (2 %)	0 (0 %)	0.64 (0.02–27.52)	
Variables at inclusion				
Heart rate (bpm)	111 ± 23	113 ± 21	1.00 (0.99–1.02)	0.71
Systolic arterial blood pressure (mmHg)	126 ± 24	126 ± 29	1.00 (0.98–1.02)	0.96
Diastolic arterial blood pressure (mmHg)	67 ± 18	67 ± 13	1.00 (0.98–1.02)	0.99
Respiratory rate (breaths/min)	28 (25–32)	30 (27–34)	1.04 (0.98–1.10)	0.19
SpO_2 (%)	96 (94–99)	94 (90–97)	0.90 (0.83–0.97)	0.01
Body temperature (°C)	38.0 ± 1.2	37.7 ± 0.9	0.82 (0.58–1.18)	0.29
pH	7.46 (7.42–7.49)	7.44 (7.40–7.49)	0.59 (0.00–21.07)	0.30
Sodium bicarbonate (mmol/l)	24 (22–27)	24 (22–27)	1.03 (0.94–1.12)	0.83
PaO_2-to-FiO_2 ratio (mmHg)	158 ± 59	141 ± 48	0.99 (0.99–1.00)	0.15
PaO_2-to-FiO_2 ratio $\leq$ 200 mmHg	62 (77 %)	29 (85 %)	1.78 (0.60–5.23)	0.29
PaO_2 (mmHg)	74 (61–88)	70 (57–93)	1.00 (0.99–1.01)	0.38
$PaCO_2$ (mmHg)	34 (31–40)	34 (31–45)	1.01 (0.97–1.06)	0.56
$PaCO_2$ > 45 mmHg	8 (10 %)	6 (18 %)	1.96 (0.62–6.14)	0.24
Bilateral lung infiltrate	69 (85 %)	27 (79 %)	0.67 (0.24–1.89)	0.45
Vasopressors within 24 h after ICU admission	10 (12 %)	13 (38 %)	2.18 (0.85–5.62)	0.11
Immunosuppressive drug during ICU stay	22 (27 %)	6 (17 %)	0.58 (0.21–1.58)	0.35
Cause of respiratory failure				0.13
Documented infection	38 (47 %)	17 (50 %)	1	
Cardiogenic pulmonary edema	10 (12 %)	0 (0 %)	0.11 (0.01–2.17)	
Specific	11 (14 %)	8 (24 %)	1.63 (0.56–4.76)	
Other identified causes	12 (15 %)	6 (18 %)	1.14 (0.37–3.54)	
Not identified cause	10 (12 %)	3 (9 %)	0.73 (0.19–2.91)	

Nominal variables are given as number (%), and continuous data are given as median (25th–75th percentile) or mean ± standard deviation (SD) according to their distribution using the Kolmogorov–Smirnov test

SAPS Simplified Acute Physiology Score, *SOFA* Sequential Organ Failure Assessment

Table 3 Multivariate analysis of variables associated with outcomes in the overall population

	Adjusted odds ratio (95 % CI)	*p* value
Variables independently associated with intubation[a]		
Simplified Acute Physiology Score II, per point	1.04 (1.00–1.08)	0.04
Noninvasive ventilation as a first-line therapy	3.25 (1.39–7.60)	0.007
Use of vasopressors within 24 h after ICU admission	4.12 (1.32–12.84)	0.02
Variables independently associated with mortality at day 28[b]		
Age (per year)	1.03 (1.00–1.07)	0.04
Use of vasopressors within 24 h after ICU admission	2.83 (1.02–7.91)	0.047
Noninvasive ventilation as a first-line therapy	3.70 (1.49–9.19)	0.005

[a] Non-collinear variables included in the logistical regression model were Simplified Acute Physiology Score II, Noninvasive ventilation as a first-line therapy, use of vasopressors within 24 h after ICU admission, SpO_2 at ICU admission, cause of respiratory failure and $PaCO_2$ as a continuous variable. The year of ICU admission was forced in the model

[b] Non-collinear variables included in the logistical regression model were age, PaO_2-to-FiO_2 ratio at ICU admission, use of noninvasive ventilation as a first-line therapy, type of immunosuppression, use of vasopressors in the 24 h after ICU admission, cause of respiratory failure and $PaCO_2 > 45$ mmHg. The year of ICU admission was forced in the model

is well established that mortality of patients with acute respiratory distress syndrome (ARDS) is lower using low tidal volumes approximating 6 ml/kg of predicted body weight [38]. Even in patients without criteria for ARDS, the use of low tidal volumes may reduce the risk of developing ARDS [39]. In our study, the majority of patients treated with NIV had clinical criteria for ARDS according to the recent definition [40], and the expiratory tidal volumes delivered to these patients under NIV were around 9.0 ml/kg of predicted body weight. Although such high volumes are similar to those reported in recent studies focusing on NIV in acute respiratory failure [20, 34], they could be particularly deleterious by worsening lung injury. Indeed, in the study by Carteaux and colleagues, an expired tidal volume above 9.5 ml/kg of predicted body weight was a strong predictor of NIV failure in hypoxemic patients [36]. Despite the absence of expired tidal volume assessment in the HFNC group, the higher intubation rate observed in the NIV group may be explained by the high proportion of patients with an expired tidal volume above 9.5 ml/kg of predicted body weight (46 % of the patients treated with NIV). In addition, any potential deleterious effect of delayed intubation in patients treated with NIV [41, 42] can be ruled out as time from ICU admission to intubation was not longer than in patients treated with HFNC alone.

Limitations

Our study has several limitations. First, the study was monocentric and performed in a unit with experience in noninvasive management of immunocompromised patients with acute respiratory failure. Indeed, each year about 15 immunocompromised patients are treated with first-line noninvasive ventilatory support, which is close to the number of patients admitted in other highly skilled centers [2, 26]. Therefore, these results could not be extrapolated to centers with less experience. Second, the retrospective nature of the study might have induced selection bias despite the careful classification of patients included in the analysis. Indeed, the baseline characteristics of patients were not similar as patients in the HFNC group were older and as there was a higher proportion of patients with respiratory acidosis in the NIV group. NIV could have been preferentially used in hypercapnic patients due to its efficacy in correction of alveolar hypoventilation [43]. Therefore, the most severe patients might have been more frequently treated with NIV than with HFNC alone. Nevertheless, functional status before ICU admission and baseline severity scores were similar between the two groups. Our intubation and mortality rates in the NIV group were similar to those reported in the literature [2, 6, 26, 27], thereby reinforcing the external validity of our results. Third, it is possible that outcomes of immunocompromised patients admitted to our ICU over this 8-year period had improved in the recent years [44]. However, even after forcing the year of ICU admission in the logistic regression model, NIV remained associated with intubation and mortality. Obviously, these results do

Table 4 Comparison of baseline characteristics and outcomes between propensity score-matched patients treated by noninvasive positive pressure ventilation (NIV) or high-flow nasal cannula (HFNC) oxygen therapy alone

	NIV ($n = 24$)	HFNC ($n = 33$)	p value
Age (years)	62 ± 11	62 ± 11	0.72
Gender (male)	18 (75 %)	17 (52 %)	0.13
Knaus chronic health status score			0.53
A	8 (33 %)	9 (27 %)	
B	6 (25 %)	11 (33 %)	
C	10 (42 %)	11 (33 %)	
D	0 (0.0 %)	2 (6.1 %)	
Mac Cabe classification			0.27
1	11 (46 %)	12 (36 %)	
2	6 (25 %)	15 (45 %)	
3	7 (29 %)	6 (18 %)	
SAPS II at ICU admission (points)	40 ± 11	44 ± 12	0.52
Modified SOFA score at inclusion (points)	1.5 (0.0–4.0)	3.0 (1.0–6.0)	0.44
Type of immunosuppression			0.19
Hematologic cancer or neutropenia	12 (50 %)	18 (55 %)	
Solid cancer	7 (29 %)	3 (9.1 %)	
Drug-induced immunosuppression	5 (21 %)	11 (33 %)	
Acquired immune deficiency syndrome	0 (0.0 %)	1 (3.0 %)	
Cause of respiratory failure			0.08
Documented infection	9 (38 %)	19 (58 %)	
Cardiogenic pulmonary edema	4 (27 %)	3 (9.1 %)	
Specific	6 (25 %)	1 (3.0 %)	
Other identified causes	2 (8.3 %)	6 (18 %)	
Not identified cause	3 (13 %)	4 (12 %)	
Clinical and biological parameters at inclusion			
Heart rate (beats/min)	107 ± 21	112 ± 21	0.55
Systolic blood pressure (mmHg)	140 ± 22	127 ± 23	0.17
Respiratory rate (breaths/min)	30 ± 6	29 ± 6	0.76
SpO_2 (%)	94 ± 5	96 ± 4	0.10
Body temperature (°C)	37.9 ± 1.1	37.9 ± 1.1	0.66
Bilateral lung infiltrates on chest X-ray	19 (79 %)	31 (93 %)	0.12
Arterial pH	7.45 ± 0.07	7.46 ± 0.06	0.43
PaO_2-to-FiO_2 ratio (mmHg)	154 ± 57	156 ± 57	0.98
PaO_2-to-FiO_2 ratio ≤ 200 mmHg	18 (75 %)	24 (73 %)	0.85
$PaCO_2$ (mmHg)	39 ± 8	33 ± 5	0.03
$PaCO_2 > 45$ mmHg	4 (17 %)	1 (3.0 %)	0.15
Sodium bicarbonate (mmol/l)	26 ± 4	24 ± 4	0.10
Vasopressors within 24 h after ICU admission	1 (4.2 %)	4 (12 %)	0.39
Time from admission to ventilatory support initiation (h)	1 (0–1)	1 (0–1)	0.98
Need for immunosuppressive drug during ICU stay	5 (21 %)	4 (12 %)	0.47
Admission before 2011	12 (50 %)	7 (21 %)	0.04
Primary outcome			
28-day mortality	10 (42 %)	5 (15 %)	0.03
Secondary outcomes			
Intubation	13 (54 %)	10 (30 %)	0.07
Mortality of intubated	10/13 (77 %)	4/10 (40 %)	0.07
Time from admission to intubation (h)	48 (20–78)	35 (22–59)	>0.99
Length of invasive mechanical ventilation (days)	8 (5–18)	5 (3–10)	>0.99

Table 4 continued

	NIV ($n = 24$)	HFNC ($n = 33$)	p value
Length of ICU stay (days)	7 (5–16)	6 (4–9)	0.13
In-ICU mortality	10 (42 %)	4 (12 %)	0.01

Nominal variables are given as number (%), and continuous data are given as median (25th–75th percentile) or mean ± standard deviation (SD) according to their distribution using the Kolmogorov–Smirnov test

SAPS Simplified Acute Physiology Score, *SOFA* Sequential Organ Failure Assessment

not allow for definitive conclusion on the deleterious effects of NIV in this population, and our findings need to be confirmed in a randomized trial.

Conclusion

Based on this retrospective cohort study, the use of high-flow oxygen therapy through nasal cannula alone may be associated with better outcomes than noninvasive ventilation in immunocompromised patients admitted to intensive care unit for acute respiratory failure.

Abbreviations

HFNC: high-flow oxygen therapy through nasal cannula; ICU: intensive care unit; NIV: noninvasive ventilation.

Authors' contributions

RC, AJ, PP, RR AWT, and JPF participated in the design of the study and performed the statistical analysis. All authors read and approved the final manuscript.

Author details

[1] Service de Réanimation Médicale, CHU de Poitiers, 2, rue de la Milétrie, 86021 Poitiers, France. [2] INSERM CIC 1402 (ALIVE Group), Université de Poitiers, Poitiers, France.

Acknowledgements

We gratefully thank Jeffrey Arsham for editing the original manuscript.

Competing interests

The authors declare they have no competing interests.

References

1. Azoulay E, Mokart D, Pene F, Lambert J, Kouatchet A, Mayaux J, et al. Outcomes of critically ill patients with hematologic malignancies: prospective multicenter data from France and Belgium–a groupe de recherche respiratoire en reanimation onco-hematologique study. J Clin Oncol. 2013;31(22):2810–8.
2. Azevedo LC, Caruso P, Silva UV, Torelly AP, Silva E, Rezende E, et al. Outcomes for patients with cancer admitted to the ICU requiring ventilatory support: results from a prospective multicenter study. Chest. 2014; Epub 2014/02/01.
3. Molina R, Bernal T, Borges M, Zaragoza R, Bonastre J, Granada RM, et al. Ventilatory support in critically ill hematology patients with respiratory failure. Crit Care. 2012;16(4):R133.
4. Adda M, Coquet I, Darmon M, Thiery G, Schlemmer B, Azoulay E. Predictors of noninvasive ventilation failure in patients with hematologic malignancy and acute respiratory failure. Crit Care Med. 2008;36(10):2766–72.
5. Antonelli M, Conti G, Bufi M, Costa MG, Lappa A, Rocco M, et al. Noninvasive ventilation for treatment of acute respiratory failure in patients undergoing solid organ transplantation: a randomized trial. JAMA. 2000;283(2):235–41.
6. Hilbert G, Gruson D, Vargas F, Valentino R, Gbikpi-Benissan G, Dupon M, et al. Noninvasive ventilation in immunosuppressed patients with pulmonary infiltrates, fever, and acute respiratory failure. N Engl J Med. 2001;344(7):481–7.
7. Keenan SP, Sinuff T, Burns KE, Muscedere J, Kutsogiannis J, Mehta S, et al. Clinical practice guidelines for the use of noninvasive positive-pressure ventilation and noninvasive continuous positive airway pressure in the acute care setting. CMAJ. 2011;183(3):E195–214.
8. Azoulay E, Lemiale V, Mokart D, Pene F, Kouatchet A, Perez P, et al. Acute respiratory distress syndrome in patients with malignancies. Intensive Care Med. 2014;40(8):1106–14.
9. Schnell D, Timsit JF, Darmon M, Vesin A, Goldgran-Toledano D, Dumenil AS, et al. Noninvasive mechanical ventilation in acute respiratory failure: trends in use and outcomes. Intensive Care Med. 2014;40(4):582–91.
10. Demoule A, Chevret S, Carlucci A, Kouatchet A, Jaber S, Meziani F, et al. Changing use of noninvasive ventilation in critically ill patients: trends over 15 years in francophone countries. Intensive Care Med. 2016;42(1):82–92.
11. Lemiale V, Mokart D, Resche-Rigon M, Pene F, Mayaux J, Faucher E, et al. Effect of noninvasive ventilation vs oxygen therapy on mortality among immunocompromised patients with acute respiratory failure: a randomized clinical trial. JAMA. 2015;314(16):1711–9.
12. Spoletini G, Alotaibi M, Blasi F, Hill NS. Heated humidified high-flow nasal oxygen in adults: mechanisms of action and clinical implications. Chest. 2015;148(1):253–61.
13. Sztrymf B, Messika J, Bertrand F, Hurel D, Leon R, Dreyfuss D, et al. Beneficial effects of humidified high flow nasal oxygen in critical care patients: a prospective pilot study. Intensive Care Med. 2011;37(11):1780–6.
14. Roca O, Riera J, Torres F, Masclans JR. High-flow oxygen therapy in acute respiratory failure. Respir Care. 2010;55(4):408–13.
15. Frat JP, Brugiere B, Ragot S, Chatellier D, Veinstein A, Goudet V, et al. Sequential application of oxygen therapy via high-flow nasal cannula and noninvasive ventilation in acute respiratory failure: an observational pilot study. Respir Care. 2015;60(2):170–8.
16. Sim MA, Dean P, Kinsella J, Black R, Carter R, Hughes M. Performance of oxygen delivery devices when the breathing pattern of respiratory failure is simulated. Anaesthesia. 2008;63(9):938–40.
17. Parke R, McGuinness S, Eccleston M. Nasal high-flow therapy delivers low level positive airway pressure. Br J Anaesth. 2009;103(6):886–90.
18. Dysart K, Miller TL, Wolfson MR, Shaffer TH. Research in high flow therapy: mechanisms of action. Respir Med. 2009;103(10):1400–5.
19. Vargas F, Saint-Leger M, Boyer A, Bui NH, Hilbert G. Physiologic effects of high-flow nasal cannula oxygen in critical care subjects. Respir Care. 2015;60(10):1369–76.
20. Frat JP, Thille AW, Mercat A, Girault C, Ragot S, Perbet S, et al. High-flow oxygen through nasal cannula in acute hypoxemic respiratory failure. N Engl J Med. 2015;372(23):2185–96.
21. Knaus WA, Zimmerman JE, Wagner DP, Draper EA, Lawrence DE. APACHE-acute physiology and chronic health evaluation: a physiologically based classification system. Crit Care Med. 1981;9(8):591–7.
22. McCabe WR, Jackson GG. Gram negative bacteremia: I. Etiology and ecology. Arch Intern Med. 1962;110:845–7.
23. Le Gall JR, Lemeshow S, Saulnier F. A new simplified acute physiology score (SAPS II) based on a European/North American multicenter study. JAMA. 1993;270(24):2957–63.
24. Vincent JL, Moreno R, Takala J, Willatts S, De Mendonca A, Bruining H, et al. The SOFA (Sepsis-related Organ Failure Assessment) score to describe organ dysfunction/failure. On behalf of the Working Group

on Sepsis-Related Problems of the European Society of Intensive Care Medicine. Intensive Care Med. 1996;22(7):707–10.
25. D'Agostino RB Jr, D'Agostino RB Sr. Estimating treatment effects using observational data. JAMA. 2007;297(3):314–6.
26. Razlaf P, Pabst D, Mohr M, Kessler T, Wiewrodt R, Stelljes M, et al. Non-invasive ventilation in immunosuppressed patients with pneumonia and extrapulmonary sepsis. Respir Med. 2012;106(11):1509–16.
27. Gristina GR, Antonelli M, Conti G, Ciarlone A, Rogante S, Rossi C, et al. Noninvasive versus invasive ventilation for acute respiratory failure in patients with hematologic malignancies: a 5-year multicenter observational survey. Crit Care Med. 2011;39(10):2232–9.
28. Mokart D, Geay C, Chow-Chine L, Brun JP, Faucher M, Blache JL, et al. High-flow oxygen therapy in cancer patients with acute respiratory failure. Intensive Care Med. 2015;41(11):2008–10.
29. Lightowler JV, Wedzicha JA, Elliott MW, Ram FS. Non-invasive positive pressure ventilation to treat respiratory failure resulting from exacerbations of chronic obstructive pulmonary disease: Cochrane systematic review and meta-analysis. BMJ. 2003;326(7382):185.
30. Lindenauer PK, Stefan MS, Shieh MS, Pekow PS, Rothberg MB, Hill NS. Outcomes associated with invasive and noninvasive ventilation among patients hospitalized with exacerbations of chronic obstructive pulmonary disease. JAMA Intern Med. 2014;174(12):1982–93.
31. Vital FM, Ladeira MT, Atallah AN. Non-invasive positive pressure ventilation (CPAP or bilevel NPPV) for cardiogenic pulmonary oedema. Cochrane Database Syst Rev. 2013;5:CD005351.
32. Contou D, Fragnoli C, Cordoba-Izquierdo A, Boissier F, Brun-Buisson C, Thille AW. Noninvasive ventilation for acute hypercapnic respiratory failure: intubation rate in an experienced unit. Respir Care. 2013;58(12):2045–52.
33. Carrillo A, Ferrer M, Gonzalez-Diaz G, Lopez-Martinez A, Llamas N, Alcazar M, et al. Noninvasive ventilation in acute hypercapnic respiratory failure caused by obesity hypoventilation syndrome and chronic obstructive pulmonary disease. Am J Respir Crit Care Med. 2012;186(12):1279–85.
34. Thille AW, Contou D, Fragnoli C, Cordoba-Izquierdo A, Boissier F, Brun-Buisson C. Non-invasive ventilation for acute hypoxemic respiratory failure: intubation rate and risk factors. Crit Care. 2013;17(6):R269.
35. Ozsancak Ugurlu A, Sidhom SS, Khodabandeh A, Ieong M, Mohr C, Lin DY, et al. Use and outcomes of noninvasive positive pressure ventilation in acute care hospitals in Massachusetts. Chest. 2014;145(5):964–71.
36. Carteaux G, Millan-Guilarte T, De Prost N, Razazi K, Abid S, Thille AW, et al. Failure of noninvasive ventilation for de novo acute hypoxemic respiratory failure: role of tidal volume. Crit Care Med. 2015.
37. Slutsky AS, Ranieri VM. Ventilator-induced lung injury. N Engl J Med. 2014;370(10):980.
38. Ventilation with lower tidal volumes as compared with traditional tidal volumes for acute lung injury and the acute respiratory distress syndrome. The acute respiratory distress syndrome network. N Engl J Med. 2000;342(18):1301–8.
39. Serpa Neto A, Cardoso SO, Manetta JA, Pereira VG, Esposito DC, Pasqualucci Mde O, et al. Association between use of lung-protective ventilation with lower tidal volumes and clinical outcomes among patients without acute respiratory distress syndrome: a meta-analysis. JAMA. 2012;308(16):1651–9.
40. The ARDS Definition Task Force. Acute respiratory distress syndrome: the Berlin definition. JAMA. 2012;307(23):2526–33.
41. Esteban A, Frutos-Vivar F, Ferguson ND, Arabi Y, Apezteguia C, Gonzalez M, et al. Noninvasive positive-pressure ventilation for respiratory failure after extubation. N Engl J Med. 2004;350(24):2452–60.
42. Carrillo A, Gonzalez-Diaz G, Ferrer M, Martinez-Quintana ME, Lopez-Martinez A, Llamas N, et al. Non-invasive ventilation in community-acquired pneumonia and severe acute respiratory failure. Intensive Care Med. 2012;38(3):458–66.
43. L'Her E, Deye N, Lellouche F, Taille S, Demoule A, Fraticelli A, et al. Physiologic effects of noninvasive ventilation during acute lung injury. Am J Respir Crit Care Med. 2005;172(9):1112–8.
44. Quaresma M, Coleman MP, Rachet B. 40-year trends in an index of survival for all cancers combined and survival adjusted for age and sex for each cancer in England and Wales, 1971–2011: a population-based study. Lancet. 2015;385(9974):1206–18.

23

Characteristics of an ideal nebulized antibiotic for the treatment of pneumonia in the intubated patient

Matteo Bassetti[1*], Charles-Edouard Luyt[2,3], David P. Nicolau[4] and Jérôme Pugin[5]

Abstract

Gram-negative pneumonia in patients who are intubated and mechanically ventilated is associated with increased morbidity and mortality as well as higher healthcare costs compared with those who do not have the disease. Intravenous antibiotics are currently the standard of care for pneumonia; however, increasing rates of multidrug resistance and limited penetration of some classes of antimicrobials into the lungs reduce the effectiveness of this treatment option, and current clinical cure rates are variable, while recurrence rates remain high. Inhaled antibiotics may have the potential to improve outcomes in this patient population, but their use is currently restricted by a lack of specifically formulated solutions for inhalation and a limited number of devices designed for the nebulization of antibiotics. In this article, we review the challenges clinicians face in the treatment of pneumonia and discuss the characteristics that would constitute an ideal inhaled drug/device combination. We also review inhaled antibiotic options currently in development for the treatment of pneumonia in patients who are intubated and mechanically ventilated.

Keywords: Hospital-acquired pneumonia, Ventilator-associated pneumonia, Gram-negative bacteria, Multidrug resistance, Systemic antibiotics, Nebulizers, Inhaled antibiotics, Clinical cure

Background

Management of pneumonia in the intensive care unit (ICU) remains challenging

Hospital-acquired pneumonia (HAP) and ventilator-associated pneumonia (VAP) remain important causes of morbidity and mortality despite advances in antimicrobial therapy [1]. Patients with severe pneumonia or critical illness often require intubation and mechanical ventilation to manage acute respiratory failure; furthermore, 9–27 % of intubated patients will develop VAP [1, 2]. In mechanically ventilated patients with VAP, attributable mortality estimates vary considerably and have been reported to range from 0 to 50 % [3, 4]; however, there are large differences between subgroups of patients, and VAP-attributable mortality may be as high as 69 % in surgical patients for example [3]. Failure to provide timely and effective therapy in the first 48 h is also linked to particularly high mortality (Fig. 1) [5]. Clearly, early initiation of appropriate antibiotics is essential for effective management.

Current treatments are typically given through the intravenous (IV) route; however, despite widespread implementation of current antibiotic guidelines for the treatment of pneumonia, clinical cure rates rarely exceed 60 %, and recurrence rates remain high [6–10]. The high prevalence of multidrug-resistant (MDR) pathogens such as the 'ESKAPE' species (in particular *Staphylococcus aureus, Klebsiella pneumoniae, Acinetobacter baumannii, Pseudomonas aeruginosa* and *Enterobacter* spp.) add to the increasing difficulty of treating VAP. Unsurprisingly, MDR pathogens are associated with significant attributable mortality [11], and their increasing prevalence has been a concern due to the limited number of new antibiotics currently in development [12, 13]; clearly, there is an urgent clinical need to optimize therapy for critically ill patients with pneumonia [14].

*Correspondence: mattba@tin.it
[1] Infectious Diseases Clinic, Santa Maria Misericordia University Hospital, Udine, Italy
Full list of author information is available at the end of the article

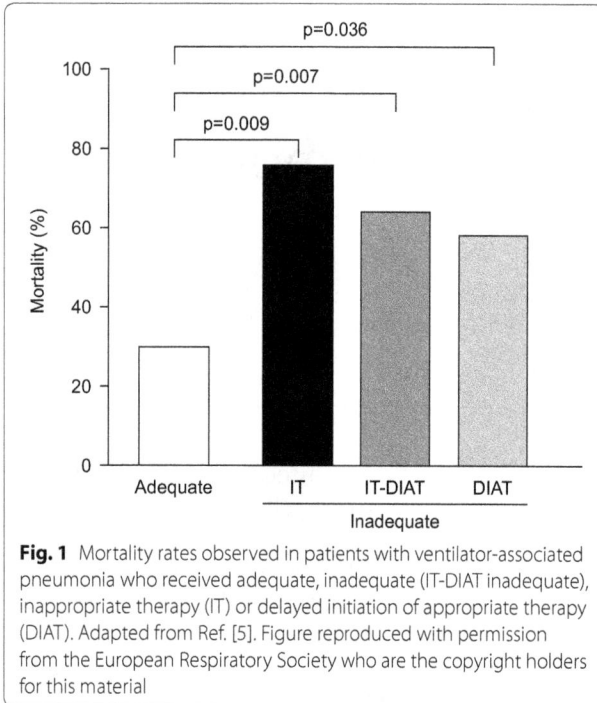

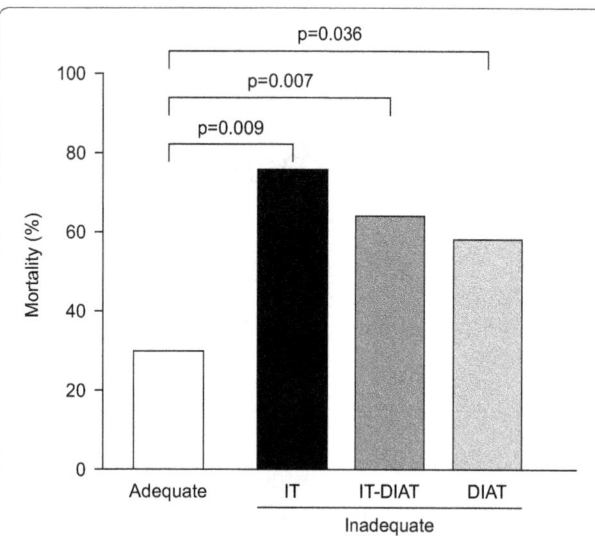

Fig. 1 Mortality rates observed in patients with ventilator-associated pneumonia who received adequate, inadequate (IT-DIAT inadequate), inappropriate therapy (IT) or delayed initiation of appropriate therapy (DIAT). Adapted from Ref. [5]. Figure reproduced with permission from the European Respiratory Society who are the copyright holders for this material

What makes antibiotics effective at the site of infection?

Effective treatment of bacterial pneumonia requires the concentration of the antibiotic in the lung to exceed the minimum inhibitory concentration (MIC) of the infecting pathogen. However, while some antimicrobial drugs such as fluoroquinolones penetrate well into lung tissue when administered intravenously [15], others (e.g., β-lactams, colistin, aminoglycosides and glycopeptides such as vancomycin) have poor lung penetration and tissue distribution [16–18]. Poor lung penetration of drugs can be overcome by dose increases, but this management approach is often limited by the associated risk of systemic adverse events; for example, high systemic concentrations of aminoglycosides are associated with nephrotoxicity and ototoxicity [19, 20]. The effectiveness of IV antibiotic therapy may be further diminished by pharmacokinetic changes in critically ill patients, including changes in absorption, distribution and elimination [21]. Such patient-specific variation makes adequate dosing of antibiotics challenging and may result in the delivery of drug concentrations that are either too low (and therefore sub-therapeutic) or too high (and therefore toxic) [22, 23].

In mechanically ventilated and intubated patients with pneumonia, targeting antibiotics to the lungs via aerosolization could offer a way to achieve high exposures of antibiotics directly at the site of infection, while minimizing systemic side effects [24, 25]. Initial treatment with aerosolized antibiotics combined with IV therapy is therefore a promising treatment strategy that could improve clinical outcomes.

Potential benefits of nebulized antibiotics

Previous approaches to nebulized antibiotic therapy have had several clinical and technical limitations, including sub-optimal delivery and lack of drugs specifically formulated for aerosolization [26, 27]. While issues such as these have hampered aerosolized delivery techniques, several recent developments suggest that these shortcomings could soon be eliminated.

Nebulized antibiotics can achieve high drug concentrations in the lung

Perhaps the key advantage of administering antibiotics by inhalation rather than via IV infusion is the potential to deliver high concentrations of antibiotic directly to the site of lung infection [28, 29]. Animal studies in ventilated piglets have demonstrated that nebulized antibiotics achieved high deposition in infected lung parenchyma with concentrations far above the MICs for most Gram-negative strains [30], and indeed, the efficiency of bacterial killing in piglets inoculated with *E. coli* was greater after nebulization compared with intravenous administration [31]. Furthermore, clinical studies have shown that inhaled tobramycin, for example, can achieve high bronchial concentrations, and inhaled amikacin can reach epithelial lining fluid (ELF) concentrations far in excess of the MICs for Gram-negative strains usually responsible for pneumonia [32, 33]. These concentrations may also exceed the MICs for MDR pathogens.

Nebulized antibiotics are associated with low systemic exposure

The high lung concentrations achieved with inhaled antibiotics are paired with low systemic absorption [34]; indeed, administering antibiotics such as aminoglycosides by aerosolization generates significantly lower peak serum concentrations compared with intravenous administration [27, 35]. One potential benefit of lower systemic concentrations is a reduced incidence of adverse events, such as nephrotoxicity [27]. In addition, low systemic concentrations may also have the benefit of falling outside the mutant selection window, thus reducing the risk of systemic resistance development [36, 37]. Studies in patients with cystic fibrosis treated with aerosolized antibiotics have not reported an increase in the emergence of resistance with inhaled therapy compared with standard therapy or placebo [38, 39]. This is supported by a recent double-blind placebo-controlled study of patients in the ICU, which demonstrated that in comparison with placebo, aerosolized antibiotics were not associated with the development of new antibiotic resistance [40].

Inhaled administration may reduce the need for systemic antibiotics

Aerosolized antibiotic therapy also provides the potential for a reduction in the overall use of systemic antibiotics [24, 41], with clear benefits for antibiotic stewardship and management of emergent resistance. Increased resistance due to frequent or excessive use of systemic antimicrobials has been documented for several drug classes. For example, between 2007 and 2011 the increased use of amoxicillin/clavulanic acid, ceftazidime and cefepime, carbapenems, and fluoroquinolones has correlated with an increase in the incidence of resistance in isolates of *K. pneumoniae*, *P. aeruginosa* and AmpC-producing *Enterobacteriaceae*, among others [42, 43]; decreasing the general use of antibiotics is therefore a key aim of antimicrobial stewardship programs. Importantly, this goal may be aided by the wider use of aerosolized therapies, and results from a Phase II study demonstrated that inhaled antibiotics could significantly reduce the use of IV antibiotics [44].

Characteristics of an 'ideal' inhaled antibiotic: what needs to be optimized?

Improving outcomes for critically ill patients with pneumonia requires the optimization of clinical factors such as ventilator settings, device usability and patient safety. An ideal inhaled antibiotic therapy should have a suitable formulation for aerosolization and consistently deliver high antibiotic concentrations to the site of infection via an efficient device; the drug should also have limited systemic penetration to prevent unwanted side effects.

Formulation of the ideal antibiotic for aerosolization

Currently available IV drug formulations are not optimized for aerosolization and often have properties that may impede drug delivery [26]. In addition, IV formulations usually contain preservatives such as phenols and many have sub-optimal osmolarity (<150 mOsm/L, >1200 mOsm/L), which can increase bronchospasm and coughing [26, 27]. To be suitable for aerosolization, the formulation should be sterile, preservative-free and non-pyrogenic. It should also be adjusted for the lung environment with a suitable pH (4.0–8.0), osmolarity (150–1200 mOsm/L) and tonicity [26, 27, 29] (Fig. 2). A solution that is specifically formulated for inhalation could minimize adverse effects, such as airway irritation, and increase delivery efficiency. Currently, the only

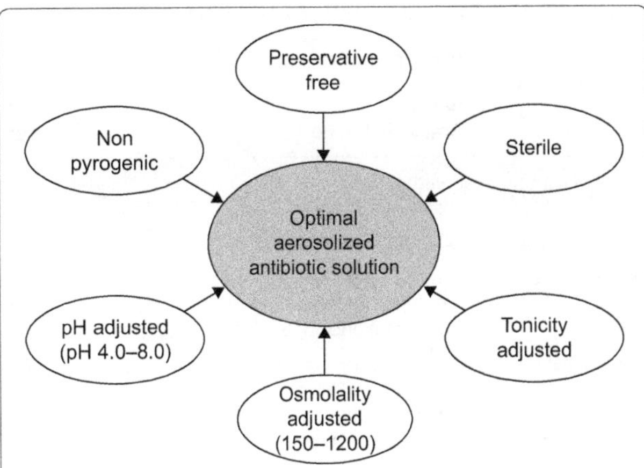

Fig. 2 Ideal properties of an antibiotic solution for aerosolization. Adapted from information in references [26, 27, 29]

antimicrobials that have a specific formulation developed for inhalation are colistin [45], aztreonam [46] and tobramycin [47], all of which are approved exclusively for use in cystic fibrosis [48].

Optimizing the dose

The choice of dose in early studies assessing aerosol delivery of antibiotics was sometimes based on the packaging of parenteral IV antibiotics, rather than on an a priori definition of the amount of drug that was needed in the lower airway [49]. Since then, studies have generally selected doses designed to achieve lung concentrations that far exceed the MIC of relevant pathogens in the lung [41, 49]. One recent study, for example, assessed two different dosing regimens of an inhaled aminoglycoside against a stringent pharmacokinetic target of achieving 25 times the highest MICs reported for *P. aeruginosa* and *Acinetobacter* spp. in North American ICUs [41].

Characteristics of the ideal delivery device

For optimal therapeutic effect, an appropriately formulated antibiotic should be used in combination with an efficient delivery device. A recent meta-analysis of inhaled treatments showed that while nebulized antibiotics (with or without IV antibiotic) may improve clinical cure rates compared with IV antibiotics alone, nebulizers themselves vary considerably in efficiency [50]. Indeed, jet nebulizers are known to have considerably lower efficiency (i.e., drug delivery rates) than vibrating mesh nebulizers (<15 vs 40–60 %, respectively) [51]. However, even within the vibrating mesh nebulizer device category, there is significant variation in delivery efficiency (Table 1). One of the primary determinants of delivery efficiency and drug deposition is particle size; a

Table 1 Technical considerations and performance characteristics of vibrating mesh nebulizers

Technical consideration	Performance characteristics vibrating mesh nebulizers		
	Bayer Amikacin Inhale	Aerogen Aeroneb Solo	PARI eFlow
Mode of action	Breath synchronized (hand-held = continuous nebulization)	Continuous nebulization	Breath enhanced
Delivered dose	On-vent: 35–58 %; hand-held: 35–64 % [54]	13–17 % [71, 72]	31–44 % [73]
Delivery time	Timing depends on patient and flow rate but has been reported to be 36 ± 16 (on-vent) and 15 ± 5 (hand-held) [54]	Dependent on medication but suggested to be around 7–10 min with 3 mL albuterol [71, 72]	Dependent on medication [63]
Humidification	Humidification does not affect delivered dose of amikacin Recommended to remove HME device	Recommended to turn humidification off during delivery Remove HME as per manufacturer's instructions	Humidification can be left on during delivery [66]

consistent and optimal particle size promotes distribution throughout the lungs and avoids condensation ('rain out') within the ventilator circuit [27, 52]. Particle size is usually measured as mass median aerodynamic diameter (MMAD) or volumetric median diameter (VMD), and a particle size in the range of 1–5 μm is considered to be suitable for deposition in the lung [36]; within this range, an MMAD or VMD of 3–5 μm is considered optimal for deposition in the bronchial conducting airways and throughout the alveoli (Fig. 3). However, currently available jet nebulizers cannot produce such small particles [52].

New drug–device combinations may hold promise in this area. The pulmonary drug delivery system (PDDS) device currently in development (NKTR-061) is an adaptive vibrating mesh nebulizer which has been combined with a specially formulated Amikacin Inhalation Solution (BAY41-6551). With this combination, approximately 60 % of the inhaled dose is delivered to the lung [53, 54]. These data indicate that specifically designed drug–device combinations have the potential to consistently generate and deliver optimally sized drug particles homogeneously throughout the lung, including to the peripheral airways. Any new drug–device combination that can deliver particles within the optimal 3–5 μm range could facilitate high drug concentrations at the site of pneumonia infection [36, 55].

Ease of use: ventilator setting adjustments

A key practical consideration for an ideal nebulizer is its ease of use in the hospital setting. For intubated and mechanically ventilated patients, the nebulizer should integrate directly into the ventilator circuit, with only minimal need to adjust ventilator settings or remove humidification [27, 52]. However, current-generation nebulizers, regardless of the drug formulation used, require careful attention to be paid to ventilator settings (e.g., choice of ventilator mode—pressure versus volume-controlled, inspiratory time, inspiratory flow, tidal volume, duty cycle and respiratory rate) to ensure optimal performance [53] and may also necessitate increased sedation of the patient as these settings are altered. Such adjustments can be complex due to the wide variety of modes and settings available, and guidelines advise avoiding heavy sedation if possible [1]. These complexities currently make the use of nebulization technically demanding; in order to optimize this route of administration, standardized aerosolization procedures are required [35]. The increased sedation of patients to enable better synchronization to ventilator settings may also be associated with longer durations of mechanical ventilation; one study reported no statistically significant difference in the duration of mechanical ventilation between patients treated with aerosolized antimicrobials compared with those treated with intravenous antimicrobials [35]. If a nebulizer device could be added to the circuit without the need for ventilator setting adjustment, this could minimize delays in treatment and reduce undesirable increases in sedation.

Synchronizing aerosol generation with the inspiratory flow of the ventilator could also enhance drug delivery [56]. An in vivo study found that levels of antibiotic delivered with breath-synchronized nebulization were four to seven times higher than with continuous nebulization, depending on the extent of ventilator humidification [57]. While humidification improves patient outcomes and prevents adverse events such as hypothermia, bronchospasm and cilia damage, studies (primarily conducted with jet nebulizers or metered-dose inhalers) have demonstrated that humidification greatly reduces drug delivery efficiency with conventional inhaled treatment approaches [53, 58]. Therefore, clinicians currently have to choose between the removal of humidification (thus improving delivery efficiency but potentially exposing the patient to adverse side effects) or the retention of humidification (protecting the patient but compromising

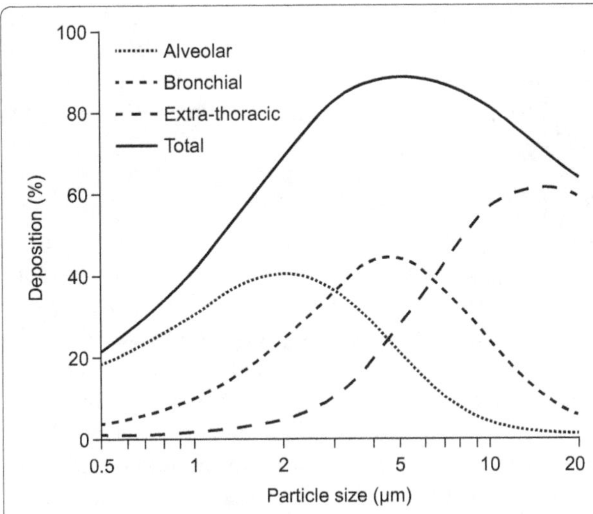

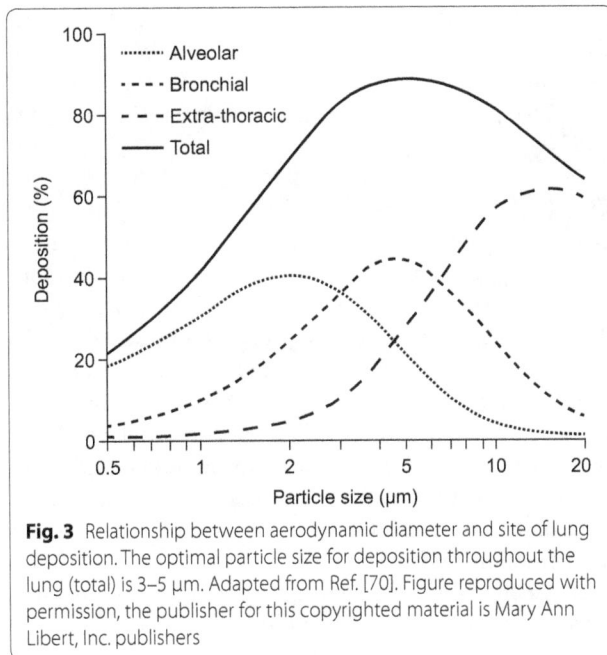

Fig. 3 Relationship between aerodynamic diameter and site of lung deposition. The optimal particle size for deposition throughout the lung (total) is 3–5 μm. Adapted from Ref. [70]. Figure reproduced with permission, the publisher for this copyrighted material is Mary Ann Libert, Inc. publishers

delivery efficiency). An ideal inhaled antibiotic should therefore achieve consistent lung delivery irrespective of humidification.

Overview of current understanding of inhaled treatments in intubated patients

The use of nebulized antibiotics has been increasing steadily since the 1970s, and inhaled antibiotic therapy is being revisited as a potential treatment option due to the surge in pneumonia caused by MDR bacteria [36]. Aerosolized therapy offers a way to administer high doses of antibiotics that exert their efficacy against pathogens directly at the site of infection while reducing systemic toxicity.

Evidence from clinical trials

Inhaled colistin has shown clinical utility in pneumonia, generating high lung concentrations and achieving efficient bacterial killing with a clinical cure rate of approximately 67 % [25, 51, 59]. Other studies have further demonstrated that nebulized antibiotics, such as specially formulated Amikacin Inhale, produce low systemic concentrations with limited toxic side effects [33], and a recent meta-analysis supports that nebulized antibiotics may improve clinical cure rates in patients with VAP, although additional clinical studies are still needed [50].

Indeed, despite some promising data, the overall number of well-designed trials examining the efficacy and tolerability of nebulized antibiotics remains low. Many studies have only involved a single center and are confounded by inadequate patient enrollment, poor methodology or failures in standardizing or reporting delivery methods and particle sizes [52]. Currently, there is no standardized technique for administration of a given aerosolized drug, and different studies have used different doses or formulations as well as differing patient cohorts. These factors make the comparison of efficiency and tolerability data difficult and pose challenges when trying to standardize this method of treatment and decide best practice. There is a clear unmet need for further multicenter studies, with standardized methodologies, consistent dosing and larger cohorts to improve the data available on the efficacy and safety of inhaled therapy.

Treatment guidelines

Aerosolized adjunctive therapy with IV antimicrobials is suggested by the ATS/IDSA guidelines (2005) as appropriate for patients with pneumonia caused by MDR Gram-negative organisms who are not responding to systemic therapy alone; however, these guidelines are now a decade old and may no longer be an accurate reflection of the bacterial landscape currently confronting clinicians in the ICU. Other more recent guidelines, such as the Canadian HAP/VAP guideline (2008), recommend the use of aerosolized vancomycin in patients infected with MRSA; other guidelines currently make no recommendations for the use of inhaled antibiotics [60, 61].

Healthcare worker perceptions and understanding

While there is now a more positive attitude toward nebulized antibiotics, clinician knowledge pertaining to the delivery of aerosolized therapy remains poor. Techniques to improve nebulizer output, such as reducing the inspiratory flow, are not regularly employed, and potentially dangerous practices (such as connecting the nebulizer to an external gas source or never changing the expiratory limb filter) were reported in a recent survey into physicians' practice, knowledge and beliefs regarding aerosol therapy [62].

Inhaled therapies currently in development

Aerosolized antibiotics have been used off-label for the treatment of pneumonia in mechanically ventilated, critically ill patients for around 40 years, but there is still no consensus, guideline or FDA-approved product available for such treatment [24]. There are, however, three aerosol-based therapies currently in development for the treatment of pneumonia in this vulnerable patient group.

The PARI eFlow rapid nebuliser system® [63] is a multiple-use, single-patient device that is placed on the inspiratory limb of the ventilator circuit [52] to deliver a combination of amikacin and fosfomycin; the two drugs are added sequentially to the nebulizer. In two Phase I studies, the PARI system generated small amikacin–fosfomycin droplets and achieved high tracheal aspirate concentrations with low systemic exposure [64–66]. When delivered using a drug ratio of 5:2 (amikacin–fosfomycin), the combination reduced resistance development, and the authors attributed this effect to synergy between the two antibiotics [64–66]. A Phase II trial with the PARI system is ongoing (NCT01969799).

Inhaled tobramycin (TOBI®) is approved by the FDA for use in patients with cystic fibrosis and is currently under investigation for use in patients with pneumonia. Early studies have suggested that TOBI® is well tolerated and effective for the treatment of VAP caused by *P. aeruginosa* or *Acinetobacter* spp., with reduced systemic side effects compared with IV tobramycin [67]. While these results are promising, the study was performed using a very small cohort, with only five patients in each group.

Amikacin Inhale, a drug–device combination being developed to treat patients who are intubated and mechanically ventilated who develop Gram-negative pneumonia, consists of a specifically formulated Amikacin Inhalation Solution and the pulmonary drug delivery system (PDDS) (NKTR-061, BAY41-6551). The PDDS synchronizes aerosolization of the antibiotic with the first 75 % of the inspiratory flow, with the aim of enhancing deposition in the lung and reducing wastage. The system can also be used in on-vent and hand-held configurations in a number of orientations to allow therapy to continue after extubation, with no need for ventilator setting or dose adjustment [54, 68]. In an in vitro study, the on-vent configuration of the PDDS (and Amikacin Inhalation Solution) achieved an estimated lung dose (ELD) of 35–58 % of the nominal dose, while the hand-held configuration achieved an ELD of 35–64 % of the nominal dose [54]. Phase II studies have demonstrated that the concentration of amikacin delivered to the lung substantially exceeded MIC values for the Gram-negative organisms primarily responsible for pneumonia (NCT01004445 and NCT01021436) [33, 41]. In the first study, the median ELF amikacin concentration, as determined by bronchoalveolar lavage, was 976.1 μg/mL [33]. In the second study, the primary endpoint of achieving both a tracheal aspirate amikacin concentration $\geq$6,400 μg/mL (25 times the reference MIC of 256 μg/mL) and a ratio of amikacin aspirate AUC_{0-24h} to MIC $\geq$ 100 at day 1 was achieved in 50 % of patients receiving Amikacin Inhale 400 mg every 12 h [41]. Amikacin Inhale can achieve consistently high drug delivery independent of humidity or humidification method [69]. Maximum concentrations of amikacin in serum remained below the recommended maximal trough concentration for systemic amikacin administration, and Amikacin Inhale was generally well tolerated [41]. Two Phase III studies are ongoing (NCT01799993 and NCT00805168).

Conclusions

Nebulizer technology continues to evolve. Improvements in nebulizer capabilities may offer new treatment options that maximize the potential benefits of inhaled antibiotic therapy. Recent advances are promising to deliver nebulized therapy options with optimal particle sizes and to achieve improved drug delivery throughout the lung, while maintaining low systemic exposures. The combination of specifically designed drug formulations and modern, high efficiency delivery devices has the potential to overcome current challenges in the aerosolized treatment of pneumonia [29].

Increasing resistance and limited efficacy of currently available IV antibiotics for the treatment of pneumonia in intubated and mechanically ventilated patients are a growing cause for concern, and the choice of effective treatments is limited. New therapy options are urgently needed; continued improvements in antibiotic formulations and nebulizer system designs provide an increasingly positive outlook for the future of inhaled antibiotics.

Abbreviations

ATS: American Thoracic Society; CAP: community-acquired pneumonia; ELD: estimated lung dose; ELF: epithelial lining fluid; FDA: food and drug administration; HAP: hospital-acquired pneumonia; ICU: intensive care unit; IDSA: Infectious Diseases Society of America; IV: intravenous; MDR: multidrug resistant; MIC: minimum inhibitory concentration; MMAD: mass median aerodynamic diameter; MRSA: methicillin-resistant staphylococcus aureus; PDDS: pulmonary drug delivery system; VAP: ventilator-associated pneumonia; VMD: volumetric median diameter.

Authors' contributions

MB, CEL, DPN and JP made substantial contributions to conception and design, or acquisition of data, or analysis and interpretation of data. MB, CEL, DPN and JP were involved in drafting the manuscript or revising it critically for important intellectual content. MB, CEL, DPN and JP gave final approval of the version to be published. MB, CEL, DPN and JP were accountable for all aspects of the work in ensuring that questions related to the accuracy or integrity of any part of the work are appropriately investigated and resolved.

Author details

[1] Infectious Diseases Clinic, Santa Maria Misericordia University Hospital, Udine, Italy. [2] Service de Réanimation, Institut de Cardiologie, Groupe Hospitalier Pitié–Salpêtrière, Assistance Publique–Hôpitaux de Paris, Paris, France. [3] Sorbonne Universités, UPMC Université Paris 06, INSERM, UMRS_1166-ICAN Institute of Cardiometabolism and Nutrition, Paris, France. [4] Center for Anti-Infective Research and Development, Hartford Hospital, Hartford, USA. [5] Service des Soins Intensifs, University Hospitals of Geneva and Faculty of Medicine, University of Geneva, Geneva, Switzerland.

Acknowledgements

Medical writing services were provided by Highfield Communication, Oxford, UK, and funded by Bayer.

Competing interests

Matteo Bassetti serves on scientific advisory boards for AstraZeneca, Astellas Pharma Inc., Basilea, Bayer, Gilead, MSD, Pfizer Inc., Tetraphase, and has received funding for travel or speaker honoraria from Astellas, AstraZeneca, Gilead/Gilead Sciences, MSD, Novartis, Pfizer Inc., and Vifor Pharma. Charles-Edouard Luyt has received research grants from Bayer and has received fees for lectures from Astellas, Bayer, Biomérieux, MSD, Novartis and ThermoFischer Brahms. He has also served on advisory boards for Bayer. David Nicolau has been a consultant, speaker bureau member or has received research funding from: Allergan, AstraZeneca, Bayer, GSK, Medicines Co., Merck, Pfizer, Tetraphase. He is also a voting member of the Clinical Laboratory Standards Institute (CLSI). Jérôme Pugin has received consulting fees from Bayer, Biomérieux and ThermoFischer.

References

1. American Thoracic Society/Infectious Diseases Society of America (ATS/IDSA). Guidelines for the management of adults with hospital-acquired, ventilator-associated, and healthcare-associated pneumonia. Am J Respir Crit Care Med. 2005;171:388–416.
2. Kalanuria AA, Zai W, Mirski M. Ventilator-associated pneumonia in the ICU. Crit Care. 2014;18:208.
3. Melsen WG, Rovers MM, Groenwold RHH, Bergmans DCJJ, Camus C, Bauer TT, Hanisch EW, Klarin B, Koeman M, Krueger WA, Lacherade JC, Lorente L, Memish ZA, Morrow LE, Nardi G, van Nieuwenhoven CA CA, O'Keefe GE, George Nakos G, Scannapieco FA, Seguin P, Staudinger T, Topeli A, Ferrer M, Bonten MJM. Attributable mortality of ventilator-associated pneumonia: a meta-analysis of individual patient data from randomised prevention studies. Lancet Infect Dis. 2013;13:665–71.
4. Koenig SM, Truwit JD. Ventilator-associated pneumonia: diagnosis, treatment, and prevention. Clin Microbiol Rev. 2006;19:637–57.
5. Luna C, Aruj P, Niederman M, Garzón J, Violi D, Prignoni A, Ríos F, Baquero S, Gando S. Appropriateness and delay to initiate therapy in ventilator-associated pneumonia. Eur Respir J. 2006;27:158–64.
6. Chastre J, Wunderink R, Prokocimer P, Lee M, Kaniga K, Friedland I. Efficacy and safety of intravenous infusion of doripenem versus imipenem in ventilator-associated pneumonia: a multicenter, randomized study. Crit Care Med. 2008;36:1089–96.
7. Jenkins S, Fisher A, Peterson J, Nicholson S, Kaniga K. Meta-analysis of doripenem vs comparators in patients with Pseudomonas infections enrolled in four phase III efficacy and safety clinical trials. Curr Med Res Opin. 2009;25:3029–36.
8. Kollef M, Chastre J, Clavel M, Restrepo M, Michiels B, Kaniga K, Cirillo I, Kimko H, Redman R. A randomized trial of 7-day doripenem versus 10-day imipenem-cilastatin for ventilator-associated pneumonia. Crit Care. 2012;16:R218.
9. Awad SS, Rodriguez AH, Chuang YC, Marjanek Z, Pareigis AJ, Reis G, Scheeren TWL, Sánchez AS, Zhou X, Saulay M, Engelhardt M. A phase 3 randomized double-blind comparison of ceftobiprole medocaril versus ceftazidime plus linezolid for the treatment of hospital-acquired pneumonia. Clin Infect Dis. 2014;59:51–61.
10. Flume P, VanDevanter D. Clinical applications of pulmonary delivery of antibiotics. Adv Drug Deliv Rev. 2015;85:1–6.
11. Bercault N, Boulain T. Mortality rate attributable to ventilator-associated nosocomial pneumonia in an adult intensive care unit: a prospective case–control study. Respir Ther. 2001;29:2303–9.
12. Boucher H, Talbot G, Bradley J, Edwards J, Gilbert D, Rice L, Scheld M, Spellberg B, Bartlett J. Bad bugs, no drugs: no ESKAPE! An update from the Infectious Diseases Society of America. Clin Infect Dis. 2009;48:1–12.
13. Spellberg B, Bartlett J, Wunderink R, Gilbert DN. Novel approaches are needed to develop tomorrow's antibacterial therapies. Am J Respir Crit Care Med. 2015;191:135–40.
14. Bassetti M, De Waele JJ, Eggimann P, Garnacho-Montero J, Kahlmeter G, Menichetti F, Nicolau DP, Paiva JA, Tumbarello M, Welte T, Wilcox M, Zahar RJ, Poulakou G. Preventive and therapeutic strategies in critically ill patients with highly resistant bacteria. Intensive Care Med. 2015;41:776–95.
15. Wise R, Honeybourne D. Pharmacokinetics and pharmacodynamics of fluoroquinolones in the respiratory tract. Eur Respir J. 1999;14:221–9.
16. Honeybourne D. Antibiotic penetration into lung tissues. Thorax. 1994;49:104–6.
17. Cruciana M, Gatti G, Lazzarini L, Furlan G, Broccali G, Malena M, Franchini C, Concia E. Penetration of vancomycin into human lung tissue. J Antimicrob Chemother. 1996;38:865–9.
18. Imberti R, Cusato M, Villani P, Carnevale L, Iotti G, Langer M, Regazzi M. Steady-state pharmacokinetics and BAL concentration of colistin in critically ill patients after IV colistin methanesulfonate administration. Chest. 2010;138:1333–9.
19. Avent ML, Rogers BA, Cheng AC, Paterson DL. Current use of aminoglycosides: indications, pharmacokinetics and monitoring for toxicity. Int Med J. 2011;41:441–9.
20. Arnold A, Brouse S, Pitcher W, Hall R. Empiric therapy for Gram-negative pathogens in nosocomial and health care-associated pneumonia: starting with the end in mind. J Intensive Care Med. 2010;25:259–70.
21. Smith B, Yogaratnam D, Levasseur-Franklin K, Forni A, Fong J. Introduction to drug pharmacokinetics in the critically ill patient. Chest. 2012;141:1327–36.
22. Blot S, Pea F, Lipman J. The effect of pathophysiology on pharmacokinetics in the critically ill patient—concepts appraised by the example of antimicrobial agents. Adv Drug Deliv Rev. 2014;77:3–11.
23. Vinks A, Derendorf H, Mouton J. Fundamentals of Antimicrobial Pharmacokinetics and Pharmacodynamics. New York/Heidelberg/Dordrecht/London: Springer; 2014. p. 63–72.
24. Palmer LB. Aerosolized antibiotics in the intensive care unit. Clinics Chest Med. 2011;32:559–74.
25. Lu Q, Luo R, Bodin L, Yang J, Zahr N, Aubry A, Golmard J, Rouby J. Efficacy of high-dose nebulized colistin in ventilator-associated pneumonia caused by multidrug-resistant *Pseudomonas aeruginosa* and *Acinetobacter baumannii*. Anesthesiology. 2012;117:1335–47.
26. Le J, Neuhauser M, Brown J, Gentry C, Klepser M, Marr A, Schiller D, Schwiesow J, Tice S, VandenBussche H, Wood C. Consensus summary of aerosolized antimicrobial agents: application of guideline criteria. Pharmacotherapy. 2010;30:562–84.
27. Wood C. Aerosolized antibiotics for treating hospital-acquired and ventilator-associated pneumonia. Exp Rev Anti-Infect Ther. 2011;9:993–1000.
28. Luyt C-E, Combes A, Nieszkowska A, Trouillet J, Chastre J. Aerosolized antibiotics to treat ventilator-associated pneumonia. Curr Opin Infect Dis. 2009;22:154–8.
29. Abu-Salah T, Dhand R. Inhaled antibiotic therapy for ventilator-associated tracheobronchitis and ventilator-associated pneumonia: an update. Adv Ther. 2011;29:728–47.
30. Goldstein I, Wallet F, Robert J, Bequemin M, Marquette C, Rouby J. Lung tissue concentrations of nebulized amikacin during mechanical ventilation in piglets with healthy lungs. Am J Respir Crit Care Med. 2002;165:171–5.
31. Goldstein I, Wallet F, Nicolas-Robin A, Ferrari F, Marquette C-H, Rouby J-J, the Experimental Intensive Care Unit Study Group. Lung deposition and efficiency of nebulized amikacin during *Escherichia coli* pneumonia in ventilated piglets. Am J Respir Crit Care Med. 2002;166:1375–81.
32. Badia J, Soy D, Adrover M, Ferrer M, Sarasa M, Alarcón A, Codina C, Torres A. Disposition of instilled versus nebulized tobramycin and imipenem in ventilated intensive care unit (ICU) patients. J Antimicrob Chemother. 2004;54:508–14.
33. Luyt C-E, Clavel M, Guntupalli K, Johannigman J, Kennedy J, Wood C, Corkery K, Gribben D, Chastre J. Pharmacokinetics and lung delivery of PDDS-aerosolized amikacin (NKTR-061) in intubated and mechanically ventilated patients with nosocomial pneumonia. Crit Care. 2009;13:R200.
34. Cooney G, Lum B, Tomaselli M, Fiel S. Absolute bioavailability and absorption characteristics of aerosolized tobramycin in adults with cystic fibrosis. Clin Pharmacol. 1994;34:255–9.
35. Lu Q, Yang J, Liu Z, Gutierrez C, Aymard G, Rouby JJ, the Nebulized Antibiotics Study Group. Nebulized ceftazidime and amikacin in ventilator-associated pneumonia caused by *Pseudomonas aeruginosa*. Am J Respir Crit Care Med. 2011;184:106–15.
36. Dhand R. The role of aerosolized antimicrobials in the treatment of ventilator-associated pneumonia. Respir Care. 2007;52:866–84.
37. Drlica K, Zhao X. Mutant selection window hypothesis updated. Clin Infect Dis. 2007;44:681–8.
38. Ramsey BW, Dorkin HL, Eisenberg JD, Gibson RL, Harwood IR, Kravitz RM,

Schidlow DV, Wilmott RW, Astley SJ, McBurnie MA, Wentz K, Smith AL. Efficacy of aerosolized tobramycin in patients with cystic fibrosis. N Engl J Med. 1993;328:1740–6.
39. Burns JL, Van Dalfsen JM, Shawar RM, Otto KL, Garber RL, Quan JM, Montgomery AB, Albers GM, Ramsey BW, Smith AL. Effect of chronic intermittent administration of inhaled tobramycin on respiratory microbial flora in patients with cystic fibrosis. J Infect Dis. 1999;179:1190–6.
40. Palmer LB, Smaldone GC. Reduction of bacterial resistance with inhaled antibiotics in the intensive care unit. Am J Respir Crit Care Med. 2014;189:1225–33.
41. Niederman M, Chastre J, Corkery K, Fink J, Luyt C-E, Sanchez Garcia M. BAY41-6551 achieves bactericidal tracheal aspirate amikacin concentrations in mechanically ventilated patients with Gram-negative pneumonia. Intensive Care Med. 2012;38:263–71.
42. Chastre J, Luyt C-E. Optimising the duration of antibiotic therapy for ventilator-associated pneumonia. Eur Respir Rev. 2007;16:40–4.
43. Fihman V, Messika J, Hajage D, Tournier V, Gaudry S, Magdoud F, Barnaud G, Billard-Pomares T, Branger C, Dreyfuss D, Ricard JD. Five-year trends for ventilator-associated pneumonia: correlation between microbiological findings and antimicrobial drug consumption. Int J Antimicrob Agents. 2015;46:518–25.
44. Niederman M, Chastre J, Corkery K, Marcantonio A, Fink J, Luyt C-E, Sanchez M and The Amikacin Study Group. NKTR-061 (inhaled amikacin) reduces intravenous antibiotic use in intubated mechanically ventilated patients during treatment of Gram-negative pneumonia. ATS 18–23 May 2007, Poster A326.
45. Colistin summary of product characteristics. https://www.medicines.org.uk/emc/medicine/27647. Accessed 25 Nov 2015.
46. Aztreonam summary of product characteristics. https://www.medicines.org.uk/emc/medicine/22358. Accessed 25 Nov 2015.
47. Tobramycin summary of product characteristics. https://www.medicines.org.uk/emc/medicine/19020. Accessed 25 Nov 2015.
48. Quon B, Goss C, Ramsey B. Inhaled antibiotics for lower airway infections. Ann Am Thorac Soc. 2014;11:425–34.
49. Geller DE. Aerosol antibiotics in cystic fibrosis. Respir Care. 2009;54:658–70.
50. Zampieri F, Nassar A Jr, Gusmao-Flores D, Taniguchi L, Torres A, Ranzani O. Nebulized antibiotics for ventilator-associated pneumonia: a systematic review and meta-analysis. Crit Care. 2015;19:150.
51. Rouby J, Bouhemad B, Monsel A, Brisson H, Arbelot C, Lu Q, the Nebulized Antibiotic Study Group. Aerosolized antibiotics for ventilator-associated pneumonia: lessons from experimental studies. Anesthesiology. 2012;117:1364–80.
52. Kollef M, Hamilton C, Montgomery A. Aerosolized antibiotics: do they add to the treatment of pneumonia? Curr Opin Infect Dis. 2013;26:538–44.
53. Dhand R. Aerosol delivery during mechanical ventilation: from basic techniques to new devices. J Aerosol Med Pulm Drug Deliv. 2008;21:45–60.
54. Kadrichu N, Boc S, Corkery K, Challoner P. In vitro efficiency of the Amikacin Inhale System, a novel integrated drug-device delivery system. ISICEM, 19–22 March 2013, Poster A384.
55. Laube B, Janssens H, de Jongh F, Devadason S, Dhand R, Diot P, Everard M, Horvath I, Navalesi P, Voshaar T, Chrystyn H. What the pulmonary specialist should know about the new inhalation therapies. Eur Respir J. 2011;37:1308–31.
56. Dhand R. Maximising aerosol delivery during mechanical ventilation: go with the flow and go slow. Intensive Care Med. 2003;29:1041–2.
57. Miller D, Amin M, Palmer L, Shah A, Smaldone G. Aerosol delivery and modern mechanical ventilation: in vitro/in vivo evaluation. Am J Respir Crit Care Med. 2003;168:1205–9.
58. Restrepo R, Walsh B. Humidification during invasive and noninvasive mechanical ventilation: 2012. Respir Care. 2012;57:782–8.
59. Lu Q, Girardi C, Zhang M, Bouhemad B, Louchahi K, Petitjean O, Wallet F, Becquemin M, Le Naour G, Marquette C, Rouby J. Nebulized and intravenous colistin in experimental pneumonia caused by *Pseudomonas aeruginosa*. Intensive Care Med. 2010;36:1147–55.
60. Mandell LA, Wunderink RG, Anzueto A, Bartlett JG, Campbell GD, Dean NC, Dowell SF, File TM Jr, Musher DM, Niederman MS, Torres A, Whitney CG. Infectious Diseases Society of America/American Thoracic Society consensus guidelines on the management of community-acquired pneumonia in adults. Clin Infect Dis. 2007;44:S27–72.
61. Masterton RG, Galloway A, French G, Street M, Armstrong E, Brown E, Cleverley J, Dilworth P, Fry C, Gascoigne AD, Knox A, Nathwani D, Spencer R, Wilcox M. Guidelines for the management of hospital-acquired pneumonia in the UK: report of the Working Party on hospital-acquired pneumonia of the British Society for Antimicrobial Chemotherapy. J Antimicrob Chemother. 2008;62:5–34.
62. Ehrmann S, Roche-Campo F, Sferrazza Papa G, Isabey D, Brochard L, Apiou-Sbirlea G, REVA research network. Aerosol therapy during mechanical ventilation: an international survey. Intensive Care Med. 2013;39:1048–56.
63. PARI eFlow rapid, Technical Data. http://www.pari.de/uk-en/products/lower-airways-1/eflow-rapid-nebuliser-system-1/. Accessed 13 Nov 2015.
64. Montgomery A, Rhomberg P, Abuan T, Walters K, Flamm R. Amikacin-fosfomycin at a five-to-two ratio: characterization of mutation rates in microbial strains causing ventilator-associated pneumonia and interactions with commonly used antibiotics. Antimicrob Agents Chemother. 2014;58:3707–13.
65. Montgomery A, Rhomberg P, Abuan T, Walters K, Flamm R. Potentiation effects of amikacin and fosfomycin against selected amikacin-nonsusceptible Gram-negative respiratory tract pathogens. Antimicrob Agents Chemother. 2014;58:3714–9.
66. Montgomery A, Vallance S, Abuan T, Tservistas M, Davies A. A randomized double-blind placebo-controlled dose-escalation Phase 1 study of aerosolized amikacin and fosfomycin delivered via the PARI Investigational eFlow® Inline Nebulizer System in mechanically ventilated patients. J Aerosol Med Pulm Drug Deliv. 2014;27:441–8.
67. Hallal A, Cohn S, Namias N, Habib F, Baracco G, Manning R, Crookes B, Schulman C. Aerosolized tobramycin in the treatment of ventilator-associated pneumonia: a pilot study. Surg Infect (Larchmt). 2007;8:73–81.
68. Kadrichu N, Corkery K, Dang T, Challoner P. Performance of amikacin inhale: impact of supplemental oxygen and device orientation. Crit Care. 2015;19(Suppl 1):P120.
69. Kadrichu N, Boc S, Corkery K and Challoner P. Influence of humidification on in vitro dose delivery for Amikacin Inhale by mechanical ventilation. ESICM, 27 September–1 October 2014, Abstract 0867.
70. Pritchard JN. The influence of lung deposition on clinical response. J Aerosol Med. 2001;14(Suppl 1):19–26.
71. Aerogen. Aeroneb® Solo datasheet. http://www.aerogen.com/uploads/datasheets/Aeroneb_Solo_Product_Datasheet_FINAL_A4.pdf. Accessed 13 Nov 2015.
72. Aerogen. Aeroneb® Solo FAQs. http://www.aerogen.com/medical-community/faq/faq-aerogen-solo.html. Accessed 13 Nov 2015.
73. Seemann S, Schmitt A, Waldner R, Hug M, Knoch M. Improving aerosol drug delivery in CF therapy. European Cystic Fibrosis Conference, 22–26 June 2005, Poster P113.

Permissions

All chapters in this book were first published in AIC, by Springer; hereby published with permission under the Creative Commons Attribution License or equivalent. Every chapter published in this book has been scrutinized by our experts. Their significance has been extensively debated. The topics covered herein carry significant findings which will fuel the growth of the discipline. They may even be implemented as practical applications or may be referred to as a beginning point for another development.

The contributors of this book come from diverse backgrounds, making this book a truly international effort. This book will bring forth new frontiers with its revolutionizing research information and detailed analysis of the nascent developments around the world.

We would like to thank all the contributing authors for lending their expertise to make the book truly unique. They have played a crucial role in the development of this book. Without their invaluable contributions this book wouldn't have been possible. They have made vital efforts to compile up to date information on the varied aspects of this subject to make this book a valuable addition to the collection of many professionals and students.

This book was conceptualized with the vision of imparting up-to-date information and advanced data in this field. To ensure the same, a matchless editorial board was set up. Every individual on the board went through rigorous rounds of assessment to prove their worth. After which they invested a large part of their time researching and compiling the most relevant data for our readers.

The editorial board has been involved in producing this book since its inception. They have spent rigorous hours researching and exploring the diverse topics which have resulted in the successful publishing of this book. They have passed on their knowledge of decades through this book. To expedite this challenging task, the publisher supported the team at every step. A small team of assistant editors was also appointed to further simplify the editing procedure and attain best results for the readers.

Apart from the editorial board, the designing team has also invested a significant amount of their time in understanding the subject and creating the most relevant covers. They scrutinized every image to scout for the most suitable representation of the subject and create an appropriate cover for the book.

The publishing team has been an ardent support to the editorial, designing and production team. Their endless efforts to recruit the best for this project, has resulted in the accomplishment of this book. They are a veteran in the field of academics and their pool of knowledge is as vast as their experience in printing. Their expertise and guidance has proved useful at every step. Their uncompromising quality standards have made this book an exceptional effort. Their encouragement from time to time has been an inspiration for everyone.

The publisher and the editorial board hope that this book will prove to be a valuable piece of knowledge for researchers, students, practitioners and scholars across the globe.

List of Contributors

Francois Beloncle
Keenan Research Centre and Li Ka Shing Knowledge Institute, St. Michael's Hospital, 30 Bond St, Toronto, ON M5B 1W8, Canada
Medical Intensive Care Unit, Hospital of Angers, University of Angers, Angers, France

Evangelia Akoumianaki
Department of Intensive Care Medicine, University Hospital of Heraklion, Crete, Greece

Nuttapol Rittayamai
Keenan Research Centre and Li Ka Shing Knowledge Institute, St. Michael's Hospital, 30 Bond St, Toronto, ON M5B 1W8, Canada
Division of Respiratory Diseases and Tuberculosis, Department of Medicine, Faculty of Medicine Siriraj Hospital, Bangkok, Thailand

Aissam Lyazidi
Institut Supérieur des Sciences de la Santé, Université Hassan 1er, Settat, Morocco

Laurent Brochard
Keenan Research Centre and Li Ka Shing Knowledge Institute, St. Michael's Hospital, 30 Bond St, Toronto, ON M5B 1W8, Canada
Interdepartmental Division of Critical Care Medicine, University of Toronto, Toronto, ON, Canada

Cheryl Elizabeth Hickmann, Diego Castanares-Zapatero, Emilie Bialais, Jonathan Dugernier, Antoine Tordeur, Lise Colmant, Xavier Wittebole, Giuseppe Tirone, Jean Roeseler and Pierre-François Laterre
Intensive Care Unit, Cliniques universitaires Saint-Luc, Université catholique de Louvain (UCL), Avenue Hippocrate 10, 1200 Brussels, Belgium

Lieuwe D. Bos, Laura R. Schouten and Marcus J. Schultz
Department of Intensive Care, Academic Medical Center, Meibergdreef 9, 1105 AZ Amsterdam, The Netherlands

Olaf L. Cremer
Department of Intensive Care Medicine, University Medical Center Utrecht, Utrecht, The Netherlands

David S. Y. Ong
Department of Intensive Care Medicine, University Medical Center Utrecht, Utrecht, The Netherlands
Department of Medical Microbiology, University Medical Center Utrecht, Utrecht, The Netherlands

Zhong Yuanbo, Wang Jin, Shi Fei, Long Liangong, Liu Xunfa, Xu Shihai and Shan Aijun
Emergency Center, Shenzhen People's Hospital, Shenzhen 518020, China

Noémie Zucman
Medico-Surgical Intensive Care Unit, Hôpital Louis Mourier, AP-HP, 178 rue des Renouillers, 92700 Colombes, France

Stéphane Gaudry
Medico-Surgical Intensive Care Unit, Hôpital Louis Mourier, AP-HP, 178 rue des Renouillers, 92700 Colombes, France
Sorbonne Paris Cité, ECEVE UMR 1123, Univ Paris Diderot, 75018 Paris, France

Samuel Tuffet
Medico-Surgical Intensive Care Unit, Hôpital Louis Mourier, AP-HP, 178 rue des Renouillers, 92700 Colombes, France
Département d'Anesthésie Réanimation, Hôpital Lariboisière, AP-HP, 75010 Paris, France
UMR U 1160, Université Paris-Diderot Paris 7, 75010 Paris, France

Anne-Claire Lukaszewicz and Didier Payen
Département d'Anesthésie Réanimation, Hôpital Lariboisière, AP-HP, 75010 Paris, France
UMR U 1160, Université Paris-Diderot Paris 7, 75010 Paris, France

Christian Laplace and Jacques Duranteau
Département d'Anesthésie Réanimation, Hôpital Bicêtre, AP-HP, 94270 Le Kremlin-Bicêtre, France

Marc Pocard
Hôpital Lariboisière, Chirurgie digestive et cancérologique, AP-HP, 75010 Paris, France
UMR U 965, Université Paris-Diderot Paris 7, 75010 Paris, France

Bruno Costaglioli
Hôpital Bicêtre, Chirurgie générale et digestive, AP-HP, 94270 Le Kremlin-Bicêtre, France

Simon Msika
Hôpital Louis Mourier, Chirurgie digestive, AP-HP, 178 rue des Renouillers, 92700 Colombes, France
UMR 1149, Univ Paris Diderot, Sorbonne Paris Cité, 75018 Paris, France

Didier Dreyfuss
Medico-Surgical Intensive Care Unit, Hôpital Louis Mourier, AP-HP, 178 rue des Renouillers, 92700 Colombes, France
IAME,UMR 1137, INSERM, 75018 Paris, France
IAME, UMR 1137, Univ Paris Diderot, Sorbonne Paris Cité, 75018 Paris, France

David Hajage
Sorbonne Paris Cité, ECEVE UMR 1123, Univ Paris Diderot, 75018 Paris, France
Epidemiology and Clinical Research Department, Hôpital Louis Mourier, AP-HP, 178 rue des Renouillers, 92700 Colombes, France

Jean-Damien Ricard
Medico-Surgical Intensive Care Unit, Hôpital Louis Mourier, AP-HP, 178 rue des Renouillers, 92700 Colombes, France
IAME, UMR 1137, INSERM, 75018 Paris, France
IAME, UMR 1137, Univ Paris Diderot, Sorbonne Paris Cité, 75018 Paris, France
Service de Réanimation Médicale, 178 rue des Renouillers, 92701 Colombes Cedex, France

Maxime Elbaz, Damien Léger and Stéphane Rio
Centre du Sommeil et de la Vigilance, Hôtel-Dieu de Paris, APHP, Université Paris Descartes, Paris, France
EA 7330 VIFASOM Sommeil-Vigilance-Fatigue et Santé Publique, Hôtel Dieu de Paris, Université Paris Descartes, 1 place du Parvis Notre Dame, 75004 Paris, France

Fabien Sauvet and Mounir Chennaoui
EA 7330 VIFASOM Sommeil-Vigilance-Fatigue et Santé Publique, Hôtel Dieu de Paris, Université Paris Descartes, 1 place du Parvis Notre Dame, 75004 Paris, France
Unité Fatigue et Vigilance, Institut de Recherche Biomédicale des Armées (IRBA), Brétigny-sur-Orge, France

Benoit Champigneulle and Jean Paul Mira
Service de Réanimation médicale, Hôpital Cochin, APHP, Université Paris Descartes, Paris, France

Mélanie Strauss
Centre du Sommeil et de la Vigilance, Hôtel-Dieu de Paris, APHP, Université Paris Descartes, Paris, France
Cognitive Neuroimaging Unit, U992, INSERM, Gif/Yvette, France
NeuroSpin Center Institute of Bioimaging, Commissariat à l'Energie Atomique (CEA), Gif/Yvette, France

Christian Guilleminault
Stanford University Sleep Disorders Clinic, Palo Alto, CA, USA

Rafael Fernandez and Carles Subira
Critical Care Department, Hospital Sant Joan de Deu- Fundacio Althaia, CIBERES, Universitat Internacional de Catalunya, Dr Joan Soler 1, 08243 Manresa, Spain

Fernando Frutos-Vivar, Amanda Lesmes and Luna Panadero
CIBERES, Hospital de Getafe, Madrid, Spain

Gemma Rialp
Hospital Son Llatzer, Majorca, Spain

Cesar Laborda
Hospital Valle Hebron, Barcelona, Spain

Joan Ramon Masclans
Hospital del Mar, CIBERES, IMIM, Pompeu Fabra University, Barcelona, Spain

Gonzalo Hernandez
Hospital Virgen de la Salud, Toledo, Spain

Alexandra Buisson, Blandine Vanel, Bruno Massenavette and Robin Pouyau
Réanimation pédiatrique, Hôpital Femme Mère Enfant, Hospices Civils de Lyon, 69500 Bron, France

Florent Baudin and Etienne Javouhey
Réanimation pédiatrique, Hôpital Femme Mère Enfant, Hospices Civils de Lyon, 69500 Bron, France
UMR T_9405, UMRESTTE, Ifsttar, Université Claude Bernard Lyon1, Univ Lyon, 69373 Lyon, France

Nicolas S. Marjanovic
Urgences Adultes/SAMU 86, CHU de Poitiers, 86000 Poitiers Cedex, France
ABS-Lab, Laboratoire d'Anatomie, Biomécanique et Simulation, Université de Poitiers, Rue de la Milétrie, 86000 Poitiers Cedex, France

Agathe De Simone and Guillaume Jegou
B-Com Technical Research Institute, 29200 Brest Cedex, France

Erwan L'Her
CeSim/LaTIM INSERM UMR 1101, Université de Bretagne Occidentale, Rue Camille Desmoulins, 29200 Brest Cedex, France
Médecine Intensive et Réanimation, CHRU de Brest, Boulevard Tanguy Prigent, 29200 Brest Cedex, France

Pedro Emmanuel Americano do Brasil
National Institute of Infectious Disease Evandro Chagas, Oswaldo Cruz Foundation (FIOCRUZ), Rio de Janeiro, Brazil

Cássia Righy
National Institute of Infectious Disease Evandro Chagas, Oswaldo Cruz Foundation (FIOCRUZ), Rio de Janeiro, Brazil
ICU, Paulo Niemeyer Brain Institute, Rio de Janeiro, Brazil

Fernando A. Bozza
National Institute of Infectious Disease Evandro Chagas, Oswaldo Cruz Foundation (FIOCRUZ), Rio de Janeiro, Brazil
IDOR, D'Or Institute for Research and Education, Rio de Janeiro, Brazil

Jordi Vallés
CIBER Enfermedades Respiratorias (CIBERES), Barcelona, Spain
Critical Care Center, CIBER Enfermedades Respiratorias, Hospital Sabadell, Sabadell, Spain

Ignacio Martin-Loeches
CIBER Enfermedades Respiratorias (CIBERES), Barcelona, Spain
Department of Clinical Medicine, Trinity Centre for Health Sciences, Multidisciplinary Intensive Care Research Organization (MICRO), Wellcome Trust, HRB Clinical Research, St James's University Hospital Dublin, Dublin, Ireland
Irish Centre for Vascular Biology (ICVB), Dublin, Ireland

Nilde Eronia
Department of Emergency and Intensive Care, San Gerardo Hospital, Via Pergolesi 33, Monza, Italy

Tommaso Mauri, Laura Alban, Antonio Pesenti and Tommaso Sasso
Department of Pathophysiology and Transplantation, University of Milan, Via Festa del Perdono 7, Milan, Italy
Department of Anesthesia, Critical Care and Emergency, Fondazione IRCCS Ca' Granda Ospedale Maggiore Policlinico, Via Francesco Sforza 28, Milan, Italy

Filippo Binda, Cristina Marenghi and Giacomo Grasselli
Department of Anesthesia, Critical Care and Emergency, Fondazione IRCCS Ca' Granda Ospedale Maggiore Policlinico, Via Francesco Sforza 28, Milan, Italy

Elisabetta Maffezzini, Stefano Gatti and Alfio Bronco
Department of Medicine, School of Medicine and Surgery, University of Milan-Bicocca, Via Cadore 48, Monza, Italy

Giacomo Bellani and Giuseppe Foti
Department of Emergency and Intensive Care, San Gerardo Hospital, Via Pergolesi 33, Monza, Italy
Department of Medicine, School of Medicine and Surgery, University of Milan-Bicocca, Via Cadore 48, Monza, Italy

Diego Orbegozo, Lokmane Rahmania, Marian Irazabal, Manuel Mendoza, Filippo Annoni, Daniel De Backer, Jacques Creteur and Jean-Louis Vincent
Department of Intensive Care, Erasme University Hospital, Université Libre de Bruxelles, Route de Lennik 808, 1070 Brussels, Belgium

Guo-guang Ma, Guang-wei Hao, Xiao-mei Yang, Du-ming Zhu, Lan Liu, Hua Liu, Guo-wei Tu and Zhe Luo
Department of Critical Care Medicine, Zhongshan Hospital, Fudan University, No. 180 Fenglin Road, Shanghai 200032, Xuhui District, People's Republic of China

Guillaume Mortamet
Pediatric Intensive Care Unit, CHU Sainte-Justine, 3175 Côte Sainte-Catherine, Montreal, QC, Canada
INSERM U 955, Equipe 13, Créteil, France
CHU Sainte-Justine Research Center, Université de Montréal, Montreal, Canada

Alexandrine Larouche, Laurence Ducharme-Crevier, Philippe Jouvet, Guillaume Emeriaud and Gabrielle Constantin
Pediatric Intensive Care Unit, CHU Sainte-Justine, 3175 Côte Sainte-Catherine, Montreal, QC, Canada
CHU Sainte-Justine Research Center, Université de Montréal, Montreal, Canada

Olivier Fléchelles
Pediatric Intensive Care Unit, CHU Fort-de-France, Fort-de-France, France

Sandrine Essouri
CHU Sainte-Justine Research Center, Université de Montréal, Montreal, Canada
Department of Pediatrics, CHU Sainte-Justine, Montreal, QC, Canada

Amélie-Ann Pellerin-Leblanc
Queen's University, Kingston, Canada

Jennifer Beck
Keenan Research Centre for Biomedical Science, Li Ka Shing Knowledge Institute, St. Michael's Hospital, Toronto, ON, Canada
Department of Pediatrics, University of Toronto, Toronto, Canada
Institute for Biomedical Engineering and Science Technology (iBEST), Ryerson University and St-Michael's Hospital, Toronto, Canada

Christer Sinderby
Keenan Research Centre for Biomedical Science, Li Ka Shing Knowledge Institute, St. Michael's Hospital, Toronto, ON, Canada
Institute for Biomedical Engineering and Science Technology (iBEST), Ryerson University and St-Michael's Hospital, Toronto, Canada
Department of Medicine, University of Toronto, Toronto, Canada

Hernan Aguirre-Bermeo, Indalecio Morán, Stefano Italiano, Francisco José Parrilla, Eugenia Plazolles and Jordi Mancebo
Servei de Medicina Intensiva, Hospital de la Santa Creu i Sant Pau, Universidad Autònoma de Barcelona (UAB), Sant Quintí, 89, 08041 Barcelona, Spain

Maurizio Bottiroli
Anestesia e Rianimazione 3, Ospedale Niguarda Ca' Granda, Milan, Italy

Ferran Roche-Campo
Servei de Medicina Intensiva, Hospital Verge de la Cinta, Tortosa, Spain

Jun Kataoka, Yosuke Homma, Shimada Yumiko, Yuiko Hoshina and Eiji Hiraoka
Department of Emergency and Critical Care Medicine, Tokyo Bay Urayasu Ichikawa Medical Center, 3-4-32 Todaijima, Urayasu, Chiba 2790001, Japan

Takaki Naito, Junpei Tsukuda, Kentaro Okamoto, Takeshi Kawaguchi and Shigeki Fujitani
Department of Emergency and Critical Care Medicine, St. Marianna University Hospital, 2-16-1 Sugao, Kawasaki, Kanagawa 2168511, Japan

Yasuhiro Norisue
Department of Emergency and Critical Care Medicine, Tokyo Bay Urayasu Ichikawa Medical Center, 3−4−32 Todaijima, Urayasu, Chiba 2790001, Japan
Department of Emergency and Critical Care Medicine, St. Marianna University Hospital, 2−16−1 Sugao, Kawasaki, Kanagawa 2168511, Japan
Department of Pulmonary and Critical Care Medicine, Tokyo Bay Urayasu Ichikawa Medical Center, 3-4-32 Todaijima, Urayasu, Chiba 2790001, Japan

Lonny Ashworth
Department of Respiratory Care, Boise State University, 1910 W University Drive, Boise, ID 83725, USA

S. Valade, V. Lemiale and E. Azoulay
AP-HP, Medical ICU, Hôpital Saint-Louis, 1 Avenue Claude Vellefaux, 75010 Paris, France
UFR de Médecine, University Paris-7 Paris-Diderot, Paris, France

L. Biard
UFR de Médecine, University Paris-7 Paris-Diderot, Paris, France
AP-HP, DBIM, Hôpital Saint-Louis, Paris, France

L. Argaud
Hôpital Edouard Herriot, Service de Réanimation Médicale, Hospices Civils de Lyon, Lyon, France

F. Pène
AP-HP, Réanimation médicale, Hôpital Cochin, Paris, France

L. Papazian
Réanimation des Détresses Respiratoires et Infections Sévères, Assistance Publique-Hôpitaux de Marseille, Hôpital Nord, Marseille, France

F. Bruneel
Service de Réanimation, Centre Hospitalier de Versailles, Le Chesnay, France

A. Seguin
Department of Medical Intensive Care, CHU de Caen, Caen, France

A. Kouatchet
Service de Réanimation Médicale et Médecine Hyperbare, Hôpital Angers, Angers, France

J. Oziel
AP-HP, Medical-Surgical Intensive Care Unit, Avicenne University Hospital, Bobigny, France

S. Rouleau
Service de Réanimation polyvalente, Angoulême, France

N. Bele
Intensive Care Unit, Draguignan Hospital, Draguignan, France

K. Razazi
AP-HP, Groupe Henri Mondor-Albert Chenevier, Service de Réanimation Médicale, Hôpital Henri Mondor, Créteil, France

O. Lesieur
Service de Réanimation, CH Saint-Louis, La Rochelle, France

F. Boissier
AP-HP, Réanimation médicale, Hôpital Européen Georges Pompidou, Paris, France

B. Megarbane
AP-HP, Department of Medical and Toxicological Critical Care, Lariboisière Hospital, Paris, France

N. Bigé
AP-HP, Medical Intensive Care Unit, Hôpital Saint-Antoine, Paris, France

N. Brulé
Medical Intensive Care Unit, Centre Hospitalier Universitaire de Nantes, Nantes, France

A. S. Moreau
Centre de réanimation, Hôpital Salengro, CHU-Lille, Lille, France

A. Lautrette
Service de Réanimation Médicale Polyvalente, CHU Gabriel Montpied, Clermont-Ferrand, France

O. Peyrony
AP-HP, Service des urgences, Hôpital Saint-Louis, Paris, France

P. Perez
Service e Réanimation médicale, Hôpital Brabois, Nancy, France

J. Mayaux
AP-HP, Pneumology and Critical Care Medicine Department, Universitary Hospital La Pitié Salpêtrière-Charles Foix, Paris, France

Byeong-Ho Jeong
Division of Pulmonary and Critical Care Medicine, Department of Medicine, Samsung Medical Center, Sungkyunkwan University School of Medicine, 81 Irwon-ro, Gangnam-gu, Seoul 06351, Republic of Korea

Kyeong Yoon Lee, Jimyoung Nam and Myeong Gyun Ko
Intensive Care Unit Nursing Department, Samsung Medical Center, Sungkyunkwan University School of Medicine, Seoul, Republic of Korea

Soo Jin Na
Department of Critical Care Medicine, Samsung Medical Center, Sungkyunkwan University School of Medicine, Seoul, Republic of Korea

Gee Young Suh and Kyeongman Jeon
Division of Pulmonary and Critical Care Medicine, Department of Medicine, Samsung Medical Center, Sungkyunkwan University School of Medicine, 81 Irwon-ro, Gangnam-gu, Seoul 06351, Republic of Korea
Department of Critical Care Medicine, Samsung Medical Center, Sungkyunkwan University School of Medicine, Seoul, Republic of Korea

François Reminiac
Médecine Intensive Réanimation, CHRU de Tours, 2, Bd Tonnellé, 37044 Tours Cedex 9, France
Centre d'étude des pathologies respiratoires, INSERM U1100, Faculté de médecine, Université de Tours, Tours, France Clinique du Mail, La Rochelle, France

Laurent Vecellio, Deborah Le Pennec and Maria Cabrera
Centre d'étude des pathologies respiratoires, INSERM U1100, Faculté de médecine, Université de Tours, Tours, France

Laetitia Bodet-Contentin and Charlotte Salmon Gandonnière
Médecine Intensive Réanimation, CHRU de Tours, 2, Bd Tonnellé, 37044 Tours Cedex 9, France
Centre d'investigation clinique, INSERM CIC 1415, CHRU de Tours, Tours, France
CRICS-TRIGGERSEP Network, Tours, France

Laurent Plantier
Centre d'étude des pathologies respiratoires, INSERM U1100, Faculté de médecine, Université de Tours, Tours, France
Service de pneumologie et d'explorations fonctionnelles respiratoires, CHRU de Tours, Tours, France

Valérie Gissot
Centre d'investigation clinique, INSERM CIC 1415, CHRU de Tours, Tours, France

Pierre-François Dequin and Stephan Ehrmann
Médecine Intensive Réanimation, CHRU de Tours, 2, Bd Tonnellé, 37044 Tours Cedex 9, France
Centre d'étude des pathologies respiratoires, INSERM U1100, Faculté de médecine, Université de Tours, Tours, France
Centre d'investigation clinique, INSERM CIC 1415, CHRU de Tours, Tours, France
CRICS-TRIGGERSEP Network, Tours, France

Renato Carneiro de Freitas Chaves, Bruno de Arruda Bravim, Ricardo Luiz Cordioli, Fabio Tanzillo Moreira, Karina Tavares Timenetsky and Murillo Santucci Cesar de Assunção
Intensive Care Unit, Hospital Israelita Albert Einstein, Av. Albert Einstein, 627/701, 5th Floor, São Paulo, SP 05651-901, Brazil

Thiago Domingos Corrêa
Intensive Care Unit, Hospital Israelita Albert Einstein, Av. Albert Einstein, 627/701, 5th Floor, São Paulo, SP 05651–901, Brazil
Intensive Care Unit, Hospital Municipal Dr. Moysés Deutsch - M'Boi Mirim, São Paulo, SP, Brazil

Ary Serpa Neto
Intensive Care Unit, Hospital Israelita Albert Einstein, Av. Albert Einstein, 627/701, 5th Floor, São Paulo, SP 05651–901, Brazil
Department of Intensive Care, Academic Medical Center, University of Amsterdam, Amsterdam, The Netherlands

Christophe Guervilly, Jean-Marie Forel, Sami Hraiech and Laurent Papazian
Aix-Marseille Univ, APHM, URMITE UMR CNRS 7278, Hôpital Nord, Réanimation des Détresses Respiratoires et Infections Sévères, Marseille, France

Antoine Roch
Aix-Marseille Univ, APHM, URMITE UMR CNRS 7278, Hôpital Nord, Réanimation des Détresses Respiratoires et Infections Sévères, Marseille, France
Service d'Accueil des Urgences, APHM, Hôpital Nord, Marseille, France

Daniel Talmor
Department of Anesthesia, Critical Care, and Pain Medicine, Beth Israel Deaconess Medical Center, 330 Brookline Ave, Boston, MA, USA

Angéline Jamet and Philippe Petua
Service de Réanimation Médicale, CHU de Poitiers, 2, rue de la Milétrie, 86021 Poitiers, France

Rémi Coudroy, René Robert, Jean-Pierre Frat and Arnaud W. Thille
Service de Réanimation Médicale, CHU de Poitiers, 2, rue de la Milétrie, 86021 Poitiers, France
INSERM CIC 1402 (ALIVE Group), Université de Poitiers, Poitiers, France

Matteo Bassetti
Infectious Diseases Clinic, Santa Maria Misericordia University Hospital, Udine, Italy

Charles-Edouard Luyt
Service de Réanimation, Institut de Cardiologie, Groupe Hospitalier Pitié–Salpêtrière, Assistance Publique–Hôpitaux de Paris, Paris, France
Sorbonne Universités, UPMC Université Paris 06, INSERM, UMRS_1166- ICAN Institute of Cardiometabolism and Nutrition, Paris, France.

David P. Nicolau
Center for Anti-Infective Research and Development, Hartford Hospital, Hartford, USA

Jérôme Pugin
Service des Soins Intensifs, University Hospitals of Geneva and Faculty of Medicine, University of Geneva, Geneva, Switzerland

Index

www.ingramcontent.com/pod-product-compliance
Lightning Source LLC
Chambersburg PA
CBHW082037190326
41458CB00010B/3392